An Evidence-Based Approach to Vitamins and Minerals

Health Benefits
and Intake Recommendations

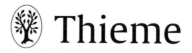 Thieme

An Evidence-Based Approach to Vitamins and Minerals

Health Benefits and Intake Recommendations

Jane Higdon, Ph.D.

The Linus Pauling Institute
Oregon State University
Corvallis, Oregon

Thieme
New York • Stuttgart

Thieme New York
333 Seventh Avenue
New York, NY 10001

Acquisitions Editor: Melissa Parsons
Director, Production and Manufacturing: Anne Vinnicombe
Production Editor: Anne Vinnicombe
Marketing Director: Phyllis Gold
Sales Director: Ross Lumpkin
Chief Financial Officer: Peter van Woerden
President: Brian Scanlan
Compositor: primustype Hurler
Printer: Triltsch

Library of Congress Cataloging-in-Publication Data is available from the publisher.

Important note: Medical knowledge is ever-changing. As new research and clinical experience broaden our knowledge, changes in treatment and drug therapy may be required. The author of the material herein has consulted sources believed to be reliable in her efforts to provide information that is complete and in accord with standards accepted at the time of publication. However, in view of the possibility of human error by the author or publisher of the work herein, or changes in medical knowledge, neither the author nor the publisher, nor any other party who has been involved in the preparation of this work, warrants that the information contained herein is in every respect accurate or complete, and they are not responsible for any errors or omissions or for the results obtained by the use of such information. Readers are advised to check the product information sheet included in the package of each drug they plan to administer to be certain that the information contained in this publication is accurate and that changes have not been made in the recommended dose or in the contraindications for administration. This recommendation is of particular importance in connection with new and infrequently used drugs.

Some of the product names, patents, and registered designs referred to in this book are in fact registered trademarks or proprietary names even though specific reference to this fact is not always made in the text. Therefore, the appearance of a name without designation as proprietary is not to be construed as a representation by the publisher that it is in the public domain.

Printed in Germany

5 4 3 2

TMP ISBN 0-58890-124-6
GTV ISBN 3-13-132451-1

Contents

Preface

During my clinical training, I learned to approach micronutrient nutrition from the perspective of preventing or treating deficiency diseases, such as scurvy or iron- deficiency anemia. In clinical practice, I became increasingly interested in the potential for micronutrients to prevent and treat chronic diseases at intakes higher than those required to prevent deficiency. However, the standard medical and nutrition texts of the day rarely provided the kind of information I was looking for. Today, scientific and medical research on the roles of micronutrients in health and disease is expanding rapidly, as are, unfortunately, exaggerated health claims from numerous supplement manufacturers. Keeping up with the explosion of contradictory information regarding the safety and efficacy of dietary supplements has become an overwhelming task for consumers as well as health care and nutrition professionals. My goal in writing this book was to provide clinicians and consumers with a practical evidence-based reference to the rapidly expanding field of micronutrient nutrition.

While my own interest in nutrition and health led me to pursue doctoral work in nutrition and biochemistry, such a step should not be necessary for health care and nutrition professionals who want more information on the health implications of dietary and supplemental micronutrients. With the support of the Linus Pauling Institute at Oregon State University (LPI), I have synthesized and organized hundreds of experimental, clinical, and epidemiologic studies, providing an overview of the current scientific knowledge of the roles of vitamins and nutritionally important minerals in human health and disease. To ensure the accuracy of the information presented, I asked at least one recognized scientific expert in the field to review each chapter. The names and affiliations of these scientists are listed in the Editorial Advisory Board.

Throughout this book, I have tried to emphasize human research published in peer-reviewed journals. Where relevant, I have included the results of experimental studies in cell culture or animal models. Although randomized clinical trials provide the strongest evidence for the effect of micronutrient intake on disease outcomes in humans, it is not always ethical or practical to perform a double-blind, placebo-controlled trial. Observational studies can also provide useful information about micronutrient intake and disease outcomes. In reviewing the epidemiologic research, I have given more weight to the results of large prospective cohort studies, such as the Nurses Health Study, than retrospective case-control or cross-sectional studies. When available, I have included the results of systematic reviews and meta-analyses, which summarize information on the findings of many similar studies.

Nearly 35 years ago Linus Pauling, Ph.D., the only individual ever to win two unshared Nobel Prizes, concluded that micronutrients could play a significant role in enhancing human health and preventing chronic disease, not just deficiency disease. The basic premise that an optimum diet is the key to optimum health continues today as the foundation of the Linus Pauling Institute at Oregon State University. Scientists at the Linus Pauling Institute investigate the roles that micronutrients and other dietary constituents play in human aging and chronic diseases, particularly cancer, cardiovascular diseases, and neurodegenerative diseases. The goals of our research are to understand the molecular mechanisms behind the effects of nutrition on health and to determine how micronutrients and other dietary factors can be used in the prevention and treatment of diseases, thereby enhancing human health and well-being. The Linus Pauling Institute is also dedicated to training and supporting new researchers in the interdisciplinary science of nutrition and optimum health, as well as to educating the public about the science of optimum nutrition.

As you read this book, it will become apparent that the Linus Pauling Institute recommendations for certain micronutrients (e.g., vitamin C) differ considerably from those of Linus Pauling himself. Dr. Pauling, for whom the Linus Pauling Institute has great respect, based his own micronutrient recommendations largely on theoretical arguments. For example, in developing his recommendations for vitamin C intake, he used cross-species comparisons, evolutionary arguments, and the amount of vitamin C likely consumed in a raw plant food diet. At the Linus Pauling Institute, we base our micronutrient recommendations on current scientific evidence, much of which was unavailable to Dr. Pauling. The Linus Pauling Institute's recommendation for a vitamin C intake of at least 200 mg/day for generally healthy adults takes into account the currently available epidemiologic, biochemical, and clinical evidence. Similarly, the Linus Pauling Institute's intake recommendation for each micronutrient in this book is based on the current scientific research available, while, in many cases, acknowledging that the intake levels most likely to promote optimum health remain to be determined.

Acknowledgments

First and foremost, I wish to thank the faculty, staff, and students of the Linus Pauling Institute for providing me with the inspiration and the opportunity to write this book. Specifically, Balz Frei, Ph.D., the director, and Stephen Lawson, the chief administrative officer of the Linus Pauling Institute, provided valuable advice and editorial assistance throughout the project. Barbara McVicar also provided much needed technical assistance and support. I am very grateful for the support of Bruce N. Ames, Ph.D., who was enthusiastic about this project from the beginning. His research and his eloquent foreword have been invaluable in laying the groundwork for this book.

I would like to thank each of the distinguished scientists listed in the Editorial Advisory Board for taking the time to carefully review each chapter of this book and provide insightful and constructive comments. I am also grateful to Aram Chobanian, M.D., for reviewing the information presented on salt. The artist, Pat Grimaldi of the Communication Media Center at Oregon State University, was both patient and skillful in creating the book's illustrations.

This project would not have been possible without the generous financial support of the donors to the Linus Pauling Institute, who deserve special thanks. Finally, although I did not know him personally, I would like to thank Dr. Linus Pauling for courageously stimulating scientific, medical, and popular interest in the roles played by micronutrients in promoting optimum health and preventing and treating disease.

Jane Higdon, Ph.D., The Linus Pauling Institute
Oregon State University
Corvallis, Oregon

Foreword

An Evidence-Based Approach to Vitamins and Minerals: Health Benefits and Intake Recommendations by Dr. Jane Higdon provides a much needed source of authoritative information on the role of micronutrients in health promotion and in disease prevention and treatment. The book is especially important because of the potential health benefits of tuning up people's micronutrient metabolism, particularly those with inadequate diets, such as the many low-income and elderly people. A metabolic tune-up is likely to have enormous health benefits but is currently not being addressed adequately by the medical community.

Maximum health and life span require metabolic harmony. It is commonly thought that Americans' intake of the more than 40 essential micronutrients (vitamins, minerals, and other biochemicals that humans require) is adequate. Classic deficiency diseases such as scurvy, beriberi, pernicious anemia, and rickets are rare, but the evidence suggests that metabolic damage occurs at intake levels between the level causing acute micronutrient deficiency diseases and the recommended dietary allowances (RDAs). When one input in the metabolic network is inadequate, repercussions are felt on a large number of systems and can lead to degenerative disease. This may, for example, result in an increase in DNA damage (and possibly cancer), neuron decay (and possibly cognitive dysfunction), or mitochondrial decay (and possibly accelerated aging and degenerative diseases). The optimum amount of folate or zinc that is truly "required" is the amount that minimizes DNA damage and maximizes a healthy life span, which is higher than the amount to prevent acute disease. Vitamin and metabolite requirements of older people are likely to differ from those of younger people, but this issue has not been seriously examined. An optimal intake of micronutrients and metabolites will also vary with genetic constitution. A tune-up of micronutrient metabolism should give a marked increase in health at little cost. It is inexcusable that anyone in the world should have an inadequate intake of a vitamin or mineral, at great cost to that person's health, when a year's supply of a daily multivitamin/multimineral pill as insurance against deficiencies costs less than a few packs of cigarettes. Low-income populations, in general, are the most likely to have poor diets and have the most to gain from multivitamin/multimineral supplementation. As Hippocrates said: "Leave your drugs in the chemist's pot if you can heal the patient with food".

Although many degenerative diseases will benefit from optimal nutrition, and optimal nutrition clearly involves more than adequate micronutrients, there are several important reasons for focusing on micronutrients and health, particularly DNA damage: (1) More than 20 years of efforts to improve the American diet have not been notably successful, though this work must continue. A parallel approach focusing on micronutrient intake is overdue and might be more successful, since it should be easier to convince people to take a multivitamin/multimineral pill as insurance against ill health than to change their diet significantly. (2) A multivitamin/multimineral pill is inexpensive, is recognized as safe, and supplies the range of vitamins and minerals that a person requires, though not the essential fatty acids. Fortification of food is another approach that is useful, but its implementation has been very slow, as with folic acid fortification. Moreover, fortification of food does not allow for differences between individuals. For example, menstruating women need more iron than men or postmenopausal women, who may be getting too much. That is why two types of vitamin pills are marketed, one with iron and one without. With better knowledge it seems likely that a broader variety of multivitamin/multimineral pills will be developed, reflecting such life stage differences.

The above issues and many others discussed in this book highlight the need to educate the public about the crucial importance of optimal nutrition and the potential health benefits of something as simple and affordable as a daily multivitamin/multimineral supplement. The numerous advances in the science of nutrition and changing ideas about optimal intakes of micronutrients make *An Evidence-Based Approach to Vitamins and Minerals: Health Benefits and Intake Recommendations* an excellent and timely resource. Dr. Higdon, who has a background in health care and nutrition science, has synthesized a large amount of recent scientific research on vitamins and nutritionally essential minerals into an organized volume that includes information on optimal micronutrient intakes to prevent and treat chronic diseases. The book also contains much needed and up-to-date information on safety and drug interactions of vitamins and minerals. The credibility of this book is enhanced by the fact that it is endorsed by the Linus Pauling Institute at Oregon State University and that each chapter has been critically reviewed by a recognized expert in the field. Tuning up the metabolism to maximize human health will require scientists, clinicians, and educators to abandon outdated paradigms of micronutrients merely preventing deficiency disease and to explore more meaningful ways to prevent chronic disease and achieve optimal health through optimal nutrition.

Bruce N. Ames, Ph.D.
University of California, Berkeley
Children's Hospital Oakland Research Institute
Oakland, California

Editorial Advisory Board

How To Use This Book

Chapter Organization

Information on individual vitamins, organic (carbon-containing) compounds that are required by humans in small amounts from the diet to maintain normal physiological function, can be found in Chapters 1 through 13, in alphabetical order by vitamin. In addition to vitamins, a number of inorganic elements (minerals) are required in the human diet to support a wide range of biological functions. Information on nutritionally important minerals can be found in Chapters 14 through 26, in alphabetical order by mineral. For ease of use, the information in each chapter is organized in the following manner:

- **Function** Current scientific understanding of the function of the micronutrient with respect to maintaining health and preventing disease.
- **Deficiency** Risk factors, signs, symptoms, and physiological effects of frank deficiency of the micronutrient.
- **Disease Prevention** Where controlled research is available, information on the role(s) of the micronutrient in the prevention of disease.
- **Disease Treatment** Where controlled research is available, information on the role(s) of the micronutrient in the treatment of disease.
- **Sources** Information on dietary, supplemental, and other sources of the micronutrient. When available, this section includes a table of dietary sources.
- **Safety** Information on toxicity and adverse effects of the micronutrient, as well as micronutrient-drug interactions.
- **The Linus Pauling Institute Recommendation** A daily intake recommendation based on relevant scientific research and reflecting an intake level aimed at the prevention of chronic disease and the promotion of optimum health in generally healthy individuals. Recommendations for adults over 65 years of age are also addressed in this section.
- **References**

In addition to the Linus Pauling Institute Recommendations, the Food and Nutrition Board (FNB) of the Institute of Medicine appoints committees of expert scientists to set Dietary Reference Intakes (DRIs), which are used to plan and evaluate diets of apparently healthy people. Three different DRIs appear regularly throughout this book:

- The *Recommended Dietary Allowance* (RDA) is defined as the average daily dietary intake level of a specific nutrient sufficient to meet the requirement of nearly all (97%-98%) healthy individuals in a particular life-stage group. Because RDAs generally reflect intake levels designed to prevent deficiency, they are presented in the **Deficiency** section of each chapter.
- An *Adequate Intake* (AI) is provided if there is insufficient evidence to determine an RDA. The AI is based on experimentally derived intake levels or observed average intake levels of apparently healthy people. For example, the AI of a nutrient for infants is generally based on the average daily intake of that nutrient supplied by human milk in healthy, full-term infants who are

exclusively breastfed. Because AIs reflect intake levels thought to prevent deficiency, they are also presented in the **Deficiency** section of each chapter.

- The *Tolerable Upper Intake Level* (UL) is defined as the highest level of a nutrient determined to pose no risk of adverse effects for almost all individuals in the general population. The UL is discussed in the **Safety** section of each chapter.

Three minerals did not have DRIs at the time this book went to press. In 1989, the FNB set only minimum requirements for potassium, sodium, and chloride, which are presented in the **Deficiency** sections of Chapter 24 (Potassium) and Chapter 26 (Sodium Chloride). The FNB has appointed a committee of experts to develop DRIs for potassium, sodium, chloride, sulfate, and water. Their report is expected in March 2003.

Appendices

Several appendices have been included to facilitate the use of this book by clinicians as well as consumers.

- **Nutrient-Drug Interactions**   A table summarizing the information on nutrient-drug interactions discussed in the book.
- **Nutrient-Nutrient Interactions**   A table summarizing the information on nutrient-nutrient interactions discussed in the book.
- **Quick Reference to Diseases**   A useful chart that allows the reader to locate micronutrient information by disease or health condition.
- **The Linus Pauling Institute Prescription for Health**   A list summarizing the Linus Pauling Institute Recommendations for a healthy diet, lifestyle, and supplement use.

1 Biotin

Biotin is a water-soluble vitamin, generally classified as a B-complex vitamin. After the initial discovery of biotin, nearly 40 years of research were required to establish it as a vitamin.[1] Biotin is required by all organisms but can only be synthesized by bacteria, yeasts, molds, algae, and some plant species.[2]

Function

Cofactor for Enzymes

In its physiologically active form biotin is attached at the active site of four important enzymes, known as carboxylases.[3] Each carboxylase catalyzes an essential metabolic reaction.

- *Acetyl-coenzyme A (CoA) carboxylase* Acetyl-CoA carboxylase catalyzes the binding of bicarbonate to acetyl-CoA to form malonyl-CoA. Malonyl-CoA is required for the synthesis of fatty acids.
- *Pyruvate carboxylase* Pyruvate carboxylase is a critical enzyme in gluconeogenesis, the formation of glucose from sources other than carbohydrates, for example, amino acids and fats.
- *Methylcrotonyl-CoA carboxylase* Methylcrotonyl-CoA carboxylase catalyzes an essential step in the metabolism of leucine, an indispensable (essential) amino acid.
- *Propionyl-CoA carboxylase* Propionyl-CoA carboxylase catalyzes essential steps in the metabolism of amino acids, cholesterol, and odd chain fatty acids.[4]

Biotinylation of Histones

Histones are proteins that bind to DNA and package it into compact structures to form chromosomes. The compact packaging of DNA must be relaxed somewhat for DNA replication and transcription to occur. Modification of histones through the attachment of acetyl or methyl groups (acetylation or methylation) has been shown to affect the structure of histones, thereby affecting replication and transcription of DNA. The attachment of biotin to another molecule, such as a protein, is known as *biotinylation*. The enzyme biotinidase has recently been shown to catalyze the biotinylation of histones, suggesting that biotin may play a role in DNA replication and transcription.[5,6]

Deficiency

Although biotin deficiency is very rare, the human requirement for dietary biotin has been demonstrated in two different situations: prolonged intravenous feeding without biotin supplementation and consumption of raw egg white for a prolonged period (many weeks to years). Avidin is a protein found in egg white, which binds biotin and prevents its absorption. Cooking egg white denatures avidin, rendering it susceptible to digestion and unable to prevent the absorption of dietary biotin.[7]

Symptoms

Symptoms of overt biotin deficiency include hair loss and a scaly red rash around the eyes, nose, mouth, and genital area. Neurologic symptoms in adults have included depression, lethargy, hallucination, and numbness and tingling of the extremities. The characteristic facial rash, together with an unusual facial fat distribution, has been termed the "biotin-deficient face" by some experts.[7] Individuals with hereditary disorders of biotin metabolism resulting in functional biotin deficiency have evidence of impaired immune system function, including increased susceptibility to bacterial and fungal infections.[8]

Table 1–1   Adequate Intake (AI) for Biotin

Life Stage	Age	Males, µg/d	Females, µg/d
Infants	0–6 months	5	5
Infants	7–12 months	6	6
Children	1–3 years	8	8
Children	4–8 years	12	12
Children	9–13 years	20	20
Adolescents	14–18 years	25	25
Adults	19 years and older	30	30
Pregnancy	all ages	–	30
Breastfeeding	all ages	–	35

Predisposing Conditions

Two hereditary disorders, biotinidase deficiency and holocarboxylase synthetase (HCS) deficiency, result in an increased biotin requirement. Biotinidase is an enzyme that catalyzes the release of biotin from small proteins and the amino acid lysine thereby recycling biotin. There are several ways in which biotinidase deficiency leads to biotin deficiency. Intestinal absorption is decreased because a lack of biotinidase inhibits the release of biotin from dietary protein. Recycling of one's own biotin bound to protein is impaired, and urinary loss of biotin is increased because the kidneys appear to excrete more rapidly biotin that is not bound to biotinidase.[5,7] Biotinidase deficiency sometimes requires supplementation of as much as 5 to 10 mg/d of oral biotin, though smaller doses are often sufficient. HCS is an enzyme that catalyzes the attachment of biotin to all four carboxylase enzymes. HCS deficiency results in decreased formation of all carboxylases at normal blood levels of biotin and requires high-dose supplementation of 40 to 100 mg of biotin per day. In general, the prognosis of both disorders is good if biotin therapy is introduced early (infancy or childhood) and continued for life.[8]

Aside from prolonged consumption of raw egg white or intravenous feedings lacking biotin, other conditions may increase the risk of biotin depletion. The rapidly dividing cells of the developing fetus require biotin for DNA replication and synthesis of essential carboxylases, thereby increasing the biotin requirement in pregnancy. Recent research suggests that a substantial number of women develop marginal or subclinical biotin deficiency during normal pregnancy.[6,9] Some types of liver disease may also increase the requirement for biotin. A recent study of 62 children with chronic liver disease and 27 healthy controls found serum biotinidase activity to be abnormally low in those with severely impaired liver function due to cirrhosis.[10] Anticonvulsant medications, used to prevent seizures in individuals with epilepsy, increase the risk of biotin depletion.[11,12]

The Adequate Intake Level

In 1998 the Food and Nutrition Board of the Institute of Medicine felt the existing scientific evidence was insufficient to calculate a recommended dietary allowance for biotin, so they set an adequate intake level (AI) (Table 1–1). The AI for biotin assumes that current average intakes of biotin (35 µg to 60 µg/d) are meeting the dietary requirement.[1]

Disease Prevention

Birth Defects

Recent research indicates that biotin is broken down more rapidly during pregnancy and that biotin nutritional status declines during the course of pregnancy.[6] Approximately half of pregnant women have abnormally high excretion of a metabolite (3-hydroxyisovaleric acid) thought to reflect decreased activity of a biotin-dependent enzyme. A recent study of 26 pregnant women found that biotin supplementation decreased the excretion of this metabolite compared with supplementation with a placebo, suggesting that marginal biotin deficiency is relatively common in pregnancy.[9] Although this level of biotin depletion is not severe enough to cause symptoms, it is reason for concern because subclinical biotin deficiency has been shown to cause birth defects in several animal species.[11] There exists no direct evidence that marginal biotin deficiency causes birth defects in humans. However, the potential risk for biotin depletion makes it prudent to ensure adequate biotin intake throughout pregnancy. As pregnant women are advised to consume supplemental folic acid prior to and during pregnancy to prevent neural tube defects, it would be easy to consume supplemental biotin (at least 30 μg/d) in the form of a multivitamin that also contains at least 400 μg of folic acid.

Disease Treatment

Diabetes Mellitus

It has been known for many years that overt biotin deficiency results in impaired utilization of glucose.[13] Blood biotin levels were significantly lower in 43 patients with non-insulin-dependent diabetes mellitus than in nondiabetic control subjects, and lower fasting blood glucose levels were associated with higher blood biotin levels.[14] After 1 month of biotin supplementation (9 mg/d) fasting blood glucose levels decreased by an average of 45 %. Reductions in blood glucose levels were also found in seven insulin-dependent diabetics after 1 week of supplementation with 16 mg of biotin daily.[15] Several mechanisms could explain the glucose-lowering effect of biotin. As a cofactor of enzymes required for fatty acid synthesis, biotin may increase the utilization of glucose to synthesize fats. Biotin has been found to stimulate glucokinase, an enzyme in the liver, resulting in increased synthesis of glycogen, the storage form of glucose. Biotin has also been found to stimulate the secretion of insulin in the pancreas of rats, which also has the effect of lowering blood glucose.[16] An effect on cellular glucose transporters (GLUTs) is also currently under investigation. Presently, studies of the effect of supplemental biotin on blood glucose levels in humans are extremely limited, but they highlight the need for further research.

Table 1–2   Food Sources of Biotin

Food	Serving	Biotin, μg
Liver, cooked	3 ounces*	27
Egg, cooked	1 large	25
Yeast, bakers active	1 packet (7 g)	14
Wheat bran, crude	1 ounce	14
Avocado	1 whole	6
Bread, whole wheat	1 slice	6
Cheese, camembert	1 ounce	6
Cauliflower, raw	1 cup	4
Salmon, cooked	3 ounces*	4
Chicken, cooked	3 ounces*	3
Artichoke, cooked	1 medium	2
Cheese, cheddar	1 ounce	2
Pork, cooked	3 ounces*	2
Raspberries	1 cup	2

*A 3-ounce serving of meat or fish is about the size of a deck of cards.

Sources

Food Sources

Biotin is found in many foods, but generally in lower amounts than other water-soluble vitamins. Egg yolk, liver, and yeast are rich sources of biotin. Large national nutritional surveys in the United States were unable to estimate biotin intake due to the scarcity of data on the biotin content of food. Smaller studies estimate average daily intakes of biotin to be from 40 to 60 μg/d in adults.[1] Table 1–2 lists some richer food sources of biotin along with their biotin content in micrograms.[17]

Bacterial Synthesis

The bacteria that normally colonize the colon (large intestine) are capable of making their own biotin. It is not yet known whether humans can absorb a meaningful amount of the biotin synthesized by their own intestinal bacteria. However, a specialized process for the uptake of biotin has been identified in cultured cells derived from the lining of the colon, suggesting that humans may be able to absorb biotin produced by the bacteria normally present in the large intestine.[18]

Safety

Toxicity

Biotin is not known to be toxic. Toxicity has not been reported with daily oral doses of up to 200 mg, used to treat hereditary disorders of biotin metabolism and biotin deficiency. Due to the lack of reports of adverse effects, the Food and Nutrition Board did not set a tolerable upper level of intake for biotin.[1]

Drug Interactions

Individuals on long-term anticonvulsant therapy have been found to have reduced levels of biotin in their blood and urinary excretion of metabolites consistent with decreased carboxylase activity.[2] The anticonvulsants primidone and carbamazepine inhibit biotin absorption in the small intestine. Phenobarbital, phenytoin, and carbamazepine appear to increase urinary excretion of biotin. Use of the anticonvulsant valproic acid has been associated with decreased biotinidase activity in children.[12] Long-term treatment with sulfa drugs or other antibiotics may decrease bacterial synthesis of biotin, potentially increasing the requirement for dietary biotin. Large doses of the nutrient pantothenic acid have the potential to compete with biotin for intestinal and cellular uptake due to their similar structures. Very high (pharmacologic) doses of lipoic acid have been found to decrease the activity of biotin-dependent carboxylases in rats, but such an effect has not been demonstrated in humans.[4,19]

LPI Recommendation

Little is known regarding the amount of dietary biotin required to promote optimal health or prevent chronic disease. The Linus Pauling Institute supports the intake recommendation by the Food and Nutrition Board of 30 μg of biotin per day for adults. A varied diet should provide enough biotin for most people. However, following the Linus Pauling Institute recommendation to take a daily multivitamin/multimineral supplement containing 10% of the daily value for biotin will ensure an intake of at least 30 μg of biotin per day.

Older Adults
Presently, there is no indication that older adults (65 years and older) have an increased requirement for biotin. If dietary biotin intake is not sufficient, a daily multivitamin/multimineral supplement will ensure an intake of at least 30 μg of biotin per day.

References

1. Food and Nutrition Board, Institute of Medicine. Biotin. *Dietary Reference Intakes: Thiamin, Riboflavin, Niacin, Vitamin B-6, Vitamin B-12, Pantothenic Acid, Biotin, and Choline.* Washington, D.C.: National Academy Press; 1998:374–389.
2. Mock DM. Biotin. In: Ziegler EE, Filer LJ, eds. *Present Knowledge in Nutrition.* 7th ed. Washington, D.C.: ILSI Press; 1996:220–236.
3. Chapman-Smith A, Cronan JE, Jr. Molecular biology of biotin attachment to proteins. *J Nutr* 1999;129(2 Suppl):477S–484S.
4. Zempleni J, Mock DM. Biotin biochemistry and human requirements. *J Nutr Biochem* 1999;10:128–138.
5. Hymes J, Wolf B. Human biotinidase isn't just for recycling biotin. *J Nutr* 1999;129(Suppl 2):485S–489S.
6. Zempleni J, Mock DM. Marginal biotin deficiency is teratogenic. *Proc Soc Exp Biol Med* 2000;223(1):14–21.
7. Mock DM. Biotin. In: Shils M, Olson JA, Shike M, Ross AC, eds. *Nutrition in Health and Disease.* 9th ed. Baltimore: Williams & Wilkins; 1999:459–466.
8. Baumgartner ER, Suormala T. Inherited defects of biotin metabolism. *Biofactors* 1999;10(2–3):287–290.
9. Mock DM, Quirk JG, Mock NI. Marginal biotin deficiency during normal pregnancy. *Am J Clin Nutr* 2002;75:295–299.
10. Pabuccuoglu A, Aydogdu S, Bas M. Serum biotinidase activity in children with chronic liver disease and its clinical significance. *J Pediatr Gastroenterol Nutr* 2002;34(1):59–62.

11. Mock DM. Biotin status: which are valid indicators and how do we know? *J Nutr* 1999;129(2 Suppl):498S–503S.

12. Schulpis KH, Karikas GA, Tjamouranis J, Regoutas S, Tsakiris S. Low serum biotinidase activity in children with valproic acid monotherapy. *Epilepsia* 2001;42(10):1359–1362.

13. Zhang H, Osada K, Sone H, Furukawa Y. Biotin administration improves the impaired glucose tolerance of streptozotocin-induced diabetic Wistar rats. *J Nutr Sci Vitaminol (Tokyo)* 1997;43(3):271–280.

14. Maebashi M, Makino Y, Furukawa Y, Ohinata K, Kimura S, Sato T. Therapeutic evaluation of the effect of biotin on hyperglycemia in patients with non-insulin-dependent diabetes mellitus. *J Clin Biochem Nutr* 1993;14:211–218.

15. Coggeshall JC, Heggers JP, Robson MC, Baker H. Biotin status and plasma glucose levels in diabetics. *Ann NY Acad Sci* 1985;447:389–392.

16. Romero-Navarro G, Cabrera-Valladares G, German MS, et al. Biotin regulation of pancreatic glucokinase and insulin in primary cultured rat islets and in biotin-deficient rats. *Endocrinology* 1999;140(10):4595–4600.

17. Briggs DR, Wahlqvist ML. *Food Facts: The Complete No-Fads-Plain-Facts Guide to Healthy Eating.* Victoria, Australia: Penguin Books; 1988.

18. Said HM, Ortiz A, McCloud E, Dyer D, Moyer MP, Rubin S. Biotin uptake by human colonic epithelial NCM460 cells: a carrier-mediated process shared with pantothenic acid. *Am J Physiol* 1998;275(5 Pt 1):C1365–1371.

19. Flodin N. *Pharmacology of Micronutrients.* New York: Alan R. Liss, Inc.; 1988.

2 Folic Acid

The terms *folic acid* and *folate* are often used interchangeably for this water-soluble, B-complex vitamin. Folic acid, the most stable form, occurs rarely in foods or the human body but is the form most often used in vitamin supplements and fortified foods. Naturally occurring folates exist in many chemical forms. Folates are found in foods as well as in metabolically active forms, in the human body.[1] In the following discussion, forms found in food or the body will be referred to as *folates*, and the form found in supplements or fortified foods will be referred to as *folic acid.*

Function

One-Carbon Metabolism

The only function of folate cofactors in the body appears to be mediating the transfer of one-carbon units.[2] Folate cofactors act as acceptors and donors of one-carbon units in a variety of reactions critical to the metabolism of nucleic acids and amino acids.[3]

Nucleic Acid Metabolism. Folate cofactors play a vital role in DNA metabolism through two different pathways (Fig. 2–1). The synthesis of DNA from its precursors is dependent on folate cofactors. A folate cofactor is required for the

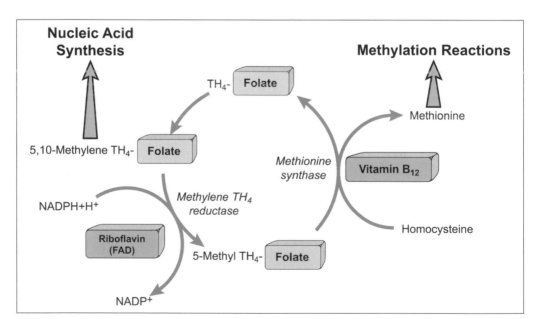

Figure 2–1. Folate and nucleic acid metabolism. 5,10-Methylene tetrahydrofolate (TH_4-folate) is required for the synthesis of nucleic acids, and 5-methyl TH_4-folate is required for the formation of methionine from homocysteine. Methionine, in the form of S-adenosylmethionine, is required for many biological methylation reactions, including DNA methylation. Methylene TH_4-folate reductase is a flavin-dependent enzyme required to catalyze the reduction of 5,10-methylene TH_4-folate to 5-methyl TH_4-folate.

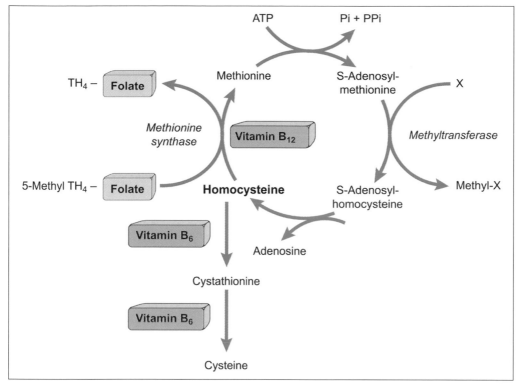

Figure 2–2. Homocysteine metabolism. S-adenosyl-homocysteine is formed during S-adenosyl-methionine-dependent methylation reactions, and the hydrolysis of S-adenosylhomocysteine results in homocysteine. Homocysteine may be remethylated to form methionine by a folate-dependent reaction that is catalyzed by methionine synthase, a vitamin B_{12}–dependent enzyme. Alternately, homocysteine may be metabolized to cysteine in reactions catalyzed by two vitamin B_6–dependent enzymes.

synthesis of methionine, and methionine is required for the synthesis of S-adenosyl-methionine (SAM). SAM is a methyl group (one-carbon unit) donor used in many biological methylation reactions, including the methylation of a number of sites within DNA and RNA. Methylation of DNA may be important in cancer prevention.

Amino Acid Metabolism. Folate cofactors are required for the metabolism of several important amino acids. The synthesis of methionine from homocysteine requires a folate cofactor as well as a vitamin B_{12}–dependent enzyme. Thus, folate deficiency can result in decreased synthesis of methionine and a buildup of homocysteine. Increased levels of homocysteine may be a risk factor for cardiovascular and other chronic diseases.

Nutrient Interactions

The metabolism of homocysteine, an intermediate in the metabolism of sulphur-containing amino acids, provides an example of the interrelationships among nutrients necessary to optimize physiological function and health. Healthy individuals utilize two different pathways to metabolize homocysteine (Fig. 2–2). One pathway results in the remethylation of homocysteine to form methionine and is dependent on a vitamin B_{12}–dependent enzyme and folate in the form of 5-methyl tetrahydrofolate. The other pathway converts homocysteine to another amino acid, cysteine, and requires two vitamin B_6–dependent enzymes. Thus, the amount of homocysteine in the blood is regulated by at least three vitamins—folic acid, vitamin B_{12}, and vitamin B_6.[4]

Deficiency

Causes

Folate deficiency occurs in a number of situations. For example, low dietary intake and diminished absorption, as in alcoholism, can result in a decreased supply of folate. Certain conditions like pregnancy or cancer result in increased rates of cell division and metabolism, leading to an increase in the body's demand for folate.[5] Several medications may also contribute to deficiency (see the section on drug interactions).

Symptoms

Individuals in the early stages of folate deficiency may not show obvious symptoms, but blood levels of homocysteine may increase. Rapidly dividing cells are most vulnerable to the effects of folate deficiency. When the folate supply to the rapidly dividing cells of the bone marrow is inadequate, blood cell division becomes abnormal, resulting in fewer but larger red blood cells. This type of anemia is called *megaloblastic* or *macrocytic* anemia, referring to the large immature red blood cells. Neutrophils, a type of white blood cell, become hypersegmented, a change that can be found by examining a blood sample microscopically. Because normal red blood cells have a lifetime in the circulation of approximately 4 months, it can take months for folate-deficient individuals to develop the characteristic megaloblastic anemia. Progression of such an anemia leads to a decreased oxygen carrying capacity of the blood and may ultimately result in symptoms of fatigue, weakness, and shortness of breath.[1] It is important to point out that megaloblastic anemia resulting from folate deficiency is identical to megaloblastic anemia resulting from vitamin B_{12} deficiency, and further clinical testing is required to diagnose the true cause of megaloblastic anemia.

Table 2–1   Recommended Dietary Allowance (RDA) for Folate in DFE

Life Stage	Age	Males, µg/d	Females, µg/d
Infants	0–6 months	65 (AI)	65 (AI)
Infants	7–12 months	80 (AI)	80 (AI)
Children	1–3 years	150	150
Children	4–8 years	200	200
Children	9–13 years	300	300
Adolescents	14–18 years	400	400
Adults	19 years and older	400	400
Pregnancy	all ages	–	600
Breast-feeding	all ages	–	500

AI, adequate intake level.
DFE, dietary folate equivalents.

The Recommended Dietary Allowance

Traditionally, the dietary folate requirement was defined as the amount needed to prevent a deficiency severe enough to cause symptoms like anemia. The most recent recommended dietary allowance (RDA) (Table 2–1) was based primarily on the adequacy of red blood cell folate concentrations at different levels of folate intake, which have been shown to correlate with liver folate stores. Maintenance of normal blood homocysteine levels, an indicator of one-carbon metabolism, was considered only as an ancillary indicator of adequate folate intake. Because pregnancy is associated with a significant increase in cell division and other metabolic processes requiring folate coenzymes, the RDA for pregnant women is considerably higher than for women who are not pregnant.[3] However, the prevention of neural tube defects (NTD) was not taken into consideration in setting the RDA for pregnant women. Rather, reducing the risk of NTD was considered in a separate recommendation for women capable of becoming pregnant because the crucial events in the development of the neural tube occur before many women are aware that they are pregnant.[6] The recommendation for women who are capable of becoming pregnant is to consume 400 µg/d of folic acid from supplements or fortified foods, in addition to dietary sources. The recommendation for NTD prevention was not expressed as dietary folate equivalents (DFE) because the studies supporting it utilized supplemental folic acid in addition to a varied diet.[1]

Dietary Folate Equivalents

When the Food and Nutrition Board of the Institute of Medicine set the new dietary recommendation for folate, they introduced a new unit, the DFE:

- 1 μg of food folate provides 1 μg of DFE
- 1 μg of folic acid (supplement) taken with meals or as fortified food provides 1.7 μg of DFE
- 1 μg of folic acid taken on an empty stomach provides 2 μg of DFE

Use of the DFE reflects the higher bioavailability of synthetic folic acid found in supplements and fortified foods compared with that of naturally occurring food folates.[6] For example, a serving of food containing 60 μg of folate would provide 60 μg of DFE, and a serving of pasta fortified with 60 μg of folic acid would provide $1.7 \times 60 = 102$ μg DFE due to the higher bioavailability of folic acid. A folic acid supplement of 400 μg taken on an empty stomach would provide 800 μg of DFE.

Genetic Variation in Folate Requirements

A common polymorphism or variation in the gene for the methylene tetrahydrofolate reductase (MTHFR) enzyme, known as the C677T MTHFR polymorphism, results in a less stable enzyme.[7] Depending on the population, 50% may have inherited one copy (C/T) and 5 to 25% may have inherited two copies (T/T) of the abnormal MTHFR gene. MTHFR plays an important role in maintaining the specific form of folate required to remethylate homocysteine to form methionine (Fig. 2–1). When folic acid intake is low, individuals who are homozygous (T/T) for the abnormal gene have lower levels of the MTHFR enzyme and higher levels of homocysteine in their blood.[8] Improved folate nutritional status appears to stabilize the MTHFR enzyme, resulting in im-proved enzyme levels and lower homocysteine levels. An important unanswered question about folate is whether the present RDA is enough to normalize MTHFR enzyme levels in individuals who are homozygous for the C677T polymorphism or whether those individuals have a higher folate requirement than the RDA.[9]

Disease Prevention

Pregnancy Complications

Neural Tube Defects. Fetal growth and development are characterized by widespread cell division. Adequate folate is critical because of its roles in DNA and RNA synthesis. NTD may result in anencephaly or spina bifida, which are devastating and sometimes fatal birth defects. The defects occur between the 21st and 27th days after conception, a time when many women do not realize they are pregnant.[10] The risk of NTD in the United States prior to fortification of foods with folic acid was estimated to be one per 1000 pregnancies.[1] Results of randomized trials have demonstrated 60 to 100% reduction in NTD cases when women consumed folic acid supplements in addition to a varied diet during the periconceptional period (about 1 month before and 1 month after conception). The results of these and other studies prompted the U.S. Public Health Service to recommend that all women capable of becoming pregnant consume 400 μg of folic acid daily to prevent NTD. The recommendation was made to all women of childbearing age because adequate folic acid must be available very early in pregnancy and because many pregnancies in the United States are unplanned. Despite the effectiveness of folic acid supplementation, it appears that less than half of women who become pregnant follow the recommendation.[11] To decrease births affected by NTD, the Food and Drug Administration (FDA) implemented legislation in 1998 requiring the fortification of all enriched grain products with folic acid. The required level of folic acid fortification in the United States was estimated to provide 100 μg of additional folic acid in the average person's diet, though it probably provides more than this due to overuse of folic acid by food manufacturers.[9]

Other Pregnancy Complications. Adequate folate status may also prevent the occurrence of other types of birth defects, including certain heart defects and limb malformations. However, the support for these findings is not as consistent or clear as support for NTD prevention.[10] Low levels of dietary folate during pregnancy have also been associated with increased risk of premature delivery and infant low birth weight. More recently, elevated blood homocysteine levels, considered an indicator of functional folate deficiency, have been associated with increased incidence of miscarriage, as well as pregnancy complications like preeclampsia and placental abruption.[12] Thus, it is reasonable to maintain folic acid supplementation throughout pregnancy, even after closure of the neural tube, to decrease the risk of other problems in pregnancy.

Cardiovascular Diseases

Homocysteine and Cardiovascular Diseases. The results of more than 80 studies indicate that even moderately elevated levels of homocysteine in the blood increase the risk of cardiovascular diseases.[4] An analysis of the observational studies on homocysteine levels and vascular disease indicated that a prolonged decrease in plasma homocysteine of only 1 μmol/L resulted in about a 10% risk reduction.[13] The mechanism by which homocysteine increases the risk of vascular disease remains the subject of a great deal of research, but may involve adverse effects on clotting, arterial vasodilation, and thickening of arterial walls.[14] Although increased homocysteine levels in the blood have been consistently associated with increased risk of cardiovascular diseases, it is not yet clear whether lowering homocysteine levels will reduce cardiovascular disease risk. Consequently, the American Heart Association recommends screening for elevated total homocysteine levels only in "high-risk" individuals, for example those with personal or family history of premature cardiovascular disease, malnutrition or malabsorption syndromes, hypothyroidism, kidney failure, or lupus, or individuals taking certain medications (nicotinic acid, theophylline, bile acid–binding resins, methotrexate, and L-dopa).[15] Most research indicates that a plasma homocysteine level of less than 10 μmol/L is associated with a lower risk of cardiovascular disease and is a reasonable treatment goal for individuals at high risk.

Folate and Homocysteine. Folate-rich diets have been associated with decreased risk of cardiovascular disease. A study that followed 1980 Finnish men for 10 years found that those who consumed the most dietary folate had only 45% the risk of an acute coronary event when compared with those who consumed the least dietary folate.[16] Of the three vitamins that regulate homocysteine levels, folic acid has been shown to have the greatest effect in lowering basal levels of homocysteine in the blood when there is no coexisting deficiency of vitamin B_{12} or vitamin B_6. Increasing folate intake through folate-rich foods or supplements has been found to lower homocysteine levels. A supplement regimen of 400 μg of folic acid, 2 mg of vitamin B_6, and 6 μg of vitamin B_{12} has been advocated by the American Heart Association for those with elevated homocysteine levels, if an initial trial of a folate-rich diet is not successful in adequately lowering homocysteine levels.[15] Although increased folic acid intake has been found to decrease homocysteine levels, it is not presently known whether increasing supplemental folic acid intake will result in decreased rates of cardiovascular disease. Several randomized placebo-controlled trials are presently being conducted to determine whether homocysteine lowering through folic acid supplementation reduces coronary, cerebral, and peripheral vascular disease risk. Since the initiation of fortification of the U.S. food supply with folic acid, blood homocysteine levels in the population have declined.[9]

Cancer

Cancer is thought to arise from DNA damage in excess of ongoing DNA repair and/or the inappropriate expression of critical genes. Because of the important roles played by folate in DNA and RNA synthesis and methylation, it is possible for folate intake to affect both DNA repair and gene expression. The consumption of at least five servings of fruits and vegetables daily has been consistently associated with a decreased incidence of cancer. Fruits and vegetables are excellent sources of folate, which may play a role in their anticarcinogenic effect. Observational studies have found diminished folate status to be associated with cancers of the cervix, colon and rectum, lung, esophagus, brain, pancreas, and breast. Intervention trials in humans have been conducted mainly with respect to cervical and colorectal cancer. Although the results in cervical cancer have been inconsistent,[2] randomized intervention trials regarding colorectal cancer have been promising.[17,18]

Colorectal Cancer. The role of folate in preventing colorectal cancer provides an example of the complexity of the interactions between genetics and the nutritional environment. In general, observational studies have found relatively low folate intake and high alcohol intake to be associated with increased incidence of colorectal cancer.[1,19,20] Alcohol interferes with the absorption and metabolism of folate.[5] In a prospective study of more than 45,000 male health professionals, current intake of more than two alcoholic drinks per day doubled the risk of colon cancer. The combination of high alcohol and low folate intake yielded an even greater risk of colon cancer. However, increased alcohol intake in individuals who consumed 650 µg or more of folate per day was not associated with an increased risk of colon cancer.[21] In some studies, individuals who are homozygous for the C677T MTHFR polymorphism (T/T) have been found to be at decreased risk for colon cancer when folate intake is adequate. However, when folate intake is low and/or alcohol intake is high, individuals with the (T/T) genotype have been found to be at increased risk of colorectal cancer.[22,23]

Breast Cancer. A number of prospective studies have found that even moderate alcohol intake is associated with an increased risk of breast cancer in women. Recently, the results of three prospective studies suggested that increased folate intake may reduce the risk of breast cancer in women who regularly consume alcohol.[24–26] A very large prospective study of over 88,000 nurses found no relationship between folic acid intake and breast cancer in women who consumed less than one alcoholic drink per day. However, in those women consuming at least one alcoholic drink per day, folic acid intake of at least 600 µg daily resulted in about half the risk of breast cancer compared with women who consumed less than 300 µg of folic acid daily.[26]

Alzheimer's Disease and Dementia

The role of folate in nucleic acid synthesis and methylation reactions is essential for normal brain function. Over the past decade several investigators have described associations between decreased folate levels and cognitive impairment in the elderly.[27] A large cross-sectional study of elderly Canadians found that those individuals with low folate levels were more likely to have dementia, be institutionalized, and be depressed.[28] However, these findings could reflect the poorer nutritional status of institutionalized elderly and individuals with dementia. In the same study, low folate levels were associated with an increased likelihood of short-term memory problems in elderly individuals who did not show signs of dementia. In a recent study of 30 elderly nuns who lived in the same convent, ate the same diet, and had similar lifestyles, researchers found a strong association between decreased blood folate levels and the severity of brain atrophy related to Alzheimer's disease after their deaths.[29] Moderately increased homocysteine levels, as well as decreased folate and vitamin B_{12} levels, have also been associated with Alzheimer's disease and vascular dementia. Low-serum vitamin B_{12} (≤ 150 pmol/L) or folate (≤ 10 nmol/L) levels were associated with a doubling of the risk of developing Alzheimer's disease in 370 elderly men and women followed over 3 years.[30] In a sample of 1092 men and women without dementia followed for an average of 10 years, those with higher plasma homocysteine levels at baseline had a significantly higher risk of developing Alzheimer's disease and other types of dementia.[31] Those with plasma homocysteine levels greater than 14 µmol/L had nearly double the risk of developing Alzheimer's disease.

Disease Treatment

Presently, there is insufficient evidence to support the use of supplemental folic acid for the treatment of diseases or health conditions other than folate deficiency. The use of folic acid supplements to treat elevated plasma homocysteine levels (hyperhomocysteinemia) is discussed in the section on disease prevention under the heading "Cardiovascular Diseases."

Sources

Food Sources

Green leafy vegetables (foliage) are rich sources of folate and provide the basis for its name. Citrus fruit juices, legumes, and fortified cereals are also excellent sources of folate.[1] To help prevent NTD, the FDA required that 1.4 mg of folic acid per kilogram of grain be added to refined grain products, which are already enriched with niacin, thiamin, riboflavin, and iron, as of January 1, 1998. The addition of nutrients to foods to prevent a nutritional deficiency or restore nutrients lost in processing is known as *fortification*. It has been estimated that this level of fortification increases dietary intake by an average of 100 μg of folic acid per day.[10] A number of folate-rich foods are listed in Table 2–2 along with their folate content in micrograms.

Supplements

The principal form of supplementary folate is folic acid. It is available in single ingredient and combination products, such as B-complex vitamins and multivitamins. Doses of 1 mg or greater require a prescription.[32]

Safety

Toxicity

No adverse effects have been associated with the consumption of excess folate from foods. Concerns regarding safety are limited to synthetic folic acid intake. Deficiency of vitamin B_{12}, though often undiagnosed, may affect a

Table 2–2   Food Sources of Folate

Food	Serving	Folate, μg DFE
Fortified breakfast cereal	1 cup	200–400*
White rice, cooked	1 cup	222*
Lentils, cooked	1/2 cup	179
Garbanzo beans, cooked	1/2 cup	141
White pasta, cooked	1 cup	141*
Asparagus, cooked	1/2 cup (~6 spears)	131
Spinach, cooked	1/2 cup	131
Orange juice from concentrate	6 ounces	82
Lima beans, cooked	1/2 cup	78
White bread	1 slice	34*

*Fortified with folic acid (1.4 mg of folic acid/kg).

significant number of people, especially older adults. One symptom of vitamin B_{12} deficiency is megaloblastic anemia, which is indistinguishable from that associated with folate deficiency. Large doses of folic acid given to an individual with an undiagnosed vitamin B_{12} deficiency could correct megaloblastic anemia without correcting the underlying vitamin B_{12} deficiency, leaving the individual at risk of developing irreversible neurological damage. Most cases of this sort of neurological progression in vitamin B_{12} deficiency have been seen at doses of folic acid of 5000 μg (5 mg) and above. To be very sure of preventing irreversible neurological damage in vitamin B_{12}–deficient individuals, the Food and Nutrition Board of the Institute of Medicine advises that all adults limit their intake of folic acid (supplements and fortification) to 1000 μg daily (Table 2–3).[1] The board also noted that vitamin B_{12} deficiency is very rare in women in their childbearing years, making the consumption of folic acid at or above 1000 μg/d unlikely to cause problems, although there is limited data on the effects of large doses.

Table 2–3   Tolerable Upper Level of Intake (UL) for Folic Acid

Life Stage	Age	UL, μg/d
Infants	0–12 months	not possible to establish*
Children	1–3 years	300
Children	4–8 years	400
Children	9–13 years	600
Adolescents	14–18 years	800
Adults	19 years and older	1000

*Source of intake should be from food and formula only.

Drug Interactions

When taken in very large therapeutic dosages, for example in the treatment of severe arthritis, nonsteroidal anti-inflammatory drugs (NSAIDs) such as aspirin or ibuprofen may interfere with the metabolism of folate. Routine low-dose use of NSAIDs has not been found to adversely affect folate status. The anticonvulsant phenytoin has been shown to inhibit the intestinal absorption of folate, and several studies have associated decreased folate status with long-term use of phenytoin, phenobarbital, and primidone.[33] However, few studies controlled for differences in folate intake between anticonvulsant users and nonusers. Taking folic acid at the same time as the cholesterol-lowering agents cholestyramine and colestipol may decrease the absorption of folic acid.[32]

Methotrexate is a folic acid antagonist used to treat a number of diseases, including rheumatoid arthritis and psoriasis. Some of the side effects of methotrexate are similar to those of severe folate deficiency, and increased dietary folate or supplemental folic acid may decrease side effects without reducing the efficacy of methotrexate. A number of other medications have been shown to have antifolate activity, including trimethoprim (an antibiotic), pyrimethamine (an antimalarial drug), triamterene (a blood pressure medication), and sulfasalazine (a treatment for ulcerative colitis). Early studies of oral contraceptives (birth control pills) containing high doses of estrogen indicated an adverse effect on folate status, which has not been supported by more recent studies on low-dose oral contraceptives in which dietary folate was controlled.[1]

LPI Recommendation

Researchers at the Linus Pauling Institute feel that there exists ample scientific evidence to suggest that adequate folate intake is helpful in lowering the risk of cardiovascular diseases, some forms of cancer, dementia, and NTD and other poor outcomes of pregnancy, especially in genetically susceptible individuals. The Linus Pauling Institute recommends that adults take a 400-μg supplement of folic acid daily, in addition to folate and folic acid consumed in the diet. A daily multivitamin/mineral supplement containing 100% of the daily value will provide 400 μg of folic acid per day. Even with a larger than average intake of folic acid from fortified foods, it is unlikely that an individual's daily folic acid intake would regularly exceed the tolerable upper intake level of 1000 μg/d established by the Food and Nutrition Board.

Older Adults

The recommendation for 400 μg/d of supplemental folic acid as part of a daily multivitamin/multimineral supplement, in addition to a folate-rich diet, is especially relevant for adults 65 years and older because plasma homocysteine levels tend to increase with age.

Women Capable of Becoming Pregnant

Because the crucial events in the development of the neural tube occur before many women are aware that they are pregnant, women who are capable of becoming pregnant should consume 400 μg/d of folic acid from supplements or fortified food in addition to dietary sources to prevent NTD.

References

1. Food and Nutrition Board, Institute of Medicine. Folic acid. *Dietary Reference Intakes: Thiamin, Riboflavin, Niacin, Vitamin B-6, Vitamin B-12, Pantothenic Acid, Biotin, and Choline.* Washington, D.C.: National Academy Press; 1998:193–305.
2. Choi SW, Mason JB. Folate and carcinogenesis: an integrated scheme. *J Nutr* 2000;130(2):129–132.

3. Bailey LB, Gregory JF, 3rd. Folate metabolism and requirements. *J Nutr* 1999;129(4):779–782.
4. Gerhard GT, Duell PB. Homocysteine and atherosclerosis. *Curr Opin Lipidol* 1999;10(5):417–428.
5. Herbert V. Folic acid. In: Shils M, Olson JA, Shike M, Ross AC, eds. *Nutrition in Health and Disease.* 9th ed. Baltimore: Williams & Wilkins; 1999:433–446.
6. Bailey LB. Dietary reference intakes for folate: the debut of dietary folate equivalents. *Nutr Rev* 1998;56(10):294–299.
7. Bailey LB, Gregory JF, 3rd. Polymorphisms of methylenetetrahydrofolate reductase and other enzymes: metabolic significance, risks and impact on folate requirement. *J Nutr* 1999;129(5):919–922.
8. Kauwell GP, Wilsky CE, Cerda JJ, et al. Methylenetetrahydrofolate reductase mutation (677C->T) negatively influences plasma homocysteine response to marginal folate intake in elderly women. *Metabolism* 2000;49(11):1440–1443.
9. Shane B. Folic acid, vitamin B-12, and vitamin B-6. In: Stipanuk M, ed. *Biochemical and Physiological Aspects of Human Nutrition.* Philadelphia: W.B. Saunders Co.; 2000:483–518.
10. Eskes TK. Open or closed? A world of difference: a history of homocysteine research. *Nutr Rev* 1998;56(8):236–244.
11. McNulty H, Cuskelly GJ, Ward M. Response of red blood cell folate to intervention: implications for folate recommendations for the prevention of neural tube defects. *Am J Clin Nutr* 2000;71(5 Suppl):1308S–1311S.
12. Scholl TO, Johnson WG. Folic acid: influence on the outcome of pregnancy. *Am J Clin Nutr* 2000;71(5 Suppl):1295S–1303S.
13. Boushey CJ, Beresford SA, Omenn GS, Motulsky AG. A quantitative assessment of plasma homocysteine as a risk factor for vascular disease: probable benefits of increasing folic acid intakes. *JAMA* 1995;274(13):1049–1057.
14. Seshadri N, Robinson K. Homocysteine, B vitamins, and coronary artery disease. *Med Clin North Am* 2000;84(1):215–237.
15. Malinow MR, Bostom AG, Krauss RM. Homocyst(e)ine, diet, and cardiovascular diseases: a statement for healthcare professionals from the Nutrition Committee, American Heart Association. *Circulation* 1999;99(1):178–182.
16. Voutilainen S, Rissanen TH, Virtanen J, Lakka TA, Salonen JT. Low dietary folate intake is associated with an excess incidence of acute coronary events: The Kuopio Ischemic Heart Disease Risk Factor Study. *Circulation* 2001;103(22):2674–2680.
17. Kim YI, Baik HW, Fawaz K, et al. Effects of folate supplementation on two provisional molecular markers of colon cancer: a prospective, randomized trial. *Am J Gastroenterol* 2001;96(1):184–195.
18. Cravo ML, Pinto AG, Chaves P, et al. Effect of folate supplementation on DNA methylation of rectal mucosa in patients with colonic adenomas: correlation with nutrient intake. *Clin Nutr* 1998;17(2):45–49.
19. Su LJ, Arab L. Nutritional status of folate and colon cancer risk: evidence from NHANES I epidemiologic follow-up study. *Ann Epidemiol* 2001;11(1):65–72.
20. Terry P, Jain M, Miller AB, Howe GR, Rohan TE. Dietary intake of folic acid and colorectal cancer risk in a cohort of women. *Int J Cancer* 2002;97(6):864–867.
21. Giovannucci E, Rimm EB, Ascherio A, Stampfer MJ, Colditz GA, Willett WC. Alcohol, low-methionine–low-folate diets, and risk of colon cancer in men. *J Natl Cancer Inst* 1995;87(4):265–273.
22. Slattery ML, Potter JD, Samowitz W, Schaffer D, Leppert M. Methylenetetrahydrofolate reductase, diet, and risk of colon cancer. *Cancer Epidemiol Biomarkers Prev* 1999;8(6):513–518.
23. Ma J, Stampfer MJ, Giovannucci E, et al. Methylenetetrahydrofolate reductase polymorphism, dietary interactions, and risk of colorectal cancer. *Cancer Res* 1997;57(6):1098–1102.
24. Rohan TE, Jain MG, Howe GR, Miller AB. Dietary folate consumption and breast cancer risk. *J Natl Cancer Inst* 2000;92(3):266–269.
25. Sellers TA, Kushi LH, Cerhan JR, et al. Dietary folate intake, alcohol, and risk of breast cancer in a prospective study of postmenopausal women. *Epidemiology* 2001;12(4):420–428.
26. Zhang S, Hunter DJ, Hankinson SE, et al. A prospective study of folate intake and the risk of breast cancer. *JAMA* 1999;281(17):1632–1637.
27. Weir DG, Molloy AM. Microvascular disease and dementia in the elderly: are they related to hyperhomocysteinemia? *Am J Clin Nutr* 2000;71(4):859–860.
28. Ebly EM, Schaefer JP, Campbell NR, Hogan DB. Folate status, vascular disease and cognition in elderly Canadians. *Age Ageing* 1998;27(4):485–491.
29. Snowdon DA, Tully CL, Smith CD, Riley KP, Markesbery WR. Serum folate and the severity of atrophy of the neocortex in Alzheimer disease: findings from the Nun study. *Am J Clin Nutr* 2000;71(4):993–998.
30. Wang HX, Wahlin A, Basun H, Fastbom J, Winblad B, Fratiglioni L. Vitamin B(12) and folate in relation to the development of Alzheimer's disease. *Neurology* 2001;56(9):1188–1194.
31. Seshadri S, Beiser A, Selhub J, et al. Plasma homocysteine as a risk factor for dementia and Alzheimer's disease. *N Engl J Med* 2002;346(7):476–483.
32. Hendler SS, Rorvik DR, eds. *PDR for Nutritional Supplements.* Montvale, NJ: Medical Economics Company, Inc.; 2001.
33. Apeland T, Mansoor MA, Strandjord RE. Antiepileptic drugs as independent predictors of plasma total homocysteine levels. *Epilepsy Res* 2001;47(1–2):27–35.

3 Niacin

Niacin is a water-soluble vitamin, also known as vitamin B_3. The term *niacin* refers to nicotinic acid and nicotinamide, which are both used by the body to form the coenzymes nicotinamide adenine dinucleotide (NAD) and nicotinamide adenine dinucleotide phosphate (NADP). Neither form is related to the nicotine found in tobacco, although their names are similar.[1]

Function

Oxidation-Reduction (Redox) Reactions

Living organisms derive most of their energy from oxidation-reduction (redox) reactions, which are processes involving the transfer of electrons. As many as 200 enzymes require the niacin coenzymes NAD and NADP, mainly to accept or donate electrons for redox reactions. NAD functions most often in reactions involving the degradation (catabolism) of carbohydrates, fats, proteins, and alcohol to produce energy. NADP functions more often in biosynthetic (anabolic) reactions, such as in the synthesis of fatty acids and cholesterol.[1,2]

Nonredox Reactions

The niacin coenzyme NAD is the substrate (reactant) for two classes of enzymes (mono-ADP-ribosyltransferases and poly-ADP-ribose polymerase) that separate the niacin moiety from NAD and transfer ADP-ribose to proteins (Fig. 3–1). Mono-ADP-ribosyltransferase enzymes were first discovered in certain bacteria where they were found to produce toxins such as those of cholera and diphtheria. These enzymes and their products, ADP-ribosylated proteins, have also been found in the cells of mammals and are thought to play a role in cell signaling by affecting G-protein activity.[3] G-proteins are proteins that bind guanosine triphosphate and act as intermediaries in a number of cell-signaling pathways. Poly-ADP-ribose polymerases (PARPs) are enzymes that catalyze the transfer of many ADP-ribose units from NAD to acceptor proteins. PARPs appear to function in DNA replication and repair, as well as cell differentiation, suggesting a possible role for NAD in cancer prevention.[2] At least five different PARPs have been identified, and although their functions are not yet well understood, their existence indicates a potential for considerable consumption of NAD.[4] A third class of enzyme (ADP-ribosyl cyclase) catalyzes the formation of cyclic ADP-ribose, a molecule that works within cells to provoke the release of calcium ions from internal storage sites, and probably also plays a role in cell signaling.[1]

Deficiency

Pellagra

The late stage of severe niacin deficiency is known as pellagra. Early records of pellagra followed the widespread cultivation of corn in Europe in the 1700s.[1] The disease was generally associated with the poorer social classes whose chief dietary staple consisted of cereals, like corn or sorghum. Pellagra was also common in the southern United States during the early 1900s where income was low and corn products were a major dietary staple.[5] Interestingly, pellagra was not known in Mexico, where corn was also an important dietary staple and much of the population was also poor. In fact, corn contains appreciable amounts of niacin, but it is present in a bound form that is not nutritionally available to humans. The traditional preparation of corn tortillas in Mexico involves soaking the corn in a lime (calcium oxide) solution prior to cooking. Heating the corn in an alkaline solution results in the release of bound niacin, increasing its bioavailability.[6]

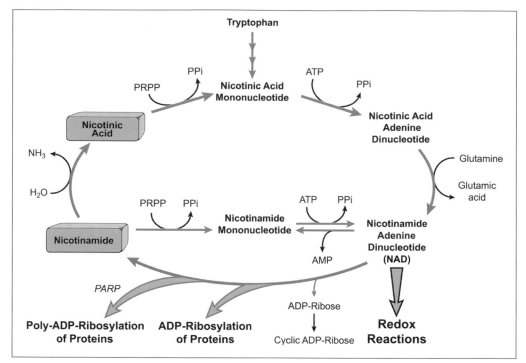

Figure 3–1. Synthesis of nicotinamide adenine dinucleotide (NAD) from nicotinic acid, nicotinamide, or tryptophan. NAD is required for numerous redox reactions. NAD is also consumed in adenosine diphosphate ribosylation reactions. Abbreviations: AMP, adenosine monophosphate; ADP, adenosine diphosphate; ATP, adenosine triphosphate; PARP, poly-ADP-ribose polymerase; PPi, inorganic pyrophosphate; PRPP, phosphoribosyl pyrophosphate.

The most common symptoms of niacin deficiency involve the skin, digestive system, and nervous system.[2] The symptoms of pellagra were commonly referred to as the four D's: dermatitis, diarrhea, dementia, and death. In the skin, a thick, scaly, darkly pigmented rash develops symmetrically in areas exposed to sunlight. The word "pellagra" comes from the Italian phrase for rough or raw skin. Symptoms related to the digestive system include a bright red tongue, vomiting, and diarrhea. Neurologic symptoms include headache, apathy, fatigue, depression, disorientation, and memory loss. If untreated, pellagra is ultimately fatal.

Nutrient Interactions

Tryptophan and Niacin. In addition to its synthesis from dietary niacin, NAD may also be synthesized in the liver from the dietary amino acid tryptophan. The synthesis of niacin from tryptophan also depends on enzymes that require vitamin B_6 and riboflavin, as well as an enzyme containing heme (iron). On average, 1 mg of niacin can be synthesized from the ingestion of 60 mg of tryptophan. Thus, 60 mg of tryptophan are considered to be 1 mg of niacin equivalents (NE). However, studies of pellagra in the southern United States during the early 20th century indicated that the diets of many individuals who suffered from pellagra contained enough NE to prevent pellagra,[3] challenging the idea that 60 mg of dietary tryptophan are equivalent to 1 mg of niacin. One study, in particular, found that the tryptophan content of the diet had no effect on the decrease in red blood cell niacin content that resulted from decreased dietary niacin in young men.[7]

Table 3–1   Recommended Dietary Allowance (RDA) for Niacin

Life Stage	Age	Males, mg NE*/d	Females, mg NE/d
Infants	0–6 months	2 (AI)[†]	2 (AI)[†]
Infants	7–12 months	4 (AI)	4 (AI)
Children	1–3 years	6	6
Children	4–8 years	8	8
Children	9–13 years	12	12
Adolescents	14–18 years	16	14
Adults	19 years and older	16	14
Pregnancy	all ages	–	18
Breastfeeding	all ages	–	17

AI, adequate intake level.
*1 mg NE = 60 mg of tryptophan = 1 mg niacin.
[†]2 mg preformed niacin/d.

Causes of Niacin Deficiency

Niacin deficiency or pellagra may result from inadequate dietary intake of niacin and/or tryptophan. As mentioned previously, other nutrient deficiencies may also contribute to the development of niacin deficiency. Patients with Hartnup's disease, a hereditary disorder resulting in defective tryptophan absorption, have developed pellagra.[2] Carcinoid syndrome, a condition of increased secretion of serotonin and other catecholamines by carcinoid tumors, may also result in pellagra due to increased utilization of dietary tryptophan for serotonin rather than niacin synthesis. Prolonged treatment with the antituberculosis drug isoniazid has also resulted in niacin deficiency.[8]

The Recommended Dietary Allowance

The recommended dietary allowance (RDA) for niacin, revised in 1998, was based on the prevention of deficiency (Table 3–1). Pellagra can be prevented by about 11 mg NE/d, but 12 to 16 mg/d has been found to normalize the urinary excretion of niacin metabolites (breakdown products) in healthy young adults. Because pellagra represents severe deficiency, the Food and Nutrition Board chose to use the excretion of niacin metabolites as an indicator of niacin status rather than symptoms of pellagra.[8] However, some researchers feel that cellular NAD and NADP content may be more relevant indicators of niacin nutritional status.[9]

Disease Prevention

Cancer

Studies of cultured cells in vitro provide evidence that NAD content influences the cellular response to DNA damage, an important risk factor for cancer. Cellular NAD is consumed in the synthesis of ADP-ribose polymers, which play a role in DNA repair, and cyclic ADP-ribose may mediate cell-signaling pathways important in the prevention of cancer.[10] Additionally, cellular NAD content has been found to influence levels of the tumor suppressor protein p53 in human breast, skin, and lung cells.[11] Neither the cellular NAD content nor the dietary intake of NAD precursors (niacin and tryptophan) necessary for optimizing protective responses following DNA damage has been determined, but they are likely to be higher than required for the prevention of pellagra. Niacin deficiency was found to decrease bone marrow NAD and poly-ADP-ribose levels and increase the risk of chemically induced leukemia in rats,[12] and niacin supplementation decreased the risk of ultraviolet light–induced skin cancers in mice.[13] However, little is known regarding cellular NAD levels and the prevention of DNA damage or cancer in humans. Elevation of NAD levels in blood lymphocytes after supplementation of two healthy individuals with 100 mg/d of nicotinic acid for 8 weeks reduced DNA strand breaks in lymphocytes exposed to free radicals in a test tube assay compared with those of nonsupplemented individuals.[14] More recently, nicotinic acid supplementation of up to 100 mg/d in 21 healthy smokers failed to provide any evidence of a decrease in cigarette smoke–induced genetic damage in blood lymphocytes compared with placebo.[15]

Generally, relationships between dietary factors and cancer are established first in epidemiologic studies and followed up by basic cancer research on the cellular level. In the case of niacin, research on biochemical and cellular aspects of DNA repair have stimulated an interest in the relationship between niacin intake and cancer risk in human populations.[16] Recently, a large case-control study found increased consumption of niacin, along with antioxidant nutrients, to be associated with decreased incidence of oral, pharyngeal, and esophageal cancers in northern Italy and Switzerland.[17,18] An increase in niacin intake of 6.2 mg was associated with about a 40% decrease in cases of cancers of the mouth and throat, and a 5.2 mg increase in niacin intake was associated with a similar decrease in cases of cancer of the esophagus.

Insulin-Dependent Diabetes Mellitus (IDDM)

Insulin-dependent diabetes mellitus in children is known to result from the autoimmune destruction of insulin-secreting β-cells in the pancreas. Prior to the onset of symptomatic diabetes, specific antibodies, including islet cell antibodies (ICA), can be detected in the blood of high-risk individuals. The ability to detect individuals at high risk for the development of IDDM has led to the enrollment of high-risk siblings of children diagnosed with IDDM into trials designed to prevent its onset. Evidence from in vitro and animal research indicates that high levels of nicotinamide protect β-cells from damage by toxic chemicals, inflammatory white blood cells, and reactive oxygen species. Pharmacologic doses of nicotinamide (up to 3 g/d) were first used to protect β-cells in patients shortly after the onset of IDDM. An analysis of 10 published trials (five placebo-controlled) found evidence of improved β-cell function after 1 year of treatment with nicotinamide but failed to find any clinical evidence of improved glycemic control.[19] Recently, high doses of nicotinamide were found to decrease insulin sensitivity in high-risk relatives of IDDM patients,[20] which might explain the finding of improved β-cell function without concomitant improvement in glycemic control. Several pilot studies for the prevention of IDDM in ICA-positive relatives of patients with IDDM yielded conflicting results. While a large randomized trial in school children that was not placebo-controlled found a significantly lower incidence of IDDM in the nicotinamide-treated group, a large multicenter, randomized, placebo-controlled trial of nicotinamide in ICA-positive siblings of IDDM patients between 3 and 12 years of age recently failed to find a difference in the incidence of IDDM after 3 years.[19] Another large multicenter trial of nicotinamide in high-risk relatives of IDDM patients is presently in progress.[21] Unlike nicotinamide, nicotinic acid has not been found effective in the prevention of IDDM.

Disease Treatment

High Cholesterol and Cardiovascular Disease

Pharmacologic doses of nicotinic acid, but not nicotinamide, have been known to reduce blood cholesterol since 1955.[22] Only one randomized placebo-controlled multicenter trial examined the effect of nicotinic acid therapy alone (3 g/d) on outcomes of cardiovascular disease. The Coronary Drug Project followed over 8000 men with a previous myocardial infarction (heart attack) for 6 years.[23] In the group that took 3 g of nicotinic acid daily, total blood cholesterol decreased by an average of 10%, triglycerides decreased by 26%, recurrent nonfatal myocardial infarction decreased by 27%, and cerebrovascular events (stroke plus transient ischemic attacks) decreased by 26% compared with the placebo group. Though nicotinic acid therapy did not decrease total deaths or deaths from cardiovascular disease during the 6-year study period, posttrial follow-up 9 years later revealed a 10% reduction in total deaths. Four of five major cardiovascular outcome trials found nicotinic acid in combination with other therapies to be of statistically significant benefit in men and women.[24] Nicotinic acid therapy has been found to result in markedly increased high-density lipoprotein (HDL) cholesterol levels, as well as decreased serum Lp(a) lipoprotein concentrations, and a shift from small, dense low-density lipoprotein (LDL) particles to large, buoyant LDL particles, all of which are considered cardioprotective changes in blood lipid profiles.

Because of the adverse side effects associated with high doses of nicotinic acid (see under "Safety"), it has most recently been used in combination with other lipid-lowering medications in slightly lower doses.[22] A recent randomized clinical trial found that a combination of nicotinic acid (2 to 3 g/d) and a cholesterol-lowering drug (simvastatin) resulted in greater benefits on serum HDL levels and cardiovascular events, such as heart attack and stroke, than placebo in patients with coronary artery disease and low HDL levels.[25,26] However, an antioxidant combination (vitamin E, vitamin C, selenium, and β-carotene) appeared to blunt the beneficial effects of niacin plus simvastatin.

Although it is a nutrient, at the pharmacologic dose required for cholesterol-lowering effects the use of nicotinic acid should be approached as if it were a drug. Individuals should only undertake cholesterol-lowering therapy with nicotinic acid under the supervision of a qualified health care provider, so that the potential for adverse effects may be minimized and treatment benefit maximized.

Human Immunodeficiency Virus

It has been hypothesized that infection with human immunodeficiency virus (HIV), the virus that causes acquired immunodeficiency syndrome (AIDS), increases the risk of niacin deficiency. Interferon-gamma (IF-γ) is a cytokine produced by cells of the immune system in response to infection. IF-γ levels are elevated in individuals infected with HIV, and higher IF-γ levels have been associated with poorer prognosis. By stimulating the enzyme, indoleamine 2,3 dioxygenase (IDO), IF-γ is known to increase the breakdown of tryptophan, a niacin precursor, supporting the idea that infection with HIV increases the risk of niacin deficiency.[27] In a very small, uncontrolled study, treatment of four HIV-positive individuals with 1000 to 1500 mg/d of nicotinamide for 2 months resulted in 40% increases in plasma tryptophan levels.[28] A study of 281 HIV-positive men found that higher levels of niacin intake were associated with decreased progression rate to AIDS and improved survival.[29]

Sources

Food Sources

Good sources of niacin include yeast, meat, poultry, fish (e.g., tuna, salmon), cereals (especially fortified cereals), legumes, and seeds. Milk, green leafy vegetables, coffee, and tea also provide some niacin.[3] In plants, especially mature cereal grains like corn and wheat, niacin may be bound to large molecules in the form of glycosides, significantly decreasing niacin bioavailability.[6]

In the United States, the average intake of niacin is about 30 mg/d for young adult men and 20 mg/d for young adult women. In a sample of adults over the age of 60, men were found to have an average dietary intake of 21 mg/d and women 17 mg/d.[8] Some foods with substantial amounts of niacin are listed in Table 3–2 along with their niacin content in milligrams. Food composition tables generally list niacin content without including NE from tryptophan or any adjustment for niacin bioavailability.

Supplements

Niacin supplements are available as nicotinamide or nicotinic acid. Nicotinamide is the form of niacin typically used in nutritional supplements and in food fortification. Nicotinic acid is available over the counter and with a prescription as a cholesterol-lowering agent.[30] The nomenclature for nicotinic acid formulations can be confusing. Nicotinic acid is available over the counter in an "immediate-release" (crystalline) and "slow-release" or "timed-release" form. A shorter-acting timed-release preparation referred to as "intermediate release" or "extended release" nicotinic acid is available by prescription.[31,32] Due to the potential for side effects, medical supervision is recommended for the use of nicotinic acid as a cholesterol-lowering agent.

Table 3–2   Food Sources of Niacin

Food	Serving	Niacin, mg
Cereal, fortified	1 cup	20–27
Tuna, light, packed in water	3 ounces*	11.3
Chicken, light meat	3 ounces,* cooked without skin	10.6
Salmon	3 ounces,* cooked	8.5
Turkey, light meat	3 ounces,* cooked without skin	5.8
Cereal, unfortified	1 cup	5–7
Peanuts	1 ounce, dry roasted	3.8
Beef, lean	3 ounces,* cooked	3.1
Pasta, enriched	1 cup, cooked	2.3
Lentils	1 cup, cooked	2.1
Lima beans	1 cup, cooked	1.8
Bread, whole wheat	1 slice	1.1
Coffee, brewed	1 cup	0.5

*A 3-ounce serving of meat or fish is about the size of a deck of cards.

Safety

Toxicity

Niacin from foods is not known to cause adverse effects. Although one study noted adverse effects from the consumption of bagels to which were added 60 times the normal amount of niacin fortification, most adverse effects have been reported with pharmacologic preparations of niacin.[8]

Nicotinic Acid. Flushing, itching, and gastrointestinal disturbances such as nausea and vomiting are common. Hepatotoxicity (liver cell damage), including elevated liver enzymes and jaundice, has been observed at intakes as low as 750 mg of nicotinic acid per day for less than 3 months.[31,32] Hepatitis has been observed with timed-release nicotinic acid on as little as 500 mg/d for 2 months, although almost all reports of severe hepatitis have been

associated with the timed-release form of nicotinic acid at doses of 3 to 9 g/d used to treat high cholesterol for months or years.[8] Immediate-release (crystalline) nicotinic acid appears to be less toxic to the liver than extended release forms. Immediate-release nicotinic acid is often used at higher doses than timed-release forms, and severe liver toxicity has occurred in individuals who substituted timed-release niacin for immediate-release niacin at equivalent doses.[30] Skin rashes and dry skin have been noted with nicotinic acid supplementation. Transient episodes of low blood pressure (hypotension) and headache have also been reported. Large doses of nicotinic acid have been observed to impair glucose tolerance, likely due to decreased insulin sensitivity. Impaired glucose-tolerance in susceptible (prediabetic) individuals could result in elevated blood glucose levels and clinical diabetes. Elevated blood levels of uric acid, occasionally resulting in attacks of gout in susceptible individuals, have also been observed with high-dose nicotinic acid therapy.[32] Nicotinic acid at doses of 1.5 to 5 g/d has resulted in a few case reports of blurred vision and other eye problems, which have generally been reversible upon discontinuation. People with abnormal liver function or a history of liver disease, diabetes, active peptic ulcer disease, gout, cardiac arrhythmias, inflammatory bowel disease, migraine headaches, and alcoholism may be more susceptible to the adverse effects of excess nicotinic acid intake than the general population.[8]

Nicotinamide. Nicotinamide is generally better tolerated than nicotinic acid. It does not generally cause flushing. However, nausea, vomiting, and signs of liver toxicity (elevated liver enzymes, jaundice) have been observed at doses of 3 g/d.[30] Nicotinamide has resulted in decreased insulin sensitivity at doses of 2 g/d in adults at high risk of IDDM.[20]

The Tolerable Upper Intake Level. Flushing of the skin primarily on the face, arms, and chest is a common side effect of nicotinic acid and may occur initially at doses as low as 30 mg/d. Although flushing on nicotinamide is rare, the Food and Nutrition Board set the tolerable upper intake level (UL) for niacin (nicotinic acid and nicotinamide) at 35 mg/d to avoid the adverse effect of flushing in the general population (Table 3–3). The UL is not meant to apply to individuals who are being treated with a nutrient under medical supervision, as should be the case with high-dose nicotinic acid for elevated blood cholesterol levels.[8]

Drug Interactions

Coadministration of nicotinic acid with lovastatin (another cholesterol-lowering medication) may have resulted in rhabdomyolysis in a small number of case reports. Rhabdomyolysis is a relatively uncommon condition in which muscle cells are broken down, releasing muscle enzymes and electrolytes into the blood, sometimes resulting in kidney failure. Sulfinpyrazone is a medication for the treatment of gout that promotes excretion of uric acid from the blood into urine. Nicotinic acid may inhibit this "uricosuric" effect of sulfinpyrazone.[30] Long-term administration of the cancer chemotherapy agent 5-fluorouracil has been reported to cause symptoms of pellagra. Niacin supplementation is recommended during long-term treatment of tuberculosis with isoniazid. Isoniazid is a niacin antagonist, and long-term treatment has resulted in pellagra-like symptoms.[33] Estrogen and estrogen-containing oral contraceptives increase the efficiency of niacin synthesis from tryptophan, resulting in a decreased dietary requirement for niacin.[2]

LPI Recommendation

The optimum intake of niacin for health promotion and chronic disease prevention is not yet known. The RDA (16 mg NE/d for men and 14 mg NE/d for women) is easily obtainable in a varied diet and should prevent deficiency in most people. Following the Linus Pauling Institute recommendation to take a daily multivitamin/mineral supplement, containing 100% of the daily value for niacin, will provide at least 20 mg of niacin daily.

Table 3–3 Tolerable Upper Level of Intake (UL) for Niacin

Life Stage	Age	UL, mg/d
Infants	0–12 months	not possible to establish*
Children	1–3 years	10
Children	4–8 years	15
Children	9–13 years	20
Adolescents	14–18 years	30
Adults	19 years and older	35

*Source of intake should be from food and formula only.

Older Adults

Dietary surveys indicate that 15 to 25% of older adults (65 years and older) do not consume enough niacin in their diets to meet the RDA (16 mg NE/d for men and 14 mg NE/d for women) and that dietary intake of niacin decreases between the ages of 60 and 90 years. Thus, it is advisable for older adults to supplement their dietary intake with a multivitamin/multimineral supplement, which will generally provide at least 20 mg of niacin daily.

References

1. Brody T. *Nutritional Biochemistry*. 2nd ed. San Diego: Academic Press; 1999.
2. Cervantes-Laurean D, McElvaney NG, Moss J. Niacin. In: Shils M, Olson JA, Shike M, Ross AC, eds. *Nutrition in Health and Disease*. 9th ed. Baltimore: Williams & Wilkins; 1999:401–411.
3. Jacob R, Swenseid M. Niacin. In: Ziegler EE, Filer LJ, eds. *Present Knowledge in Nutrition*. 7th ed. Washington, D.C.: ILSI Press; 1996:185–190.
4. Jacobson MK, Jacobson EL. Discovering new ADP-ribose polymer cycles: protecting the genome and more. *Trends Biochem Sci* 1999;24(11):415–417.
5. Park YK, Sempos CT, Barton CN, Vanderveen JE, Yetley EA. Effectiveness of food fortification in the United States: the case of pellagra. *Am J Public Health* 2000;90(5):727–738.
6. Gregory JF, 3rd. Nutritional properties and significance of vitamin glycosides. *Annu Rev Nutr* 1998;18:277–296.
7. Jacobson EL, Jacobson MK. Tissue NAD as a biochemical measure of niacin status in humans. *Methods Enzymol* 1997;280:221–230.

8. Food and Nutrition Board, Institute of Medicine. Niacin. *Dietary Reference Intakes: Thiamin, Riboflavin, Niacin, Vitamin B-6, Vitamin B-12, Pantothenic Acid, Biotin, and Choline.* Washington, D.C.: National Academy Press; 1998:123–149.

9. Fu CS, Swendseid ME, Jacob RA, McKee RW. Biochemical markers for assessment of niacin status in young men: levels of erythrocyte niacin coenzymes and plasma tryptophan. *J Nutr* 1989;119(12):1949–1955.

10. Hageman GJ, Stierum RH. Niacin, poly(ADP-ribose) polymerase-1 and genomic stability. *Mutat Res* 2001; 475(1–2):45–56.

11. Jacobson EL, Shieh WM, Huang AC. Mapping the role of NAD metabolism in prevention and treatment of carcinogenesis. *Mol Cell Biochem* 1999;193(1–2):69–74.

12. Boyonoski AC, Spronck JC, Gallacher LM, et al. Niacin deficiency decreases bone marrow poly(ADP-ribose) and the latency of ethylnitrosourea-induced carcinogenesis in rats. *J Nutr* 2002;132(1):108–114.

13. Gensler HL, Williams T, Huang AC, Jacobson EL. Oral niacin prevents photocarcinogenesis and photoimmunosuppression in mice. *Nutr Cancer* 1999;34(1): 36–41.

14. Weitberg AB. Effect of nicotinic acid supplementation in vivo on oxygen radical-induced genetic damage in human lymphocytes. *Mutat Res* 1989;216(4):197–201.

15. Hageman GJ, Stierum RH, van Herwijnen MH, van der Veer MS, Kleinjans JC. Nicotinic acid supplementation: effects on niacin status, cytogenetic damage, and poly(ADP-ribosylation) in lymphocytes of smokers. *Nutr Cancer* 1998;32(2):113–120.

16. Jacobson EL. Niacin deficiency and cancer in women. *J Am Coll Nutr* 1993;12(4):412–416.

17. Negri E, Franceschi S, Bosetti C, et al. Selected micronutrients and oral and pharyngeal cancer. *Int J Cancer* 2000;86(1):122–127.

18. Franceschi S, Bidoli E, Negri E, et al. Role of macronutrients, vitamins and minerals in the aetiology of squamous-cell carcinoma of the oesophagus. *Int J Cancer* 2000;86(5):626–631.

19. Lampeter EF, Klinghammer A, Scherbaum WA, et al. The Deutsche Nicotinamide Intervention Study: an attempt to prevent type 1 diabetes. DENIS Group. *Diabetes* 1998;47(6):980–984.

20. Greenbaum CJ, Kahn SE, Palmer JP. Nicotinamide's effects on glucose metabolism in subjects at risk for IDDM. *Diabetes* 1996;45(11):1631–1634.

21. Schatz DA, Bingley PJ. Update on major trials for the prevention of type 1 diabetes mellitus: the American Diabetes Prevention Trial (DPT-1) and the European Nicotinamide Diabetes Intervention Trial (ENDIT). *J Pediatr Endocrinol Metab* 2001;14(Suppl 1):619–622.

22. Knopp RH. Drug treatment of lipid disorders. *N Engl J Med* 1999;341(7):498–511.

23. Canner PL, Berge KG, Wenger NK, et al. Fifteen year mortality in Coronary Drug Project patients: long-term benefit with niacin. *J Am Coll Cardiol* 1986;8(6):1245–1255.

24. Guyton JR, Capuzzi DM. Treatment of hyperlipidemia with combined niacin-statin regimens. *Am J Cardiol* 1998;82(12A):82U–84U; discussion 85U–86U.

25. Cheung MC, Zhao XQ, Chait A, Albers JJ, Brown BG. Antioxidant supplements block the response of HDL to simvastatin-niacin therapy in patients with coronary artery disease and low HDL. *Arterioscler Thromb Vasc Biol* 2001;21(8):1320–1326.

26. Brown BG, Zhao XQ, Chait A, et al. Simvastatin and niacin, antioxidant vitamins, or the combination for the prevention of coronary disease. *N Engl J Med* 2001;345(22):1583–1592.

27. Brown RR, Ozaki Y, Datta SP, Borden EC, Sondel PM, Malone DG. Implications of interferon-induced tryptophan catabolism in cancer, auto-immune diseases and AIDS. *Adv Exp Med Biol* 1991;294:425–435.

28. Murray MF, Langan M, MacGregor RR. Increased plasma tryptophan in HIV-infected patients treated with pharmacologic doses of nicotinamide. *Nutrition* 2001;17(7–8):654–656.

29. Tang AM, Graham NM, Saah AJ. Effects of micronutrient intake on survival in human immunodeficiency virus type 1 infection. *Am J Epidemiol* 1996;143(12):1244–1256.

30. Hendler SS, Rorvik DR, eds. *PDR for Nutritional Supplements.* Montvale, NJ: Medical Economics Company, Inc.; 2001.

31. Knopp RH. Evaluating niacin in its various forms. *Am J Cardiol* 2000;86(12A):51L–56L.

32. Vitamins. *Drug Facts and Comparisons.* St. Louis: Facts and Comparisons; 2000:6–33.

33. Flodin N. *Pharmacology of Micronutrients.* New York: Alan R. Liss, Inc.; 1988.

4 Pantothenic Acid

Pantothenic acid, also known as vitamin B_5, is a component of coenzyme A (CoA) and acyl carrier protein.[1] In these roles, pantothenic acid is essential to virtually all forms of life.[2]

Function

Coenzyme A

As a component of coenzyme A (CoA), pantothenic acid is essential to a variety of chemical reactions that sustain life. CoA is required for the generation of energy in the form of adenosine triphosphate (ATP) from fats, carbohydrates, and proteins. The synthesis of essential fats, cholesterol, and steroid hormones requires CoA, as does the synthesis of the neurotransmitter, acetylcholine, and the hormone melatonin. Heme, a component of hemoglobin, requires a CoA-containing compound for its synthesis. Metabolism of a number of drugs and toxins by the liver requires CoA.[3] Coenzyme A was named for its role in acetylation reactions. Most acetylated proteins in the body have been modified by the addition of an acetate group that was donated by CoA. Protein acetylation affects the three-dimensional structure of proteins, potentially altering protein function and peptide hormone activity, in addition to playing a role in cell division and DNA replication. Protein acetylation also affects gene expression by facilitating the transcription of messenger RNA. A number of proteins are also modified by the attachment of long-chain fatty acids donated by CoA. These modifications are known as protein acylation and appear to play a central role in cell signaling.[1]

Acyl-Carrier Protein

The acyl-carrier protein requires pantothenic acid in the form of 4′-phosphopantetheine for its activity as an enzyme.[1,4] Both CoA and the acyl-carrier protein are required for the syn-thesis of fatty acids. Fatty acids are a component of some lipids, which are fat molecules essential for normal physiological function. Among these essential fats are sphingolipids, which are a component of the myelin sheath that enhances nerve transmission, and phospholipids in cell membranes.

Deficiency

Naturally occurring pantothenic acid deficiency in humans is very rare and has been observed only in cases of severe malnutrition. World War II prisoners in the Philippines, Burma, and Japan experienced numbness and painful burning and tingling in their feet, which was relieved specifically by pantothenic acid.[1] Pantothenic acid deficiency in humans has been induced experimentally by administering a pantothenic acid antagonist together with a pantothenic acid–deficient diet. Participants in this experiment complained of headache, fatigue, insomnia, intestinal disturbances, and numbness and tingling of their hands and feet.[5] In a more recent study, participants fed only a pantothenic acid–free diet did not develop clinical signs of deficiency, though some appeared listless and complained of fatigue.[6] Homopantothenate is a pantothenic acid antagonist with cholinergic effects (similar to those of the neurotransmitter acetylcholine). It was used in Japan to enhance mental function, especially in Alzheimer's disease. A rare side effect was the development of hepatic encephalopathy, a condition of abnormal brain function resulting from the failure of the liver to eliminate toxins. The encephalopathy was reversed by pantothenic acid supplementation, suggesting but not proving it was due to pantothenic acid deficiency caused by the antagonist.[4]

Because it is so rare, most information regarding the effects of pantothenic acid deficiency comes from experimental research in

Table 4–1   Adequate Intake (AI) for Pantothenic Acid

Life Stage	Age	Males, mg/d	Females, mg/d
Infants	0–6 months	1.7	1.7
Infants	7–12 months	1.8	1.8
Children	1–3 years	2	2
Children	4–8 years	3	3
Children	9–13 years	4	4
Adolescents	14–18 years	5	5
Adults	19 years and older	5	5
Pregnancy	all ages	–	6
Breast-feeding	all ages	–	7

animals. The diversity of symptoms emphasizes the numerous functions of pantothenic acid in its coenzyme forms. Pantothenic acid–deficient rats developed damage to the adrenal glands, and monkeys developed anemia due to decreased synthesis of heme, a component of hemoglobin. Dogs with pantothenic acid deficiency developed low blood glucose, rapid breathing and heart rates, and convulsions. Chickens developed skin irritation, feather abnormalities, and spinal nerve damage associated with the degeneration of the myelin sheath. Pantothenic acid–deficient mice showed decreased exercise tolerance and diminished storage of glucose (in the form of glycogen) in muscle and liver. Mice also developed skin irritation and graying of the fur, which was reversed by administering pantothenic acid. This finding led to the idea of adding pantothenic acid to shampoo, although it has not been successful in restoring hair color in humans.[7]

The Adequate Intake Level

The Food and Nutrition Board of the Institute of Medicine felt the existing scientific evidence was insufficient to calculate a recommended dietary allowance for pantothenic acid, so they set an adequate intake level (AI). The AI for pantothenic acid (Table 4–1) was based on estimated dietary intakes in healthy population groups.[8]

Disease Prevention

Presently, there is insufficient evidence to support the use of pantothenic acid to prevent diseases or health conditions other than frank pantothenic acid deficiency, which appears to be quite rare in humans. (See "Deficiency.")

Disease Treatment

Wound Healing

Administration of pantothenic acid orally and application of pantothenol ointment to the skin have been shown to accelerate the closure of skin wounds and increase the strength of scar tissue in animals. Adding calcium-D-pantothenate to cultured human skin cells given an artificial wound increased the number of migrating skin cells and their speed of migration, effects likely to accelerate wound healing.[9] However, little data exist in humans to support the findings of accelerated wound healing in cell culture and animal studies. A randomized, double-blind study examining the effect of supplementing patients undergoing surgery for tattoo removal with 1000 mg of vitamin C and 200 mg of pantothenic acid could not document any significant improvement in the wound healing process in those who received the supplements.[10]

High Cholesterol

A pantothenic acid derivative called *pantethine* has been reported by a number of investigators to have a cholesterol-lowering effect. Pantethine is actually two molecules of pantetheine joined by a disulfide bond (chemical bond between two molecules of sulfur). In the synthetic pathway of CoA, pantetheine is closer to CoA than pantothenic acid and is the functional component of CoA and acyl-carrier proteins. Several studies found doses of 900 mg of pantethine daily (300 mg, three times daily) to be significantly more effective than placebo in lowering total cholesterol and triglyceride levels in the blood of both diabetic and nondiabetic individuals.[11] Pantethine was also found to lower cholesterol and triglyceride levels in diabetic patients on hemodialysis without adverse side effects. The low side effect profile of pantethine was especially attractive for hemodialysis patients because of the increased risk of drug toxicity in patients with renal (kidney) failure.[12] Pantethine is not a vitamin; it is a derivative of pantothenic acid. The decision to use pantethine to treat elevated blood cholesterol or triglycerides should be made in collaboration with a qualified health care provider who can provide appropriate follow-up.

Sources

Food Sources

Pantothenic acid is available in a variety of foods. Rich sources of pantothenic acid include liver and kidney, yeast, egg yolk, and broccoli. Fish, shellfish, chicken, milk, yogurt, legumes, mushrooms, avocado, and sweet potatoes are also good sources. Whole grains are good sources of pantothenic acid, but processing and refining grains may result in a 35 to 75% loss. Freezing and canning of foods have been found to result in similar losses.[8] Large national nutritional surveys were unable to estimate pantothenic acid intake due to the scarcity of data on the pantothenic acid content of food. Smaller studies estimate average daily intakes of pantothenic acid to be from 5 to 6 mg/d in adults. Table 4–2 lists some rich sources of pantothenic acid along with their content in milligrams.

Intestinal Bacteria

The bacteria that normally colonize the colon (large intestine) are capable of making their own pantothenic acid. It is not yet known whether humans can absorb the pantothenic acid synthesized by their own intestinal bacteria in meaningful amounts. However, a specialized process for the uptake of biotin and pantothenic acid was recently identified in cultured cells derived from the lining of the colon, suggesting that humans may be able to absorb pantothenic acid and biotin produced by the bacteria normally present in the colon.[13]

Table 4–2 Food Sources of Pantothenic Acid

Food	Serving	Pantothenic Acid, mg
Avocado, California	1 whole	1.68
Yogurt	8 ounces	1.35
Chicken, cooked	3 ounces*	0.98
Milk	1 cup (8 ounces)	0.79
Sweet potato, cooked	1 medium (1/2 cup)	0.74
Lentils, cooked	1/2 cup	0.64
Egg, cooked	1 large	0.61
Split peas, cooked	1/2 cup	0.59
Mushrooms, raw	1/2 cup, chopped	0.51
Broccoli, steamed	1/2 cup, chopped	0.40
Lobster, cooked	3 ounces*	0.24
Fish, cod, cooked	3 ounces*	0.15
Tuna, canned	3 ounces*	0.18
Bread, whole wheat	1 slice	0.16

*A 3-ounce serving of meat or fish is about the size of a deck of cards.

Supplements

Pantothenic Acid. Supplements commonly contain pantothenol, a more stable alcohol derivative, which is rapidly converted by humans to pantothenic acid. Calcium and sodium D-pantothenate, the calcium and sodium salts of pantothenic acid, are also available as supplements.[1]

Pantethine. Although it is used as a cholesterol-lowering agent in Europe and Japan, pantethine is available in the United States as a dietary supplement.[14]

Safety

Toxicity

Pantothenic acid is not known to be toxic in humans. The only adverse effect noted was diarrhea resulting from very high intakes of 10 to 20 g/d of calcium D-pantothenate.[15] Due to the lack of reports of adverse effects, the Food and Nutrition Board did not set a tolerable upper level of intake for pantothenic acid.[8] Pantethine is generally well tolerated in doses up to 1200 mg/d. However, gastrointestinal side effects like nausea and heartburn have been reported.[14]

Drug Interactions

Oral contraceptives (birth control pills) containing estrogen and progestin may increase the requirement for pantothenic acid.[15] Use of pantethine in combination with HMG-CoA reductase inhibitors (statins) or nicotinic acid may produce additive effects on blood lipids.[14]

LPI Recommendation

Little is known regarding the amount of dietary pantothenic acid required to promote optimal health or prevent chronic disease. The Linus Pauling Institute supports the recommendation by the Food and Nutrition Board of 5 mg/d of pantothenic acid for adults. A varied diet should provide enough pantothenic acid for most people. Following the Linus Pauling Institute recommendation to take a daily multivitamin/multimineral supplement, containing 100% of the daily value, will ensure an intake of at least 5 mg/d of pantothenic acid.

Older Adults

Presently there is little evidence that older adults (65 years and older) differ in their intake or requirement for pantothenic acid. Most multivitamin/multimineral supplements provide at least 5 mg/d of pantothenic acid.

References

1. Plesofsky-Vig N. Pantothenic acid. In: Shils M, Olson JA, Shike M, Ross AC. eds. *Nutrition in Health and Disease*. 9th ed. Baltimore: Williams & Wilkins; 1999:423–432.
2. Tahiliani AG, Beinlich CJ. Pantothenic acid in health and disease. *Vitam Horm* 1991;46:165–228.
3. Brody T. *Nutritional Biochemistry*. 2nd ed. San Diego: Academic Press; 1999.
4. Bender DA. Optimum nutrition: thiamin, biotin and pantothenate. *Proc Nutr Soc* 1999;58(2):427–433.
5. Hodges RE, Ohlson MA, Bean WB. Pantothenic acid deficiency in man. *J Clin Invest* 1958;37:1642–1657.
6. Fry PC, Fox HM, Tao HG. Metabolic response to a pantothenic acid deficient diet in humans. *J Nutr Sci Vitaminol (Tokyo)* 1976;22(4):339–346.
7. Plesofsky-Vig N. Pantothenic acid. In: Ziegler EE, Filer LJ, eds. *Present Knowledge in Nutrition*. 7th ed. Washington, D.C.: ILSI Press; 1996.
8. Food and Nutrition Board, Institute of Medicine. Pantothenic acid. *Dietary Reference Intakes: Thiamin, Riboflavin, Niacin, Vitamin B-6, Vitamin B-12, Pantothenic Acid, Biotin, and Choline*. Washington, D.C.: National Academy Press; 1998:357–373.
9. Weimann BI, Hermann D. Studies on wound healing: effects of calcium D-pantothenate on the migration, proliferation and protein synthesis of human dermal fibroblasts in culture. *Int J Vitam Nutr Res* 1999;69(2):113–119.
10. Vaxman F, Olender S, Lambert A, et al. Effect of pantothenic acid and ascorbic acid supplementation on human skin wound healing process. A double-blind, prospective and randomized trial. *Eur Surg Res* 1995;27(3):158–166.
11. Gaddi A, Descovich GC, Noseda G, et al. Controlled evaluation of pantethine, a natural hypolipidemic compound, in patients with different forms of hyperlipoproteinemia. *Atherosclerosis* 1984;50(1):73–83.
12. Coronel F, Tornero F, Torrente J, et al. Treatment of hyperlipemia in diabetic patients on dialysis with a physiological substance. *Am J Nephrol* 1991;11(1):32–36.
13. Said HM, Ortiz A, McCloud E, Dyer D, Moyer MP, Rubin S. Biotin uptake by human colonic epithelial NCM460 cells: a carrier-mediated process shared with pantothenic acid. *Am J Physiol* 1998;275(5 Pt 1):C1365–C1371.
14. Hendler SS, Rorvik DR, eds. *PDR for Nutritional Supplements*. Montvale, NJ: Medical Economics Company, Inc; 2001.
15. Flodin N. *Pharmacology of Micronutrients*. New York: Alan R. Liss, Inc.; 1988.

5 Riboflavin

Riboflavin is a water-soluble B-complex vitamin, also known as vitamin B_2. In the body, riboflavin is primarily found as an integral component of the coenzymes flavin adenine dinucleotide (FAD) and flavin mononucleotide (FMN).[1] Coenzymes derived from riboflavin are also called *flavins*. Enzymes that use a flavin coenzyme are called *flavoproteins*.[2]

Function

Oxidation-Reduction (Redox) Reactions

Living organisms derive most of their energy from oxidation-reduction (redox) reactions, which are processes involving the transfer of electrons. Flavin coenzymes participate in redox reactions in numerous metabolic pathways.[3] Flavins are critical for the metabolism of carbohydrates, fats, and proteins. FAD is part of the electron transport (respiratory) chain, which is central to energy production. In conjunction with cytochrome P450 enzymes, flavins also participate in the metabolism of drugs and toxins.[4]

Antioxidant Functions

Glutathione reductase is an FAD-dependent enzyme that participates in the redox cycle of glutathione. The glutathione redox cycle plays a major role in protecting organisms from reactive oxygen species, such as hydroperoxides. Glutathione peroxidase, a selenium-containing enzyme, requires two molecules of reduced glutathione to break down hydroperoxides (Fig. 5–1). Glutathione reductase requires FAD to regenerate two molecules of reduced glutathione from oxidized glutathione. Riboflavin deficiency has been associated with increased oxidative stress.[4] Measurement of glutathione reductase activity in red blood cells is commonly used to assess riboflavin nutritional status.[5]

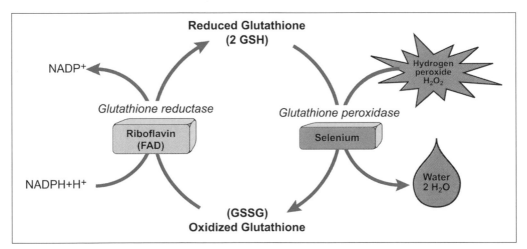

Figure 5–1. The glutathione oxidation-reduction (redox) cycle. One molecule of hydrogen peroxide is reduced to two molecules of water, and two molecules of glutathione (GSH) are oxidized in a reaction catalyzed by the selenoenzyme glutathione peroxidase. Oxidized glutathione (GSSG) may be reduced by the flavin adenine dinucleotide (FAD)-dependent enzyme glutathione reductase.

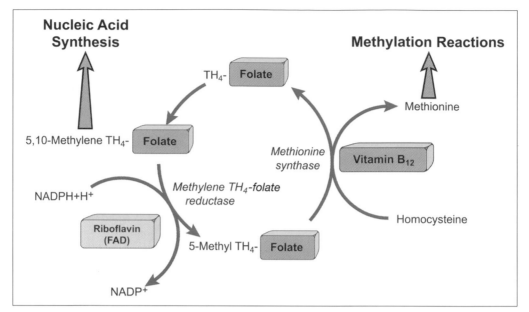

Figure 5–2. Methylene tetrahydrofolate (TH$_4$-folate) reductase. Methylene TH$_4$-folate reductase is a flavin adenine dinucleotide (FAD)–dependent enzyme required to catalyze the reduction of 5,10-methylene TH$_4$-folate to 5-methyl TH$_4$-folate, the specific folate coenzyme required to form methionine from homocysteine.

Xanthine oxidase, another FAD-dependent enzyme, catalyzes the oxidation of hypoxanthine and xanthine to uric acid. Uric acid is one of the most effective water-soluble antioxidants in the blood. Riboflavin deficiency can result in decreased xanthine oxidase activity, reducing blood uric acid levels.[6]

Nutrient Interactions

B-Complex Vitamins. Because flavoproteins are involved in the metabolism of several other vitamins (vitamin B$_6$, niacin, and folic acid), severe riboflavin deficiency may impact many enzyme systems. Conversion of most naturally available vitamin B$_6$ to its coenzyme form, pyridoxal 5′-phosphate (PLP), requires the FMN-dependent enzyme, pyridoxine 5′-phosphate oxidase.[7] At least two studies in the elderly have documented significant interactions between indicators of vitamin B$_6$ and riboflavin nutritional status.[8,9] The synthesis of the niacin-containing coenzymes, nicotinamide adenine dinucleotide (NAD) and nicotinamide adenine dinucleotide phosphate (NADP) from the amino acid tryptophan requires the FAD-dependent enzyme kynurenine mono-oxygenase. Severe riboflavin deficiency can decrease the conversion of tryptophan to NAD and NADP, increasing the risk of niacin deficiency.[3] Methylene tetrahydrofolate reductase (MTHFR) is an FAD-dependent enzyme that plays an important role in maintaining the specific folate coenzyme required to form methionine from homocysteine (Fig. 5–2). Along with other B-vitamins, increased riboflavin intake has been associated with decreased plasma homocysteine levels.[10] Recently, increased plasma riboflavin levels were associated with decreased plasma homocysteine levels mainly in those individuals who were homozygous (T/T) for the C677T polymorphism of the MTHFR gene and whose folate intake was low.[11] Such results illustrate the potential for complex interactions between genetic and dietary factors on chronic disease risk.

Iron. Riboflavin deficiency alters iron metabolism. Although the mechanism is not clear, research in animals suggests that riboflavin deficiency may impair iron absorption, increase intestinal loss of iron, and/or impair iron utilization for the synthesis of hemoglobin. In humans, improving riboflavin nutritional status has been found to increase circulating hemoglobin levels. Correction of riboflavin deficiency in individuals who are both riboflavin-deficient and iron-deficient improves the response of iron-deficiency anemia to iron therapy.[12]

Deficiency

Ariboflavinosis is the medical name for clinical riboflavin deficiency. Riboflavin deficiency is rarely found in isolation; it occurs frequently in combination with deficiencies of other water-soluble vitamins. Symptoms of riboflavin deficiency include sore throat; redness and swelling of the lining of the mouth and throat; cracks or sores on the outsides of the lips (cheliosis) and at the corners of the mouth (angular stomatitis); inflammation and redness of the tongue (magenta tongue); a moist, scaly skin inflammation (seborrheic dermatitis); the formation of blood vessels in the clear covering of the eye (vascularization of the cornea); and decreased red blood cell count in which the existing red blood cells contain normal levels of hemoglobin and are of normal size (normochromic normocytic anemia).[1,3] Severe riboflavin deficiency may result in decreased conversion of vitamin B_6 to its coenzyme form (PLP) and decreased conversion of tryptophan to niacin.

Risk Factors for Riboflavin Deficiency

The use of specialized light therapy to treat jaundice in newborns increases the destruction of riboflavin and is a recognized cause of riboflavin deficiency.[6] Alcoholics are at increased risk for riboflavin deficiency due to decreased intake, decreased absorption, and impaired utilization of riboflavin. Anorexic individuals rarely consume adequate riboflavin. Lactose intolerance may prevent people from

Table 5–1 Recommended Dietary Allowance (RDA) for Riboflavin

Life Stage	Age	Males, mg/d	Females, mg/d
Infants	0–6 months	0.3 (AI)	0.3 (AI)
Infants	7–12 months	0.4 (AI)	0.4 (AI)
Children	1–3 years	0.5	0.5
Children	4–8 years	0.6	0.6
Children	9–13 years	0.9	0.9
Adolescents	14–18 years	1.3	1.0
Adults	19 years and older	1.3	1.1
Pregnancy	all ages	–	1.4
Breast-feeding	all ages	–	1.6

AI, adequate intake level.

consuming milk or dairy products, which are good sources of riboflavin. The conversion of riboflavin into FAD and FMN is impaired by hypothyroidism and adrenal insufficiency.[3,4] People who are very active physically (athletes, laborers) may have a slightly increased riboflavin requirement. However, riboflavin supplementation has not generally been found to increase exercise tolerance or performance.[13]

The Recommended Dietary Allowance

The recommended dietary allowance (RDA) for riboflavin, revised in 1998, was based on the prevention of deficiency (Table 5–1). Clinical signs of deficiency in adults appear at intakes of less than 0.5 to 0.6 mg/d, and excess urinary excretion of riboflavin is seen at intake levels of approximately 1 mg/d.[1]

Disease Prevention

Cataracts

Age-related cataracts are the leading cause of visual disability in the United States and other developed countries. Research has focused on the role of nutritional antioxidants because of evidence that oxidative damage of lens proteins from light may lead to age-related cataracts. Two case-control studies found significantly decreased risk of age-related cataracts (33 to 51%) in men and women in the highest quintile (one fifth of the study population) of dietary riboflavin intakes (1.6 to 2.2 mg/d) compared with those in the lowest quintile (0.08 mg/d).[14] Individuals in the highest quintile of riboflavin nutritional status, as measured by red blood cell glutathione reductase activity, had approximately one half the occurrence of age-related cataracts as those in the lowest quintile of riboflavin status, though the results were not statistically significant.[15] Recently, a cross-sectional study of 2900 Australian men and women 49 years of age and older found that those in the highest quintile of intake for riboflavin were 50% less likely to have cataracts than those in the lowest quintile.[16] A prospective study of more than 50,000 women did not observe a difference between rates of cataract extraction between women in the highest quintile of riboflavin intake (1.5 mg/d) and those in the lowest quintile (1.2 mg/d).[17] However, the range between the highest and lowest quintiles was small, and median intake levels for both were above the current RDA for riboflavin. Although these observational studies provide support for the role of riboflavin in the prevention of cataracts, placebo-controlled intervention trials are needed to confirm the relationship.

Disease Treatment

Migraine Headaches

Some evidence indicates that impaired mitochondrial oxygen metabolism in the brain may play a role in the pathology of migraine headaches. As the precursor of the two flavin coenzymes (FAD and FMN) required by the flavoproteins of the mitochondrial electron transport chain, supplemental riboflavin has been investigated as a treatment for migraine. A randomized placebo-controlled trial examined the effect of 400 mg of riboflavin per day for 3 months on migraine prevention in 54 men and women with a history of recurrent migraine headaches.[18] Riboflavin was signifi-

cantly better than placebo in reducing attack frequency and the number of headache days, though the beneficial effect was most pronounced during the third month of treatment. It should be noted, however, that only about 25 mg of riboflavin can be absorbed in a single oral dose.[19] A more recent study by the same investigators found that treatment with either a beta-adrenergic-receptor–blocking agent or high-dose riboflavin resulted in clinical improvement, but each therapy appeared to act on a distinct pathological mechanism—betablockers on abnormal cortical information processing and riboflavin on decreased brain mitochondrial energy reserve. Though these findings are preliminary, they suggest that riboflavin supplementation might be a useful adjunct to pharmacologic therapy with betablockers in migraine prevention.[20]

Sources

Food Sources

Most plant- and animal-derived foods contain at least small quantities of riboflavin. White flour and bread have been enriched with riboflavin (as well as thiamin, niacin, and iron) since 1943 in the United States. Data from large dietary surveys indicate that the average intake of riboflavin for men is about 2 mg/d and for women is about 1.5 mg/d, well above the RDA. Intake levels were similar for a population of elderly men and women.[1] Riboflavin is easily destroyed by exposure to light. Up to 50% of the riboflavin in milk contained in a clear glass bottle can be destroyed after 2 hours of exposure to bright sunlight.[6] Some foods with substantial amounts of riboflavin are listed in Table 5–2 along with their riboflavin content in milligrams.

Supplements

The most common forms of riboflavin available in supplements are riboflavin and riboflavin 5′-monophosphate. Riboflavin is most commonly found in multivitamin and vitamin B-complex preparations.[21]

Table 5–2 Food Sources of Riboflavin

Food	Serving	Riboflavin, mg
Fortified cereal	1 cup	0.59–2.27
Milk, nonfat	1 cup (8 ounces)	0.34
Egg, cooked	1 large	0.27
Almonds	1 ounce	0.24
Beef, cooked	3 ounces*	0.19
Chicken, dark meat, roasted	3 ounces*	0.18
Asparagus, boiled or steamed	6 spears	0.13
Salmon, broiled	3 ounces*	0.13
Cheese, cheddar	1 ounce	0.11
Chicken, light meat, roasted	3 ounces*	0.10
Broccoli, boiled or steamed	1/2 cup, chopped	0.09
Halibut, broiled	3 ounces*	0.08
Bread, white, enriched	1 slice	0.09
Spinach, boiled or steamed	1/2 cup	0.09
Bread, whole wheat	1 slice	0.07

*A 3-ounce serving of meat or fish is about the size of a deck of cards.

Safety

Toxicity

No toxic or adverse effects of high riboflavin intake in humans are known. Studies in cell culture indicate that excess riboflavin may increase the risk of DNA strand breaks in the presence of chromium (IV), a known carcinogen.[22] This may be of concern to workers exposed to chrome, but no data in humans are available. High-dose riboflavin therapy has been found to intensify urine color to a bright yellow (flavinuria), but this is a harmless side effect. The Food and Nutrition Board did not establish a tolerable upper level of intake when the RDA was revised in 1998.[1]

Drug Interactions

Several early reports indicated that women taking high-dose oral contraceptives (OC) had diminished riboflavin nutritional status. However, when investigators controlled for dietary riboflavin intake, no differences between OC users and nonusers were found.[1] Phenothiazine derivatives, like the antipsychotic medication chlorpromazine, and tricyclic antidepressants, inhibit the incorporation of riboflavin into FAD and FMN, as do the antimalarial medication quinacrine and the cancer chemotherapy agent adriamycin.[4] Long-term use of the anticonvulsant phenobarbital may increase destruction of riboflavin by liver enzymes, increasing the risk of deficiency.[3]

LPI Recommendation

The RDA for riboflavin (1.3 mg/d for men and 1.1 mg/d for women) is easily met by eating a varied diet and should prevent deficiency in most individuals. Consuming a varied diet should supply 1.5 mg to 2 mg of riboflavin a day. Following the Linus Pauling Institute recommendation to take a multivitamin/multimineral supplement containing 100% of the daily values will ensure an intake of at least 1.7 mg of riboflavin per day.

Older Adults

Some experts in nutrition and aging feel that the RDA (1.3 mg/d for men and 1.1 mg/d for women) leaves little margin for error in people over 50 years of age.[23,24] A recent study of independently living people between 65 and 90 years of age found that almost 25% consumed less than the recommended riboflavin intake and 10% had biochemical evidence of deficiency.[25] Additionally, epidemiologic studies of cataract prevalence indicate that riboflavin intakes of 1.6 to 2.2 mg/d may reduce the risk of developing age-related cataracts. Individuals whose diets may not supply adequate riboflavin, especially those over 50, should consider taking a multivitamin/multimineral supplement, which generally provides at least 1.7 mg of riboflavin per day.

References

1. Food and Nutrition Board, Institute of Medicine. Riboflavin. *Dietary Reference Intakes: Thiamin, Riboflavin, Niacin, Vitamin B-6, Vitamin B-12, Pantothenic Acid, Biotin, and Choline*. Washington, D.C.: National Academy Press; 1998:87–122.
2. Brody T. *Nutritional Biochemistry*. 2nd ed. San Diego: Academic Press; 1999.
3. McCormick DB. Riboflavin. In: Shils M, Olson JA, Shike M, Ross AC, eds. *Nutrition in Health and Disease*. 9th ed. Baltimore: Williams & Wilkins; 1999:391–399.
4. Rivlin RS. Riboflavin. In: Ziegler EE, Filer LJ, eds. *Present Knowledge in Nutrition*. 7th ed. Washington, D.C.: ILSI Press; 1996:167–173.
5. Powers HJ. Current knowledge concerning optimum nutritional status of riboflavin, niacin and pyridoxine. *Proc Nutr Soc* 1999;58(2):435–440.
6. Bohles H. Antioxidative vitamins in prematurely and maturely born infants. *Int J Vitam Nutr Res* 1997;67(5):321–328.
7. McCormick DB. Two interconnected B vitamins: riboflavin and pyridoxine. *Physiol Rev* 1989;69(4):1170–1198.
8. Lowik MR, van den Berg H, Kistemaker C, Brants HA, Brussaard JH. Interrelationships between riboflavin and vitamin B6 among elderly people (Dutch Nutrition Surveillance System). *Int J Vitam Nutr Res* 1994;64(3):198–203.
9. Madigan SM, Tracey F, McNulty H, et al. Riboflavin and vitamin B-6 intakes and status and biochemical response to riboflavin supplementation in free-living elderly people. *Am J Clin Nutr* 1998;68(2):389–395.
10. Jacques PF, Bostom AG, Wilson PW, Rich S, Rosenberg IH, Selhub J. Determinants of plasma total homocysteine concentration in the Framingham Offspring cohort. *Am J Clin Nutr* 2001;73(3):613–621.
11. Jacques PF, Kalmbach R, Bagley PJ, et al. The relationship between riboflavin and plasma total homocysteine in the Framingham Offspring cohort is influenced by folate status and the C677T transition in the methylenetetrahydrofolate reductase gene. *J Nutr* 2002;132(2):283–288.
12. Powers HJ. Riboflavin-iron interactions with particular emphasis on the gastrointestinal tract. *Proc Nutr Soc* 1995;54(2):509–517.
13. Soares MJ, Satyanarayana K, Bamji MS, Jacob CM, Ramana YV, Rao SS. The effect of exercise on the riboflavin status of adult men. *Br J Nutr* 1993;69(2):541–551.
14. Jacques PF. The potential preventive effects of vitamins for cataract and age-related macular degeneration. *Int J Vitam Nutr Res* 1999;69(3):198–205.
15. Leske MC, Wu SY, Hyman L, et al. Biochemical factors in the lens opacities. Case-control study. The Lens Opacities Case-Control Study Group. *Arch Ophthalmol* 1995;113(9):1113–1119.
16. Cumming RG, Mitchell P, Smith W. Diet and cataract: the Blue Mountains Eye Study. *Ophthalmology* 2000;107(3):450–456.
17. Hankinson SE, Stampfer MJ, Seddon JM, et al. Nutrient intake and cataract extraction in women: a prospective study. *BMJ* 1992;305(6849):335–339.
18. Schoenen J, Jacquy J, Lenaerts M. Effectiveness of high-dose riboflavin in migraine prophylaxis: a randomized controlled trial. *Neurology* 1998;50(2):466–470.
19. Zempleni J, Galloway JR, McCormick DB. Pharmacokinetics of orally and intravenously administered riboflavin in healthy humans. *Am J Clin Nutr* 1996;63(1):54–66.
20. Sandor PS, Afra J, Ambrosini A, Schoenen J. Prophylactic treatment of migraine with beta-blockers and riboflavin: differential effects on the intensity dependence of auditory evoked cortical potentials. *Headache* 2000;40(1):30–35.
21. Hendler SS, Rorvik DR, eds. *PDR for Nutritional Supplements*. Montvale, NJ: Medical Economics Company, Inc; 2001.
22. Sugiyama M. Role of physiological antioxidants in chromium(VI)-induced cellular injury. *Free Radic Biol Med* 1992;12(5):397–407.
23. Blumberg J. Nutritional needs of seniors. *J Am Coll Nutr* 1997;16(6):517–523.
24. Russell RM, Suter PM. Vitamin requirements of elderly people: an update. *Am J Clin Nutr* 1993;58(1):4–14.
25. Lopez-Sobaler AM, Ortega RM, Quintas ME, et al. The influence of vitamin B2 intake on the activation coefficient of erythrocyte glutation reductase in the elderly. *J Nutr Health Aging* 2002;6(1):60–62.

6 Thiamin

Thiamin (also spelled *thiamine*) is a water-soluble, B-complex vitamin, previously known as vitamin B_1 or aneurine.[1] Isolated and characterized in the 1930s, thiamin was one of the first organic compounds to be recognized as a vitamin.[2] Thiamin occurs in the human body as free thiamin and its phosphorylated forms: thiamin monophosphate (TMP), thiamin triphosphate (TTP), and thiamin pyrophosphate (TPP), which is also known as thiamin diphosphate.

Function

Coenzyme Function

TPP is a required coenzyme for a small number of very important enzymes. The synthesis of TPP from free thiamin requires magnesium, adenosine triphosphate (ATP), and the enzyme thiamin pyrophosphokinase.

Pyruvate dehydrogenase, α-ketoglutarate dehydrogenase, and branched chain ketoacid dehydrogenase each comprise a different enzyme complex found within cellular organelles called *mitochondria*. They catalyze the decarboxylation of pyruvate, α-ketoglutarate, and branched-chain amino acids to form acetyl-coenzyme A, succinyl-coenzyme A, and derivatives of branched chain amino acids, respectively, all of which play critical roles in the production of energy from food.[2] In addition to the thiamin coenzyme (TPP), each dehydrogenase complex requires a niacin-containing coenzyme, a riboflavin-containing coenzyme, and lipoic acid.

Transketolase catalyzes critical reactions in another metabolic pathway known as the pentose phosphate pathway. One of the most important intermediates of this pathway is ribose-5-phosphate, a phosphorylated 5-carbon sugar required for the synthesis of the high-energy ribonucleotides, ATP and guanosine triphosphate (GTP), the nucleic acids, DNA and RNA, and the niacin-containing coenzyme nicotinamide adenine dinucleotide phosphate (NADP), which is essential for a number of biosynthetic reactions.[1,3] Because transketolase decreases early in thiamin deficiency, measurement of its activity in red blood cells has been used to assess thiamin nutritional status.[2]

Noncoenzyme Function

TTP is concentrated in nerve and muscle cells. Research in animals indicates that TTP activates membrane ion channels, possibly by phosphorylating them.[4] The flow of electrolytes like sodium and chloride in or out of nerve and muscle cells through membrane ion channels plays a role in nerve impulse conduction and voluntary muscle action. Impaired formation of TTP may play a role in the neurologic symptoms of severe thiamin deficiency.

Deficiency

Beriberi, the disease resulting from severe thiamin deficiency, was described in Chinese literature as early as 2600 B.C. Thiamin deficiency affects the cardiovascular, nervous, muscular, and gastrointestinal systems.[2] Beriberi has been termed *dry*, *wet*, and *cerebral*, depending on the systems affected by severe thiamin deficiency.[1]

The main feature of dry (paralytic or nervous) beriberi is peripheral neuropathy. Early in the course of the neuropathy "burning feet syndrome" may occur. Other symptoms include abnormal (exaggerated) reflexes, diminished sensation, and weakness in the legs and arms. Muscle pain and tenderness and difficulty rising from a squatting position have also been observed. Severely thiamin-deficient individuals may experience seizures.

In addition to neurologic symptoms, wet (cardiac) beriberi is characterized by cardiovascular manifestations of thiamin deficiency, which include rapid heart rate, enlargement of the heart, severe swelling (edema), difficulty breathing, and ultimately congestive heart failure.

Cerebral beriberi may lead to Wernicke encephalopathy and Korsakoff psychosis. The diagnosis of Wernicke's encephalopathy is based on a triad of signs, which include abnormal eye movements, stance and gait abnormalities, and abnormalities in mental function, which may include a confused apathetic state or a profound memory disorder termed Korsakoff's amnesia or Korsakoff's psychosis. Thiamin deficiency affecting the central nervous system is referred to as Wernicke's disease when the amnesic state is not present and Wernicke-Korsakoff syndrome (WKS) when the amnesic symptoms are present along with the eye movement and gait disorders. Most WKS sufferers are alcoholics, although it has been observed in other disorders of gross malnutrition, including stomach cancer and acquired immune deficiency syndrome (AIDS). Administration of intravenous thiamin to WKS patients generally results in prompt improvement of the eye symptoms, but improvements in motor coordination and memory may be less noticeable, depending on how long the symptoms have been present. Recent evidence of increased immune cell activation and increased free radical production in the areas of the brain that are selectively damaged suggests that oxidative stress plays an important role in the neurologic pathology of thiamin deficiency.[5]

Causes of Thiamin Deficiency

Thiamin deficiency may result from inadequate thiamin intake, an increased requirement for thiamin, excessive loss of thiamin from the body, consumption of antithiamin factors in food, or a combination of factors.

Inadequate Intake. Inadequate consumption of thiamin is the main cause of thiamin deficiency in underdeveloped countries.[2] Thiamin deficiency is common in low-income populations whose diets are high in carbohydrate and low in thiamin (e.g., milled or polished rice). Breast-fed infants whose mothers are thiamin-deficient are vulnerable to developing infantile beriberi. Alcoholism, which is associated with low intake of thiamin among other nutrients, is the primary cause of thiamin deficiency in industrialized countries.

Increased Requirement. Conditions resulting in an increased requirement for thiamin include strenuous physical exertion, fever, pregnancy, breast-feeding, and adolescent growth. Such conditions place individuals with marginal thiamin intake at risk for developing symptomatic thiamin deficiency. Recently, malaria patients in Thailand were found to be severely thiamin-deficient more frequently than noninfected individuals. Malarial infection leads to a large increase in the metabolic demand for glucose, as well as increased demand for the disposal of lactate. The stresses induced by malarial infection could exacerbate thiamin deficiency in individuals already predisposed.[6] Human immunodeficiency virus (HIV)-infected individuals, whether or not they had developed AIDS, were also found to be at increased risk for thiamin deficiency.[7] The lack of association between thiamin intake and evidence of deficiency in these HIV-infected individuals suggested they had an increased requirement for thiamin.

Excessive Loss. Excessive loss of thiamin may precipitate thiamin deficiency. Individuals with kidney failure requiring hemodialysis lose thiamin at an increased rate and are at risk for thiamin deficiency.[8] By increasing urinary flow, diuretics may prevent reabsorption of thiamin by the kidney and increase its excretion in the urine.[9,10] Alcoholics who maintain a high fluid intake and urine flow rate may also experience increased loss of thiamin, exacerbating the effects of low thiamin intake.[11]

Antithiamin Factors. The presence of antithiamin factors (ATF) in foods also contributes to the risk of thiamin deficiency. Certain plants contain ATF, which react with thiamin to form a product that is oxidized in the body, rendering it inactive. Consuming large amounts of tea and coffee (including decaffeinated), as well as chewing tea leaves and betel nut, have been associated with thiamin depletion in humans

Table 6–1 Recommended Dietary Allowance (RDA) for Thiamin

Life Stage	Age	Males, mg/d	Females, mg/d
Infants	0–6 months	0.2 (AI)	0.2 (AI)
Infants	7–12 months	0.3 (AI)	0.3 (AI)
Children	1–3 years	0.5	0.5
Children	4–8 years	0.6	0.6
Children	9–13 years	0.9	0.9
Adolescents	14–18 years	1.2	1.0
Adults	19 years and older	1.2	1.1
Pregnancy	all ages	–	1.4
Breast-feeding	all ages	–	1.4

AI, adequate intake level.

due to the presence of ATF. Vitamin C and other antioxidants can protect thiamin in some foods by preventing its oxidation to an inactive form.[1] Thiaminases are enzymes that break down thiamin in food. Individuals who habitually eat certain raw freshwater fish, raw shellfish, and ferns are at higher risk of thiamin deficiency because these foods contain a thiaminase, which would normally be inactivated by the heat used for cooking. An acute neurologic syndrome (seasonal ataxia) in Nigeria has been associated with thiamin deficiency precipitated by a thiaminase in African silkworms, a traditional high-protein food for some Nigerians.[12]

The Recommended Dietary Allowance

The recommended dietary allowance for thiamin, revised in 1998, was based on the prevention of deficiency in generally healthy individuals (Table 6–1).[13]

Disease Prevention

Presently, there is insufficient evidence to support the use of thiamin to prevent diseases or health conditions other than frank thiamin deficiency.

Disease Treatment

Alzheimer's Disease

Because thiamin deficiency can result in a form of dementia (Wernicke-Korsakoff syndrome), its relationship to Alzheimer's disease and other forms of dementia has been investigated. Several investigators found evidence of decreased activity of the thiamin pyrophosphate–dependent enzymes, α-ketoglutarate dehydrogenase and transketolase, in the brains of patients who died of Alzheimer's disease.[4] Such findings are consistent with evidence of reduced glucose metabolism found on positron emission tomography (PET) scans of the brains of Alzheimer's disease patients.[14] The finding of decreased brain levels of TPP in the presence of normal levels of free thiamin and TMP suggests that the decreased enzyme activity is not likely to be the result of thiamin deficiency but rather of impaired synthesis of TPP.[15,16]

Presently, there is only slight evidence that thiamin supplements are of benefit in Alzheimer's disease. A double-blind placebo-controlled study of 15 patients (10 completed the study) reported no beneficial effect of 3 g of thiamin per day on cognitive decline over a 12-month period. A preliminary report from another study claimed a mild benefit of 3 to 8 g of thiamin per day in dementia of Alzheimer's type in 1993, but no additional data from that study are available.[17] A mild beneficial effect in patients with Alzheimer's disease was reported after 12 weeks of treatment with 100 mg/d of a thiamin derivative (thiamin tetrahydrofurfuryl disulfide), but this study was not placebo-controlled.[18] A recent systematic review of randomized, double-blind, placebo-controlled trials of thiamin in patients with dementia of Alzheimer's type found no evidence that thiamin was a useful treatment for the symptoms of Alzheimer's disease.[19]

Congestive Heart Failure

Severe thiamin deficiency (wet beriberi) can lead to impaired cardiac function and ultimately congestive heart failure (CHF). Although cardiac manifestations of beriberi are rarely encountered in industrialized countries,

CHF due to other causes is common, especially in the elderly. Diuretics used in the treatment of CHF, notably furosemide (Lasix), have been found to increase thiamin excretion, potentially leading to marginal thiamin deficiency. A number of studies have examined thiamin nutritional status in CHF patients, and most found a fairly low incidence of thiamin deficiency, as measured by assays of transketolase activity. As in the general population, older CHF patients were found to be at higher risk of thiamin deficiency.[20]

An important measure of cardiac function in CHF is the left ventricular ejection fraction (LVEF), which can be assessed by echocardiography. In a randomized double-blind study of 30 CHF patients, all of whom had been taking furosemide for at least 3 months, intravenous (IV) thiamin therapy (200 mg/d) for 7 days resulted in an improved LVEF compared with IV placebo.[21] When all 30 of the CHF patients in that study subsequently received 6 weeks of oral thiamin therapy (200 mg/d) the average LVEF improved by 22%. This finding may be significant because improvements in LVEF have been associated with improved survival in CHF patients.[22] Conclusions that can be drawn from the studies published to date are limited due to small sample sizes, lack of randomization in some studies, and a need for more precise assays of thiamin status. Presently, the role of thiamin supplementation in maintaining cardiac function in CHF patients remains controversial.

Cancer

Thiamin deficiency has been observed in some cancer patients with rapidly growing tumors. Recent research in cell culture and animal models indicates that rapidly dividing cancer cells have a high requirement for thiamin.[23] All rapidly dividing cells require nucleic acids at an increased rate, but some cancer cells appear to rely heavily on the TPP–dependent enzyme transketolase to provide the ribose-5-phosphate necessary for nucleic acid synthesis. Thiamin supplementation in cancer patients is common to prevent thiamin deficiency, but some investigators caution that too much thiamin may fuel the growth of some malignant tumors. These investigators suggest that thiamin supplementation be reserved for those cancer patients that are actually thiamin-deficient.[24] Presently, there is no evidence available from studies in humans to support or refute this theory. However, it would be prudent for individuals with cancer who are considering thiamin supplementation to discuss this issue with the clinician managing their cancer therapy.

Sources

Food Sources

A varied diet should provide most individuals with adequate thiamin to prevent deficiency. In the United States the average dietary thiamin intake is about 2 mg/d for young adult men and 1.2 mg/d for young adult women. A survey of people over the age of 60 found an average dietary thiamin intake of 1.4 mg/d for men and 1.1 mg/d for women.[13] However, institutionalization and poverty increase the likelihood of inadequate thiamin intake in the elderly.[25] Whole-grain cereals, legumes (e.g., beans and lentils), nuts, lean pork, and yeast are rich sources of thiamin.[1] Because most of the thiamin is lost during the production of white flour and polished (milled) rice, white rice and foods made from white flour (e.g., bread and pasta) are fortified with thiamin. A number of thiamin-rich foods are listed in Table 6–2 along with their thiamin content in milligrams.

Supplements

Thiamin is available in nutritional supplements and for fortification as thiamin hydrochloride and thiamin nitrate.[26]

Table 6–2 Food Sources of Thiamin

Food	Serving	Thiamin, mg
Wheat germ breakfast cereal	1 cup	1.89
Pork, lean, cooked	3 ounces*	0.74
Fortified breakfast cereal	1 cup	0.5–2.0
Brazil nuts	1 ounce	0.28
Long grain white rice, enriched, cooked	1 cup	0.26
Peas, cooked	$^1/_2$ cup	0.21
Long grain brown rice, cooked	1 cup	0.19
Lentils, cooked	$^1/_2$ cup	0.17
Pecans	1 ounce	0.13
White bread, enriched	1 slice	0.12
Orange	1 fruit	0.11
Whole wheat bread	1 slice	0.10
Cantaloupe	1/2 fruit	0.10
Milk	1 cup	0.10
Spinach, cooked	$^1/_2$ cup	0.09
Egg, cooked	1 large	0.03
Long grain white rice, unenriched, cooked	1 cup	0.03

*A 3-ounce serving of meat or fish is about the size of a deck of cards.

Safety

Toxicity

The Food and Nutrition Board did not set a tolerable upper level of intake for thiamin because there are no known toxic effects from the consumption of excess thiamin in food or through long-term oral supplementation (up to 200 mg/d). A small number of life-threatening anaphylactic reactions have been observed with large intravenous doses of thiamin. However, anaphylactic reactions are the result of an overwhelming allergic response rather than a toxic effect of thiamin.[13]

Drug Interactions

Reduced blood levels of thiamin have been reported in individuals with seizure disorders (epilepsy) taking the anticonvulsant medication phenytoin for long periods of time.[27] 5-Fluorouracil, a drug used in cancer therapy, inhibits the phosphorylation of thiamin to TPP.[28] Diuretics, especially furosemide (Lasix), may increase the risk of thiamin deficiency in individuals with marginal thiamin intake due to increased urinary excretion of thiamin.[9]

LPI Recommendation

The Linus Pauling Institute supports the recommendation by the Food and Nutrition Board of 1.2 mg of thiamin per day for men and 1.1 mg/d for women. A varied diet should provide enough thiamin for most people. Following the Linus Pauling Institute recommendation to take a daily multivitamin/multimineral supplement, containing 100 % of the daily values, will ensure an intake of at least 1.5 mg of thiamin per day.

Older Adults

Presently, there is no evidence that the requirement for thiamin is increased in older adults (65 and older), but some studies have found inadequate dietary intake and thiamin insufficiency to be more common in elderly populations. Thus, it would be prudent for older adults to take a multivitamin/multimineral supplement, which will generally provide at least 1.5 mg of thiamin per day.

References

1. Tanphaichitr V. Thiamin. In: Shils M, Olson JA, Shike M, Ross AC, eds. *Nutrition in Health and Disease.* 9th ed. Baltimore: Williams & Wilkins; 1999:381–389.
2. Rindi G. Thiamin. In: Ziegler EE, Filer LJ, eds. *Present Knowledge in Nutrition.* 7th ed. Washington, D.C.: ILSI Press; 1996:160–166.
3. Brody T. *Nutritional Biochemistry.* 2nd ed. San Diego: Academic Press; 1999.
4. Bender DA. Optimum nutrition: thiamin, biotin and pantothenate. *Proc Nutr Soc* 1999;58(2):427–433.
5. Todd K, Butterworth RF. Mechanisms of selective neuronal cell death due to thiamine deficiency. *Ann NY Acad Sci* 1999;893:404–411.
6. Krishna S, Taylor AM, Supanaranond W, et al. Thiamine deficiency and malaria in adults from southeast Asia. *Lancet* 1999;353(9152):546–549.

7. Muri RM, Von Overbeck J, Furrer J, Ballmer PE. Thiamin deficiency in HIV-positive patients: evaluation by erythrocyte transketolase activity and thiamin pyrophosphate effect. *Clin Nutr* 1999;18(6):375–378.

8. Hung SC, Hung SH, Tarng DC, Yang WC, Chen TW, Huang TP. Thiamine deficiency and unexplained encephalopathy in hemodialysis and peritoneal dialysis patients. *Am J Kidney Dis* 2001;38(5):941–947.

9. Rieck J, Halkin H, Almog S, et al. Urinary loss of thiamine is increased by low doses of furosemide in healthy volunteers. *J Lab Clin Med* 1999;134(3):238–243.

10. Suter PM, Haller J, Hany A, Vetter W. Diuretic use: a risk for subclinical thiamine deficiency in elderly patients. *J Nutr Health Aging* 2000;4(2):69–71.

11. Wilcox CS. Do diuretics cause thiamine deficiency? *J Lab Clin Med* 1999;134(3):192–193.

12. Nishimune T, Watanabe Y, Okazaki H, Akai H. Thiamin is decomposed due to Anaphe spp. entomophagy in seasonal ataxia patients in Nigeria. *J Nutr* 2000;130(6):1625–1628.

13. Food and Nutrition Board, Institute of Medicine. Thiamin. In: *Dietary Reference Intakes: Thiamin, Riboflavin, Niacin, Vitamin B-6, Vitamin B-12, Pantothenic Acid, Biotin, and Choline.* Washington, D.C.: National Academy Press; 1998:58–86.

14. Kish SJ. Brain energy metabolizing enzymes in Alzheimer's disease: alpha-ketoglutarate dehydrogenase complex and cytochrome oxidase. *Ann NY Acad Sci* 1997;826:218–228.

15. Heroux M, Raghavendra Rao VL, Lavoie J, Richardson JS, Butterworth RF. Alterations of thiamine phosphorylation and of thiamine-dependent enzymes in Alzheimer's disease. *Metab Brain Dis* 1996;11(1):81–88.

16. Mastrogiacoma F, Bettendorff L, Grisar T, Kish SJ. Brain thiamine, its phosphate esters, and its metabolizing enzymes in Alzheimer's disease. *Ann Neurol* 1996;39(5):585–591.

17. Meador K, Loring D, Nichols M, et al. Preliminary findings of high-dose thiamine in dementia of Alzheimer's type. *J Geriatr Psychiatry Neurol* 1993; 6(4):222–229.

18. Mimori Y, Katsuoka H, Nakamura S. Thiamine therapy in Alzheimer's disease. *Metab Brain Dis* 1996;11(1): 89–94.

19. Rodriguez-Martin JL, Qizilbash N, Lopez-Arrieta JM. Thiamine for Alzheimer's disease (Cochrane Review). *Cochrane Database Syst Rev* 2001;2:CD001498.

20. Wilkinson TJ, Hanger HC, George PM, Sainsbury R. Is thiamine deficiency in elderly people related to age or co-morbidity? *Age Ageing* 2000;29(2):111–116.

21. Shimon I, Almog S, Vered Z, et al. Improved left ventricular function after thiamine supplementation in patients with congestive heart failure receiving long-term furosemide therapy. *Am J Med* 1995;98(5): 485–490.

22. Leslie D, Gheorghiade M. Is there a role for thiamine supplementation in the management of heart failure? *Am Heart J* 1996;131(6):1248–1250.

23. Comin-Anduix B, Boren J, Martinez S, et al. The effect of thiamine supplementation on tumour proliferation: a metabolic control analysis study. *Eur J Biochem* 2001;268(15):4177–4182.

24. Boros LG, Brandes JL, Lee WN, et al. Thiamine supplementation to cancer patients: a double edged sword. *Anticancer Res* 1998;18(1B):595–602.

25. Russell RM, Suter PM. Vitamin requirements of elderly people: an update. *Am J Clin Nutr* 1993;58(1):4–14.

26. Hendler SS, Rorvik DR, eds. *PDR for Nutritional Supplements.* Montvale, NJ: Medical Economics Company, Inc; 2001.

27. Flodin N. *Pharmacology of Micronutrients.* New York: Alan R. Liss, Inc.; 1988.

28. Schumann K. Interactions between drugs and vitamins at advanced age. *Int J Vitam Nutr Res* 1999; 69(3):173–178.

7 Vitamin A

Vitamin A is a generic term for a large number of related compounds. Retinol (an alcohol) and retinal (an aldehyde) are often referred to as *preformed vitamin A*. Retinal can be converted by the body to retinoic acid (RA), the form of vitamin A known to affect gene transcription. Retinol, retinal, RA, and related compounds are known as *retinoids*. β-carotene and other carotenoids that can be converted by the body into retinol are referred to as *provitamin A carotenoids*. Hundreds of different carotenoids are synthesized by plants, but only about 10% of them are provitamin A carotenoids.[1] The following discussion will focus mainly on preformed vitamin A and RA.

Function

Vision

The retina is located at the back of the eye. When light passes through the lens, it is sensed by the retina and converted to a nerve impulse for interpretation by the brain. Retinol is transported to the retina via the circulation, where it moves into retinal pigment epithelial cells (Fig. 7–1). There, retinol is esterified to form a retinyl ester, which can be stored. When needed, retinyl esters are broken apart (hydrolyzed) and isomerized to form 11-*cis* retinol, which can be oxidized to form 11-*cis* retinal. 11-*cis* retinal can be shuttled across the inter-

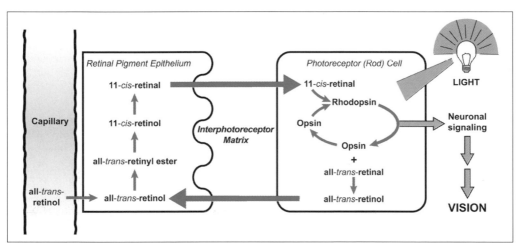

Figure 7–1. The visual cycle. Retinol is transported to the retina via the circulation, where it moves into retinal pigment epithelial cells. There, retinol is esterified to form a retinyl ester that can be stored. When needed, retinyl esters are broken apart (hydrolyzed) and isomerized to form 11-*cis* retinol, which can be oxidized to form 11-*cis* retinal. 11-*cis* retinal can be shuttled to the rod cell, where it binds to a protein called *opsin* to form the visual pigment rhodopsin (visual purple). Absorption of a photon of light cata- lyzes the isomerization of 11-*cis* retinal to all-*trans* retinal and results in its release. This isomerization triggers a cascade of events, leading to the generation of an electrical signal to the optic nerve. The nerve impulse generated by the optic nerve is conveyed to the brain where it can be interpreted as vision. Once released all-*trans* retinal is converted to all-*trans* retinol, which can be transported across the interphotoreceptor matrix to the retinal epithelial cell to complete the visual cycle.

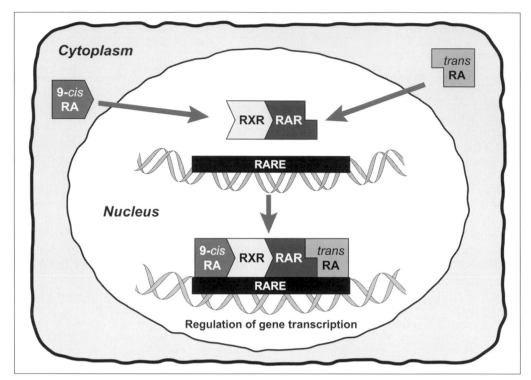

Figure 7–2. A simplified model of the regulation of gene expression by retinoic acid (RA) isomers. All-*trans* RA and 9-*cis* RA are transported to the nucleus of the cell bound to cytoplasmic retinoic acid-binding proteins. Within the nucleus, all-*trans* RA binds to retinoic acid receptors (RAR) and 9-*cis* RA binds to reti-noid receptors (RXR). RAR and RXR form RAR/RXR het-erodimers, which bind to regulatory regions of the chromosome called *retinoic acid response elements* (RARE). Binding of all-*trans* RA and 9-*cis* RA to RAR and RXR, respectively, allows the complex to regulate the rate of gene transcription.

photoreceptor matrix to the rod cell, where it binds to a protein called *opsin* to form the visual pigment rhodopsin (visual purple). Rod cells with rhodopsin can detect very small amounts of light, making them important for night vision. Absorption of a photon of light catalyzes the isomerization of 11-*cis* retinal to all-*trans* retinal and results in its release. This isomerization triggers a cascade of events, leading to the generation of an electrical signal to the optic nerve. The nerve impulse generated by the optic nerve is conveyed to the brain where it can be interpreted as vision. Once released all-*trans* retinal is converted to all-*trans* retinol, which can be transported across the interphotoreceptor matrix to the retinal epithelial cell to complete the visual cycle.[2] Inadequate retinol available to the ret-ina results in impaired dark adaptation, known as "night blindness."

Regulation of Gene Expression

RA and its isomers act as hormones to affect gene expression and thereby influence numer-ous physiological processes. All-*trans* RA and 9-*cis* RA are transported to the nucleus of the cell bound to cytoplasmic retinoic acid-bind-ing proteins. Within the nucleus, RA binds to retinoic acid receptor proteins (Fig. 7–2). All-*trans* RA binds to retinoic acid receptors (RAR) and 9-*cis* RA binds to retinoid receptors (RXR). RAR and RXR form RAR/RXR heterodimers, which bind to regulatory regions of the chro-mosome called retinoic acid response ele-ments (RARE). A dimer is a complex of two protein molecules. Heterodimers are complexes of two different proteins, while homodimers are complexes of two of the same protein. Binding of all-*trans* RA and 9-*cis* RA to RAR and RXR respectively allows the complex to regulate the rate of gene transcription, thereby influencing the synthesis of certain proteins used throughout the body. RXR may also form heterodimers with thyroid hormone receptors or vitamin D receptors. In this way, vitamin A, thyroid hormone, and vitamin D may interact to influence gene transcription.[3] Through the stimulation and inhibition of transcription of specific genes, RA plays a major role in cellular differentiation, the specialization of cells for highly specific physiological roles. Most of the physiological effects attributed to vitamin A appear to result from its role in cellular differentiation.

Immunity

Vitamin A is commonly known as the anti-infective vitamin, because it is required for normal functioning of the immune system.[4] The skin and mucosal cells (cells that line the airways, digestive tract, and urinary tract) function as a barrier and form the body's first line of defense against infection. Retinol and its metabolites are required to maintain the integrity and function of these cells.[5] Vitamin A and RA play a central role in the development and differentiation of white blood cells, such as lymphocytes, that play critical roles in the immune response. Activation of T lymphocytes, the major regulatory cells of the immune system, appears to require all-*trans* RA binding of RAR.[3]

Growth and Development

Both vitamin A excess and deficiency are known to cause birth defects. Retinol and RA are essential for embryonic development.[4] During fetal development, RA functions in limb development and formation of the heart, eyes, and ears.[6] Additionally, RA has been found to regulate expression of the gene for growth hormone.

Red Blood Cell Production

Red blood cells, like all blood cells, are derived from precursor cells called *stem cells*. These stem cells are dependent on retinoids for normal differentiation into red blood cells. Additionally, vitamin A appears to facilitate the mobilization of iron from storage sites to the developing red blood cell for incorporation into hemoglobin, the oxygen carrier in red blood cells.[2,7]

Nutrient Interactions

Zinc and Vitamin A. Zinc deficiency is thought to interfere with vitamin A metabolism in several ways: (1) Zinc deficiency results in decreased synthesis of retinol binding protein (RBP), which transports retinol through the circulation to tissues (e.g., the retina). (2) Zinc deficiency results in decreased activity of the enzyme that releases retinol from its storage form, retinyl palmitate, in the liver. (3) Zinc is required for the enzyme that converts retinol into retinal.[8,9] At present, the health consequences of zinc deficiency on vitamin A nutritional status in humans are unclear.[10]

Iron and Vitamin A. Vitamin A deficiency may exacerbate iron-deficiency anemia. Vitamin A supplementation has been shown to have beneficial effects on iron-deficiency anemia and improve iron status among children and pregnant women. The combination of vitamin A and iron seems to reduce anemia more effectively than either iron or vitamin A alone.[11]

Deficiency

Vitamin A Deficiency and Vision

Vitamin A deficiency among children in developing nations is the leading preventable cause of blindness.[12] The earliest evidence of vitamin A deficiency is impaired dark adaptation or night blindness. Mild vitamin A deficiency may result in changes in the conjunctiva (corner of the eye) called *Bitot's spots*. Severe or prolonged vitamin A deficiency causes a condition called *xerophthalmia* (dry eye), character-

Table 7–1 Recommended Dietary Allowance (RDA) for Vitamin A as Preformed Vitamin A (Retinol)

Life Stage	Age	Males, µg/d	Females, µg/d
Infants	0–6 months	400 (AI)	400 (AI)
Infants	7–12 months	500 (AI)	500 (AI)
Children	1–3 years	300	300
Children	4–8 years	400	400
Children	9–13 years	600	600
Adolescents	14–18 years	900	700
Adults	19 years and older	900	700
Pregnancy	18 years and younger	–	750
Pregnancy	19 years and older	–	770
Breast-feeding	18 years and younger	–	1200
Breast-feeding	19 years and older	–	1300

AI, adequate intake level.

ized by changes in the cells of the cornea (clear covering of the eye) that ultimately result in corneal ulcers, scarring, and blindness.[4,8]

Vitamin A Deficiency and Infectious Disease

Vitamin A deficiency can be considered a nutritionally acquired immunodeficiency disease.[13] Even children who are only mildly deficient in vitamin A have a higher incidence of respiratory disease and diarrhea, as well as a higher rate of mortality from infectious disease, than children who consume sufficient vitamin A.[14] Supplementation of vitamin A has been found to decrease the severity of and deaths from diarrhea and measles in developing countries, where vitamin A deficiency is common.[15] Human immunodeficiency virus (HIV)-infected women who were vitamin A–deficient were three to four times more likely to transmit HIV to their infants.[16]

The onset of infection reduces blood retinol levels very rapidly. This phenomenon is generally believed to be related to decreased synthesis of RBP by the liver. In this manner, infection stimulates a vicious cycle, because inadequate vitamin A nutritional status is related to increased severity and likelihood of death from infectious disease.[17]

The Recommended Dietary Allowance

The recommended dietary allowance (RDA) for vitamin A was revised by the Food and Nutrition Board (FNB) of the Institute of Medicine in 2001. The latest RDA is based on the amount needed to ensure adequate stores of vitamin A in the body to support normal reproductive function, immune function, gene expression, and vision (Table 7–1).[18]

Disease Prevention

Cancer

Studies in cell culture and animal models have documented the capacity for natural and synthetic retinoids to reduce carcinogenesis significantly in skin, breast, liver, colon, prostate, and other sites.[2] However, the results of human studies examining the relationship between the consumption of preformed vitamin A and cancer are less clear.

Lung Cancer. At least 10 prospective studies have compared blood retinol levels at baseline among people who subsequently developed lung cancer and those who did not. Only one of those studies found a statistically significant inverse association between serum retinol and lung cancer risk.[19] The results of the β-Carotene and Retinol Efficacy Trial suggest that high-dose supplementation of vitamin A and β-carotene should be avoided in people at high risk of lung cancer. About 9000 people (smokers and people with asbestos exposure) were assigned a daily regimen of 25,000 IU of retinol and 30 mg of β-carotene, while a similar number of people were assigned a placebo. After 4 years of follow-up the incidence of lung cancer was 28 % higher in the supplemented group.[20] Presently, it seems unlikely that increased retinol intake decreases the risk of lung cancer, although the effects of retinol may be different for nonsmokers compared with smokers.[19]

Breast Cancer. Retinol and its metabolites have been found to reduce the growth of breast cancer cells in the test tube, but observational studies of dietary retinol intake in humans have been less optimistic.[21] The majority of epidemiologic studies have failed to find significant associations between retinol intake and breast cancer risk in women,[22–25] although one large prospective study found total vitamin A intake to be inversely associated with the risk of breast cancer in premenopausal women with a family history of breast cancer.[26] Blood levels of retinol reflect the intake of both preformed vitamin A and provitamin A carotenoids like β-carotene. Although a recent case-control study found serum retinol levels and serum antioxidant levels to be inversely related to the risk of breast cancer,[27] two recent prospective studies did not observe significant associations between serum retinol levels and the subsequent risk of developing breast cancer.[28,29] Presently, there is little evidence in humans that increased intake of preformed vitamin A or retinol reduces breast cancer risk.

Disease Treatment

Pharmacologic Doses of Retinoids

It is important to note that treatment with high doses of natural or synthetic retinoids overrides the body's own control mechanisms and therefore carries with it risks of side effects and toxicity. Additionally, all of these compounds have been found to cause birth defects. Women who have a chance of becoming pregnant should avoid treatment with these medications. Retinoids tend to be very long acting; side effects and birth defects have been reported to occur months after discontinuing retinoid therapy.[2] The retinoids discussed in the following are prescription drugs and should not be used without medical supervision.

Diseases of the Skin

Both natural and synthetic retinoids have been used as pharmacologic agents to treat disorders of the skin. Etretinate and acitretin are retinoids that have been useful in the treatment of psoriasis, while tretinoin (Retin-A) and isotretinoin (Accutane) have been used successfully to treat severe acne. Retinoids most likely affect the transcription of skin growth factors and their receptors.[2]

Acute Promyelotic Leukemia

Normal differentiation of myeloid stem cells in the bone marrow gives rise to platelets, red blood cells, and white cells, which are important for the immune response. Altered differentiation of those stem cells results in the proliferation of immature leukemic cells, giving rise to leukemia. A mutation of the retinoic acid receptor RAR has been discovered in patients with a specific type of leukemia called acute promyelotic leukemia (APL). Treatment with all-*trans* retinoic acid or high doses of all-*trans* retinyl palmitate restores normal differentiation and leads to improvement in some APL patients.[2,17]

Sources

Retinol Activity Equivalency

Different dietary sources of vitamin A have different potencies. For example, β-carotene is less easily absorbed than retinol and must be converted to retinal and retinol by the body. The most recent international standard of measure for vitamin A is retinol activity equivalency (RAE), which represents vitamin A activity as retinol. Two micrograms of β-carotene in oil provided as a supplement can be converted by the body to 1 μg of retinol, giving it an RAE ratio of 2:1. However, 12 μg of β-carotene from foods are required to provide the body with 1 μg of retinol, giving dietary β-carotene an RAE ratio of 12:1. Other provitamin A carotenoids in foods are less easily absorbed than β-carotene, resulting in RAE ratios of 24:1. The RAE ratios for β-carotene and other provitamin A carotenoids are shown in Table 7–2.[18]

Table 7–2 Retinol Activity Equivalency (RAE) Ratios for β-Carotene and Other Provitamin A Carotenoids

Quantity Consumed	Quantity Bioconverted to Retinol	Retinol Activity Equivalency (RAE) Ratio
1 μg of dietary or supplemental vitamin A	1 μg of retinol	1:1
2 μg of supplemental β-carotene	1 μg of retinol	2:1
12 μg of dietary β-carotene	1 μg of retinol	12:1
24 μg of dietary α-carotene	1 μg of retinol	24:1
24 μg of dietary β-cryptoxanthin	1 μg of retinol	24:1

An older international standard, still commonly used, is the international unit; 1 IU is equivalent to 0.3 μg of retinol.

Food Sources

Free retinol is not generally found in foods. Retinyl palmitate, a precursor and storage form of retinol, is generally found in foods from animals. Plants contain carotenoids, some of which are precursors for vitamin A (e.g., α-carotene and β-carotene). Yellow and orange vegetables contain significant quantities of carotenoids. Green vegetables also contain carotenoids, though the pigment is masked by the green pigment of chlorophyll.[1] A number of good food sources of vitamin A are listed in Table 7–3 along with their vitamin A content in retinol activity equivalents (μg RAE). In those foods where retinol activity comes mainly from provitamin A carotenoids, the carotenoid content and the retinol activity equivalents are presented.

Table 7–3   Food Sources of Vitamin A

Food	Serving	Vitamin A, μg RAE	α-Carotene, μg	α-Carotene, μg RAE	β-Carotene, μg	β-Carotene, μg RAE
Cod liver oil	1 tablespoon	4080	0	0	0	0
Fortified cereal	1 serving	140–375	0	0	0	0
Egg	1 large	119	0	0	0	0
Butter	1 tablespoon	107	0	0	0	0
Margarine	1 tablespoon	113	0	0	68	6
Skim milk	1 cup (8 oz.)	76	0	0	0	0
Sweet potato	1/2 cup	1136	0	0	13,635	1136
Carrot, raw	1/2 cup, diced	595	2975	124	5655	471
Cantaloupe	1/2 medium	370	75	3	4402	367
Spinach, cooked	1/2 cup	393	0	0	4717	393
Apricot	1 medium	74	0	0	893	74
Squash, butternut	1/2 cup, cooked	42	0	0	505	42
Zucchini, summer	1/2 cup, cooked	31	0	0	369	31

Supplements

The principal forms of preformed vitamin A in supplements are retinyl palmitate and retinyl acetate. Multivitamin preparations generally provide a combination of vitamin A and β-carotene. Multivitamins commonly provide 5000 IU of vitamin A, some of which is in the form of β-carotene; 5000 IU is equivalent to 1500 μg of retinol or less, depending on how much is in the form of β-carotene. Note: 2 μg of supplemental β-carotene is equivalent to 1 μg of preformed vitamin A or retinol.[30]

Table 7–4   Tolerable Upper Level of Intake (UL) for Preformed Vitamin A (Retinol)

Life Stage	Age	UL, μg/d
Infants	0–12 months	600 (2000 IU)
Children	1–3 years	600 (2000 IU)
Children	4–8 years	900 (3000 IU)
Children	9–13 years	1700 (5667 IU)
Adolescents	14–18 years	2800 (9333 IU)
Adults	19 years and older	3000 (10,000 IU)

Safety

Toxicity

The condition caused by vitamin A toxicity is called *hypervitaminosis A*. It is caused by over-consumption of preformed vitamin A, not carotenoids. Preformed vitamin A is rapidly absorbed and slowly cleared from the body, so toxicity may result acutely from high-dose exposure over a short period of time or chronically from much lower intake.[2] Vitamin A toxicity is relatively rare. Symptoms include nausea, headache, fatigue, loss of appetite, dizziness, and dry skin. Signs of chronic toxicity include dry itchy skin, loss of appetite, headache, and bone and joint pain. Severe cases of hypervitaminosis A may result in liver damage, hemorrhage, and coma. Generally, signs of toxicity are associated with long-term consumption of vitamin A in excess of 10 times the RDA (8000 to 10,000 μg/d or 25,000 to 33,000 IU/d). However, there is evidence that some populations may be more susceptible to toxicity at lower doses, including the elderly, chronic alcohol users, and some people with a genetic predisposition to high cholesterol.[9] In January 2001, the FNB of the Institute of Medicine set the tolerable upper level (UL) of vitamin A intake for adults at 3000 μg (10,000 IU)/d of preformed vitamin A (Table 7–4).[18]

Safety in Pregnancy

Because excess preformed vitamin A consumed during pregnancy is known to cause birth defects, pregnant women who are not at risk of vitamin A deficiency are advised not to consume more than 800 μg/d (2600 IU/d) of retinol as a supplement.[31] Additionally, etretinate and isotretinoin (Accutane), synthetic derivatives of retinol, are known to cause birth defects and should not be taken during pregnancy or if there is a possibility of becoming pregnant. Tretinoin (Retin-A), another retinol derivative, is prescribed as a topical preparation that is applied to the skin. Because of the potential for systemic absorption of topical tretinoin, its use during pregnancy is not recommended.

Drug Interactions

Chronic alcohol consumption results in depletion of liver stores of vitamin A and may contribute to alcohol-induced liver damage.[32] However, the liver toxicity of vitamin A (retinol) is enhanced by chronic alcohol consumption, thus narrowing the therapeutic window for vitamin A supplementation in alcoholics.[33] Oral contraceptives that contain estrogen and progestin increase RBP synthesis by the liver, increasing the export of RBP-retinol complex in the blood. Whether this increases the dietary requirement of vitamin A is not known. Etretinate and isotretinoin (Accutane), retinol derivatives, should not be used in combination with vitamin A supplementation because they may increase the risk of vitamin A toxicity.[34]

LPI Recommendation

Following the Linus Pauling Institute recommendation of taking a multivitamin/mineral supplement daily will generally supply more than the RDA (900 μg/d for men and 700 μg/d for women) for vitamin A. There is no need for additional vitamin A supplementation, and high-potency vitamin A supplements should be avoided due to the risk of toxicity.

Older Adults

Presently there is little evidence that the requirement for vitamin A in older adults (65 years and older) differs from that of younger adults. Although vitamin A insufficiency does not appear to be more common in older adults, vitamin A toxicity may occur at lower doses than in younger adults. In individuals already taking a multivitamin/mineral supplement daily, there is no need for additional vitamin A supplementation. Older adults should be especially careful to avoid vitamin A intakes above the upper intake level (UL of 3000 μg (10,000 IU)/d.

References

1. Groff JL. *Advanced Nutrition and Human Metabolism.* 2nd ed. St. Paul: West Publishing; 1995.
2. Ross AC. Vitamin A and retinoids. In: Shils M, Olson JA, Shike M, Ross AC, eds. *Nutrition in Health and Disease.* 9th ed. Baltimore: Williams & Wilkins; 1999:305–327.
3. Semba RD. The role of vitamin A and related retinoids in immune function. *Nutr Rev* 1998;56(1 Pt 2):S38–S48.
4. Semba RD. Impact of vitamin A on immunity and infection in developing countries. In: Bendich A, Decklebaum RJ, eds. *Preventive Nutrition: The Comprehensive Guide for Health Professionals.* 2nd ed. Totowa, NJ: Humana Press Inc; 2001:329–346.
5. McCullough FS, Northrop-Clewes CA, Thurnham DI. The effect of vitamin A on epithelial integrity. *Proc Nutr Soc* 1999;58(2):289–293.
6. Olson JA. Vitamin A. In: Ziegler EE, Filer LJ, eds. *Present Knowledge in Nutrition.* 7th ed. Washington, D.C.: ILSI Press; 1996:109–118.
7. Lynch SR. Interaction of iron with other nutrients. *Nutr Rev* 1997;55(4):102–110.
8. Brody T. *Nutritional Biochemistry.* 2nd ed. San Diego: Academic Press; 1999.
9. Russell RM. The vitamin A spectrum: from deficiency to toxicity. *Am J Clin Nutr* 2000;71(4):878–884.
10. Christian P, West KP Jr. Interactions between zinc and vitamin A: an update. *Am J Clin Nutr* 1998;68(2 Suppl):435S–441S.
11. Suharno D, West CE, Muhilal, Karyadi D, Hautvast JG. Supplementation with vitamin A and iron for nutritional anaemia in pregnant women in West Java, Indonesia. *Lancet* 1993;342(8883):1325–1328.
12. Underwood BA, Arthur P. The contribution of vitamin A to public health. *FASEB J* 1996;10(9):1040–1048.
13. Semba RD. Vitamin A and human immunodeficiency virus infection. *Proc Nutr Soc* 1997;56(1B):459–469.
14. Field CJ, Johnson IR, Schley PD. Nutrients and their role in host resistance to infection. *J Leukoc Biol* 2002;71(1):16–32.
15. West CE. Vitamin A and measles. *Nutr Rev* 2000;58(2 Pt 2):S46–S54.
16. Semba RD, Miotti PG, Chiphangwi JD, et al. Maternal vitamin A deficiency and mother-to-child transmission of HIV-1. *Lancet* 1994;343(8913):1593–1597.
17. Thurnham DI, Northrop-Clewes CA. Optimal nutrition: vitamin A and the carotenoids. *Proc Nutr Soc* 1999;58(2):449–457.
18. Food and Nutrition Board, Institute of Medicine. Vitamin A. *Dietary Reference Intakes for Vitamin A, Vitamin K, Arsenic, Boron, Chromium, Copper, Iodine, Iron, Manganese, Molybdenum, Nickel, Silicon, Vanadium, and Zinc.* Washington, D.C.: National Academy Press; 2001:82–161.
19. Comstock GW, Helzlsouer KJ. Preventive nutrition and lung cancer. In: Bendich A, Decklebaum RJ, eds. *Preventive Nutrition: The Comprehensive Guide for Health Professionals.* 2nd ed. Totowa, NJ: Humana Press Inc; 2001:97–129.
20. Omenn GS, Goodman GE, Thornquist MD, et al. Effects of a combination of beta carotene and vitamin A on lung cancer and cardiovascular disease. *N Engl J Med* 1996;334(18):1150–1155.
21. Prakash P, Krinsky NI, Russell RM. Retinoids, carotenoids, and human breast cancer cell cultures: a review of differential effects. *Nutr Rev* 2000;58(6):170–176.
22. Bohlke K, Spiegelman D, Trichopoulou A, Katsouyanni K, Trichopoulos D. Vitamins A, C and E and the risk of breast cancer: results from a case-control study in Greece. *Br J Cancer* 1999;79(1):23–29.
23. Franceschi S. Micronutrients and breast cancer. *Eur J Cancer Prev* 1997;6(6):535–539.
24. Longnecker MP, Newcomb PA, Mittendorf R, Greenberg ER, Willett WC. Intake of carrots, spinach, and supplements containing vitamin A in relation to risk of breast cancer. *Cancer Epidemiol Biomarkers Prev* 1997;6(11):887–892.
25. Michels KB, Holmberg L, Bergkvist L, Ljung H, Bruce A, Wolk A. Dietary antioxidant vitamins, retinol, and breast cancer incidence in a cohort of Swedish women. *Int J Cancer* 2001;91(4):563–567.
26. Zhang S, Hunter DJ, Forman MR, et al. Dietary carotenoids and vitamins A, C, and E and risk of breast cancer. *J Natl Cancer Inst* 1999;91(6):547–556.
27. Ching S, Ingram D, Hahnel R, Beilby J, Rossi E. Serum levels of micronutrients, antioxidants and total antioxidant status predict risk of breast cancer in a case control study. *J Nutr* 2002;132(2):303–306.
28. Dorgan JF, Sowell A, Swanson CA, et al. Relationships of serum carotenoids, retinol, alpha-tocopherol, and selenium with breast cancer risk: results from a prospective study in Columbia, Missouri (United States). *Cancer Causes Control* 1998;9(1):89–97.
29. Hulten K, Van Kappel AL, Winkvist A, et al. Carotenoids, alpha-tocopherols, and retinol in plasma and breast cancer risk in northern Sweden. *Cancer Causes Control* 2001;12(6):529–537.

30. Hendler SS, Rorvik DR, eds. *PDR for Nutritional Supplements*. Montvale, NJ: Medical Economics Company, Inc; 2001.

31. Binkley N, Krueger D. Hypervitaminosis A and bone. *Nutr Rev* 2000;58(5):138–144.

32. Wang XD. Chronic alcohol intake interferes with retinoid metabolism and signaling. *Nutr Rev* 1999;57(2): 51–59.

33. Leo MA, Lieber CS. Alcohol, vitamin A, and beta-carotene: adverse interactions, including hepatotoxicity and carcinogenicity. *Am J Clin Nutr* 1999;69(6):1071–1085.

34. Flodin N. *Pharmacology of Micronutrients*. New York: Alan R. Liss, Inc.; 1988.

8 Vitamin B$_6$

Vitamin B$_6$ is a water-soluble vitamin that was first isolated in the 1930s. There are six forms of vitamin B$_6$: pyridoxal (PL), pyridoxine, pyridoxamine, and their phosphate derivatives: pyridoxal 5′-phosphate (PLP), pyridoxine 5′-phosphate, and pyridoxamine 5′-phosphate. PLP is the active coenzyme form and has the most importance in human metabolism.[1]

Function

Vitamin B$_6$ must be obtained from the diet because humans cannot synthesize it, and the coenzyme PLP plays a vital role in the function of approximately 100 enzymes that catalyze essential chemical reactions in the human body.[1,2] For example, PLP functions as a coenzyme for glycogen phosphorylase, an enzyme that catalyzes the release of glucose stored in the muscle as glycogen. Much of the PLP in the human body is found in muscle bound to glycogen phosphorylase. PLP is also a coenzyme for reactions used to generate glucose from amino acids, a process known as *gluconeogenesis*.

Nervous System Function

The synthesis of the neurotransmitter serotonin from the amino acid tryptophan in the brain is catalyzed by a PLP-dependent enzyme. Other neurotransmitters such as dopamine, norepinephrine, and gamma-aminobutyric acid are also synthesized using PLP-dependent enzymes.[2]

Red Blood Cell Formation and Function

PLP functions as a coenzyme in the synthesis of heme, a component of hemoglobin. Hemoglobin is found in red blood cells and is critical to their ability to transport oxygen throughout the body. Both PL and PLP are able to bind to the hemoglobin molecule and affect its ability to pick up and release oxygen. However, the impact of this on normal oxygen delivery to tissues is not known.[2]

Niacin Formation

The human requirement for another vitamin, niacin, can be met in part by the conversion of the dietary amino acid tryptophan to niacin, as well as through dietary intake. PLP is a coenzyme for a critical reaction in the synthesis of niacin from tryptophan. Thus, adequate vitamin B$_6$ decreases the requirement for niacin in the diet.[2]

Hormone Function

Steroid hormones, such as estrogen and testosterone, exert their effects in the body by binding to steroid hormone receptors in the nucleus of the cell and altering gene transcription. PLP binds to steroid receptors in such a manner as to inhibit the binding of steroid hormones, thus decreasing their effects. The binding of PLP to steroid receptors for estrogen, progesterone, testosterone, and other steroid hormones suggests that the vitamin B$_6$ status of an individual may have implications for diseases affected by steroid hormones, such as breast cancer and prostate cancer.[2]

Nucleic Acid Synthesis

PLP serves as a coenzyme for a key enzyme involved in the mobilization of single-carbon functional groups (one-carbon metabolism). Such reactions are involved in the synthesis of nucleic acids. The effect of B$_6$ deficiency on immune system function may be partly related to the role of PLP in one-carbon metabolism.

Table 8–1 Recommended Dietary Allowance (RDA) for Vitamin B$_6$

Life Stage	Age	Males, mg/d	Females, mg/d
Infants	0–6 months	0.1 (AI)	0.1 (AI)
Infants	7–12 months	0.3 (AI)	0.3 (AI)
Children	1–3 years	0.5	0.5
Children	4–8 years	0.6	0.6
Children	9–13 years	1.0	1.0
Adolescents	14–18 years	1.3	1.2
Adults	19–50 years	1.3	1.3
Adults	51 years and older	1.7	1.5
Pregnancy	all ages	–	1.9
Breast-feeding	all ages	–	2.0

AI, adequate intake level.

Deficiency

Severe deficiency of vitamin B$_6$ is uncommon. Alcoholics are thought to be most at risk of vitamin B$_6$ deficiency, due to a low intake and impaired metabolism of the vitamin. In the early 1950s seizures were observed in infants as a result of severe vitamin B$_6$ deficiency due to an error in the manufacture of infant formula. Abnormal electroencephalogram patterns have been noted in some studies of vitamin B$_6$ deficiency. Other neurologic symptoms noted in severe vitamin B$_6$ deficiency include irritability, depression, and confusion; additional symptoms include inflammation of the tongue, sores or ulcers of the mouth, and ulcers of the skin at the corners of the mouth.[1]

The Recommended Dietary Allowance

Because vitamin B$_6$ is involved in so many aspects of metabolism, several factors are likely to affect an individual's requirement for vitamin B$_6$. Of those factors, protein intake has been studied the most. Increased dietary protein results in an increased requirement for vitamin B$_6$, probably because PLP is a coenzyme for many enzymes involved in amino acid metabolism.[3] Unlike previous recommendations, the Food and Nutrition Board (FNB) of the Institute of Medicine did not express the most recent recommended dietary allowance (RDA) for vitamin B$_6$ in terms of protein intake, although the relationship was considered in setting the RDA.[4] The current RDA was revised by the FNB in 1998 (Table 8–1).

Disease Prevention

Cardiovascular Diseases

Even moderately elevated levels of homocysteine in the blood have been associated with increased risk for cardiovascular diseases, such as heart disease and stroke.[5] When we digest protein, amino acids, including methionine, are released. Homocysteine is an intermediate in the metabolism of methionine. Healthy individuals utilize two different pathways to metabolize homocysteine. One pathway results in the conversion of homocysteine back to methionine and is dependent on folic acid and vitamin B$_{12}$. The other pathway converts homocysteine to another amino acid, cysteine, and requires two vitamin B$_6$ (PLP)-dependent enzymes. Thus, the amount of homocysteine in the blood is regulated by at least three vitamins: folic acid, vitamin B$_{12}$, and vitamin B$_6$ (Fig. 8–1). Several large observational studies have demonstrated an association between low vitamin B$_6$ intake or status with increased blood homocysteine levels and increased risk of cardiovascular diseases. A large prospective study found the risk of heart disease in women who consumed, on average, 4.6 mg of vitamin B$_6$ daily to be only 67% of the risk in women who consumed an average of 1.1 mg daily.[6] Another large prospective study found higher plasma levels of PLP to be associated with decreased risk of cardiovascular disease, independent of homocysteine levels.[7] In contrast to folic acid supplementation, studies of vitamin B$_6$ supplementation alone have not resulted in significant decreases of basal (fasting) levels of homocysteine. However, vitamin B$_6$ supplementation has been found effective in lowering blood homocysteine levels after an oral dose of methionine (methionine load test) was given,[8] suggesting it may play a role in the metabolism of homocysteine after meals.

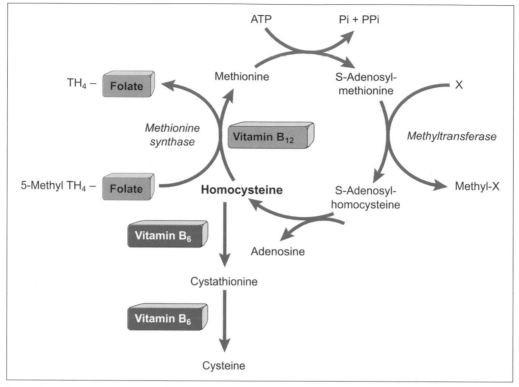

Figure 8–1. Homocysteine metabolism. S-adenosyl-homocysteine is formed during S-adenosyl-methionine-dependent methylation reactions, and the hydrolysis of S-adenosylhomocysteine results in homocysteine. Homocysteine may be remethylated to form methionine by a folate-dependent reaction that is catalyzed by methionine synthase, a vitamin B_{12}–dependent enzyme. Alternately, homocysteine may be metabolized to cysteine in reactions catalyzed by two vitamin B_6–dependent enzymes.

Immune Function

Low vitamin B_6 intake and status have been associated with impaired immune function, especially in the elderly. Decreased production of immune system cells known as lymphocytes, as well as decreased production of an important immune system protein called interleukin-2, have been measured in vitamin B_6-deficient individuals. Restoration of adequate vitamin B_6 status resulted in normalization of lymphocyte proliferation and interleukin-2 production, suggesting that adequate vitamin B_6 intake is important for optimal immune system function in older individuals.[9,10] However, one study found that the amount of vitamin B_6 required to reverse these immune system impairments in the elderly was 2.9 mg/d for men and 1.9 mg/d for women, more than the current RDA.[9]

Cognitive Function

A few recent studies have demonstrated an association between declines in cognitive function or Alzheimer's disease in the elderly and inadequate nutritional status of folic acid, vitamin B_{12}, and vitamin B_6 and thus elevated levels of homocysteine.[11] One observational study found higher plasma vitamin B_6 levels to be associated with better performance on two measures of memory but unrelated to performance on 18 other cognitive tests.[12] It is presently unclear whether marginal B vitamin deficiencies, which are relatively common in the elderly, contribute to age-associated declines in cognitive function or whether both result from processes associated with aging and/or disease.

Kidney Stones

A large prospective study examined the relationship between vitamin B_6 intake and the occurrence of symptomatic kidney stones in women. In a group of more than 85,000 women without a prior history of kidney stones, followed over 14 years, those who consumed 40 mg or more of vitamin B_6 daily had only two thirds the risk of developing kidney stones compared with those who consumed 3 mg or less.[13] However, in a group of more than 45,000 men followed over 6 years no association was found between vitamin B_6 intake and the occurrence of kidney stones.[14] Limited data have shown that supplementation of vitamin B_6 at levels higher than the tolerable upper intake level (100 mg) decreased elevated urinary oxalate levels, an important determinant of calcium oxalate kidney stone formation, in some individuals. However, it is less clear that supplementation actually resulted in decreased formation of calcium oxalate kidney stones. Presently, the relationship between vitamin B_6 intake and the risk of developing kidney stones requires further study before any recommendation can be made.

Disease Treatment

Vitamin B_6 supplements at pharmacologic doses (i.e., doses much larger than those needed to prevent deficiency) have been used in an attempt to treat a wide variety of conditions, some of which are discussed below. In general, well-designed, placebo-controlled studies have shown little evidence of benefit from large supplemental doses of vitamin B_6.[15]

Side Effects of Oral Contraceptives

Because vitamin B_6 is required for the metabolism of the amino acid tryptophan, the tryptophan load test (an assay of tryptophan metabolites after an oral dose of tryptophan) was used as a functional assessment of vitamin B_6 status. Abnormal tryptophan load tests in women taking high-dose oral contraceptives in the 1960s and 1970s suggested that these women were vitamin B_6-deficient. The abnormal results in the tryptophan load test led a number of clinicians to prescribe high doses (100 to 150 mg/d) of vitamin B_6 to women to relieve depression and other side effects sometimes experienced with oral contraceptives. However, most other indices of vitamin B_6 status were normal in women on high-dose oral contraceptives, and it is likely that the abnormality in tryptophan metabolism was not due to vitamin B_6 deficiency.[15] A more recent study of women on the low-dose oral contraceptives prescribed currently showed no benefit of up to 150 mg/d of vitamin B_6 (pyridoxine) over a placebo in the prevention of side effects, such as nausea, vomiting, dizziness, depression, and irritability.[16]

Premenstrual Syndrome

The use of vitamin B_6 to relieve the side effects of high-dose oral contraceptives led to the use of vitamin B_6 in the treatment of premenstrual syndrome (PMS). PMS refers to a cluster of symptoms, including but not limited to fatigue, irritability, moodiness/depression, fluid retention, and breast tenderness, that begin sometime after ovulation (midcycle) and subside with the onset of menstruation (the monthly period). A review of 12 placebo-controlled double-blind trials of vitamin B_6 in PMS concluded that evidence for a beneficial effect was weak.[17] A more recent review of 25 studies of vitamin B_6 and PMS suggested that doses of vitamin B_6 up to 100 mg/d may be of value, but conclusions were limited by the poor quality of most of the studies evaluated.[18]

Depression

Because key enzymes in the synthesis of the neurotransmitters, serotonin and norepinephrine, are PLP-dependent, it has been suggested that vitamin B_6 deficiency may lead to depression. However, clinical trials have not provided evidence that vitamin B_6 supplementation is effective in the treatment of depression.[15]

Nausea and Vomiting in Pregnancy

Vitamin B$_6$ has been used since the 1940s to treat nausea during pregnancy. Vitamin B$_6$ was included in the medication Bendectin, which was prescribed for the treatment of morning sickness, and later withdrawn from the market due to unproven concerns that it increased the risk of birth defects. Vitamin B$_6$ itself is considered safe during pregnancy and has been used in pregnant women without any evidence of fetal harm.[19] The results of two double-blind placebo-controlled trials (25 mg of pyridoxine every 8 hours for 3 days[20] and 10 mg of pyridoxine every 8 hours for 5 days[19]) suggest vitamin B$_6$ may be beneficial in alleviating morning sickness. Each study found a slight but significant reduction in nausea or vomiting in pregnant women. A recent systematic review of placebo-controlled trials for nausea of early pregnancy found vitamin B$_6$ to be somewhat effective.[21] However, it should be noted that morning sickness also resolves without any treatment, making it difficult to perform well-controlled trials.

Carpal Tunnel Syndrome

Carpal tunnel syndrome causes numbness, pain, and weakness of the hand and fingers due to compression of the median nerve at the wrist. It may result from repetitive stress injury of the wrist or from soft tissue swelling, which sometimes occurs with pregnancy or hypothyroidism. Several early studies by the same investigator suggested that vitamin B$_6$ status was low in individuals with carpal tunnel syndrome and that supplementation with 100 to 200 mg/d over several months was beneficial.[22,23] A recent study found decreased blood levels of PLP to be associated with increased pain, tingling, and nocturnal wakening, all symptoms of carpal tunnel syndrome, in men who were not taking vitamin supplements.[24] Studies using electrophysiological measurements of median nerve conduction have generally failed to find an association between vitamin B$_6$ deficiency and carpal tunnel syndrome. Although a few trials have noted some symptomatic relief with vitamin B$_6$ supplementation, double-blind placebo-controlled trials have not generally found vitamin B$_6$ to be effective in treating carpal tunnel syndrome.[15,25]

Sources

Food Sources

Surveys in the United States have shown that dietary intake of vitamin B$_6$ averages about 2 mg/d for men and 1.5 mg/d for women. A survey of elderly individuals found that men and women over 60 consumed about 1.2 mg/d and 1.0 mg/d, respectively, both less than the current RDA. Certain plant foods contain a unique form of vitamin B$_6$ called *pyridoxine glucoside*. This form of vitamin B$_6$ appears to be only about half as bioavailable as vitamin B$_6$ from other food sources or supplements. Vitamin B$_6$ in a mixed diet has been found to be approximately 75% bioavailable.[4] In most cases, including foods in the diet that are rich in vitamin B$_6$ should supply enough to prevent deficiency. However, those who follow a very restricted vegetarian diet might need to increase their vitamin B$_6$ intake by eating food fortified with vitamin B$_6$ or by taking a supplement. Some foods that are relatively rich in vitamin B$_6$ and their vitamin B$_6$ content in milligrams are listed in Table 8–2.

Table 8–2   Food Sources of Vitamin B$_6$

Food	Serving	Vitamin B$_6$, mg
Potato, baked with skin	1 medium	0.70
Banana	1 medium	0.68
Fortified cereal	1 cup	0.5–2.5
Salmon	3 ounces*	0.48
Chicken, light meat without skin	3 ounces*	0.46
Spinach, cooked	1 cup	0.44
Turkey, without skin	3 ounces*	0.39
Vegetable juice cocktail	6 ounces	0.25
Hazelnuts, dry roasted	1 ounce	0.18

*A 3-ounce serving of meat or fish is about the size of a deck of cards.

Supplements

Vitamin B_6 is available as pyridoxine hydrochloride in multivitamin, vitamin B-complex, and vitamin B_6 supplements.[26]

Safety

Toxicity

Because adverse effects have only been documented from vitamin B_6 supplements and never from food sources, only the supplemental form of vitamin B_6 (pyridoxine) is discussed with respect to safety. Although vitamin B_6 is a water-soluble vitamin and is excreted in the urine, very high doses of pyridoxine over long periods of time may result in painful neurological symptoms known as sensory neuropathy. Symptoms include pain and numbness of the extremities and in severe cases difficulty walking. Sensory neuropathy typically develops at doses of pyridoxine in excess of 1000 mg per day. However, there have been a few case reports of individuals who developed sensory neuropathies at doses of less than 500 mg daily over a period of months. None of the studies, in which an objective neurological examination was performed, found evidence of sensory nerve damage at intakes of pyridoxine below 200 mg/d.[15] To prevent sensory neuropathy in virtually all individuals, the Food and Nutrition Board of the Institute of Medicine set the tolerable upper intake level (UL) for pyridoxine at 100 mg/d for adults (Table 8–3).[4] Because placebo-controlled studies have generally failed to show therapeutic benefits of high doses of pyridoxine, there is little reason to exceed the UL of 100 mg/d.

Drug Interactions

Certain medications interfere with the metabolism of vitamin B_6 and may result in deficiency if individuals taking such medications are not given supplemental vitamin B_6. The antituberculosis medications isoniazid and cycloserine, the metal chelator penicillamine, and anti-Parkinsonian drugs, including levodopa, form complexes with vitamin B_6, creating a functional deficiency. The efficacy of other medications may be altered by high doses of vitamin B_6. High doses of vitamin B_6 have been found to decrease the efficacy of the anticonvulsants phenobarbital and phenytoin and levodopa.[2,15]

Table 8–3   Tolerable Upper Intake Level (UL) for Vitamin B_6

Life Stage	Age	UL, mg/d
Infants	0–12 months	not possible to establish*
Children	1–3 years	30
Children	4–8 years	40
Children	9–13 years	60
Adolescents	14–18 years	80
Adults	19 years and older	100

*Source of intake should be from food and formula only.

LPI Recommendation

Metabolic studies suggest that young women require 0.02 mg of vitamin B_6 per gram of protein consumed daily.[3,27,28] Using the upper boundary for acceptable levels of protein intake for women (100 g per day), the daily requirement for young women would be calculated at 2.0 mg daily. Older adults may also require at least 2.0 mg/d.[29] For these reasons, the Linus Pauling Institute recommends that all adults consume at least 2.0 mg of vitamin B_6 daily. Following the Linus Pauling Institute recommendation to take a daily multivitamin/multimineral supplement, containing 100 % of the daily value for vitamin B_6, will ensure an intake of at least 2.0 mg/d of vitamin B_6. Although a vitamin B_6 intake of 2.0 mg daily is slightly higher than the most recent RDA, it is 50 times less than the UL set by the Food and Nutrition Board (Table 8–3).

Older Adults

Metabolic studies have indicated that the requirement for vitamin B$_6$ in adults 65 years and older is approximately 2.0 mg daily[29] and could be higher if the effects of marginally deficient intakes of vitamin B$_6$ on immune function and homocysteine levels are clarified. Despite evidence that the requirement for vitamin B$_6$ may be slightly higher in older adults, several surveys have found that over half of individuals over age 60 consume less than the current RDA (1.7 mg/d for men and 1.5 mg/d for women). For these reasons, the Linus Pauling Institute recommends that older adults take a multivitamin/multimineral supplement, which generally provides at least 2.0 mg of vitamin B$_6$ daily.

References

1. Leklem JE. Vitamin B-6. In: Machlin L, ed. *Handbook of Vitamins*. New York: Marcel Decker Inc; 1991:341–378.
2. Leklem JE. Vitamin B-6. In: Shils M, Olson JA, Shike M, Ross AC, eds. *Nutrition in Health and Disease*, 9th ed. Baltimore: Williams & Wilkins; 1999:413–422.
3. Hansen CM, Leklem JE, Miller LT. Vitamin B-6 status of women with a constant intake of vitamin B-6 changes with three levels of dietary protein. *J Nutr* 1996;126(7):1891–1901.
4. Food and Nutrition Board, Institute of Medicine. Vitamin B6. *Dietary Reference Intakes: Thiamin, Riboflavin, Niacin, Vitamin B-6, Vitamin B-12, Pantothenic Acid, Biotin, and Choline*. Washington, D.C.: National Academy Press; 1998:150–195.
5. Boushey CJ, Beresford SA, Omenn GS, Motulsky AG. A quantitative assessment of plasma homocysteine as a risk factor for vascular disease: probable benefits of increasing folic acid intakes. *JAMA* 1995;274(13): 1049–1057.
6. Rimm EB, Willett WC, Hu FB, et al. Folate and vitamin B6 from diet and supplements in relation to risk of coronary heart disease among women. *JAMA* 1998;279(5):359–364.
7. Folsom AR, Nieto FJ, McGovern PG, et al. Prospective study of coronary heart disease incidence in relation to fasting total homocysteine, related genetic polymorphisms, and B vitamins: the Atherosclerosis Risk in Communities (ARIC) study. *Circulation* 1998;98(3):204–210.
8. Ubbink JB, Vermaak WJ, van der Merwe A, Becker PJ, Delport R, Potgieter HC. Vitamin requirements for the treatment of hyperhomocysteinemia in humans. *J Nutr* 1994;124(10):1927–1933.
9. Meydani SN, Ribaya-Mercado JD, Russell RM, Sahyoun N, Morrow FD, Gershoff SN. Vitamin B-6 deficiency impairs interleukin 2 production and lymphocyte proliferation in elderly adults. *Am J Clin Nutr* 1991;53(5):1275–1280.

10. Talbott MC, Miller LT, Kerkvliet NI. Pyridoxine supplementation: effect on lymphocyte responses in elderly persons. *Am J Clin Nutr* 1987;46(4):659–664.
11. Selhub J, Bagley LC, Miller J, Rosenberg IH. B vitamins, homocysteine, and neurocognitive function in the elderly. *Am J Clin Nutr* 2000;71(2):614S–620S.
12. Riggs KM, Spiro A, 3rd, Tucker K, Rush D. Relations of vitamin B-12, vitamin B-6, folate, and homocysteine to cognitive performance in the Normative Aging Study. *Am J Clin Nutr* 1996;63(3):306–314.
13. Curhan GC, Willett WC, Speizer FE, Stampfer MJ. Intake of vitamins B6 and C and the risk of kidney stones in women. *J Am Soc Nephrol* 1999;10(4):840–845.
14. Curhan GC, Willett WC, Rimm EB, Stampfer MJ. A prospective study of the intake of vitamins C and B6, and the risk of kidney stones in men. *J Urol* 1996;155(6): 1847–1851.
15. Bender DA. Non-nutritional uses of vitamin B6. *Br J Nutr* 1999;81(1):7–20.
16. Villegas-Salas E, Ponce de Leon R, Juarez-Perez MA, Grubb GS. Effect of vitamin B6 on the side effects of a low-dose combined oral contraceptive. *Contraception* 1997;55(4):245–248.
17. Kleijnen J, Ter Riet G, Knipschild P. Vitamin B6 in the treatment of the premenstrual syndrome—a review. *Br J Obstet Gynaecol* 1990;97(9):847–852.
18. Wyatt KM, Dimmock PW, Jones PW, Shaughn O'Brien PM. Efficacy of vitamin B-6 in the treatment of premenstrual syndrome: systematic review. *BMJ* 1999;318(7195):1375–1381.
19. Vutyavanich T, Wongtra-ngan S, Ruangsri R. Pyridoxine for nausea and vomiting of pregnancy: a randomized, double-blind, placebo-controlled trial. *Am J Obstet Gynecol* 1995;173(3 Pt 1):881–884.
20. Sahakian V, Rouse D, Sipes S, Rose N, Niebyl J. Vitamin B6 is effective therapy for nausea and vomiting of pregnancy: a randomized, double-blind placebo-controlled study. *Obstet Gynecol* 1991;78(1):33–36.
21. Jewell D, Young G. Interventions for nausea and vomiting in early pregnancy (Cochrane Review). *Cochrane Database Syst Rev* 2002(1):CD000145.
22. Ellis JM, Kishi T, Azuma J, Folkers K. Vitamin B6 deficiency in patients with a clinical syndrome including the carpal tunnel defect. Biochemical and clinical response to therapy with pyridoxine. *Res Commun Chem Pathol Pharmacol* 1976;13(4):743–757.
23. Ellis J, Folkers K, Watanabe T, et al. Clinical results of a cross-over treatment with pyridoxine and placebo of the carpal tunnel syndrome. *Am J Clin Nutr* 1979;32(10):2040–2046.
24. Keniston RC, Nathan PA, Leklem JE, Lockwood RS. Vitamin B6, vitamin C, and carpal tunnel syndrome. A cross-sectional study of 441 adults. *J Occup Environ Med* 1997;39(10):949–959.
25. Spooner GR, Desai HB, Angel JF, Reeder BA, Donat JR. Using pyridoxine to treat carpal tunnel syndrome. Randomized control trial. *Can Fam Physician* 1993;39:2122–2127.
26. Hendler SS, Rorvik DR, eds. *PDR for Nutritional Supplements*. Montvale, NJ: Medical Economics Company, Inc; 2001.
27. Hansen CM, Shultz TD, Kwak HK, Memon HS, Leklem JE. Assessment of vitamin B-6 status in young women consuming a controlled diet containing four levels of vitamin B-6 provides an estimated average requirement and recommended dietary allowance. *J Nutr* 2001;131(6):1777–1786.

28. Kretsch MJ, Sauberlich HE, Skala JH, Johnson HL. Vitamin B-6 requirement and status assessment: young women fed a depletion diet followed by a plant- or animal-protein diet with graded amounts of vitamin B-6. *Am J Clin Nutr* 1995;61(5):1091–1101.

29. Ribaya-Mercado JD, Russell RM, Sahyoun N, Morrow FD, Gershoff SN. Vitamin B-6 requirements of elderly men and women. *J Nutr* 1991;121(7):1062–1074.

9 Vitamin B$_{12}$

Vitamin B$_{12}$ is the largest and most complex of all the vitamins. It is unique among vitamins in that it contains a metal ion, cobalt. For this reason *cobalamin* is the term used to refer to compounds having B$_{12}$ activity. Methylcobalamin and 5-deoxyadenosyl cobalamin are the forms of vitamin B$_{12}$ used in the human body.[1] The form of cobalamin used in most supplements, cyanocobalamin, is readily converted to 5-deoxyadenosyl and methylcobalamin.

Function

Cofactor for Methionine Synthase

Methylcobalamin is required for the function of the folate-dependent enzyme methionine synthase. This enzyme is required for the synthesis of the amino acid methionine from homocysteine. Methionine is required for the synthesis of S-adenosylmethionine, a methyl group donor used in many biological methylation reactions, including the methylation of a number of sites within DNA and RNA.[2] Methylation of DNA may be important in cancer prevention. Inadequate function of methionine synthase can lead to an accumulation of homocysteine, which has been associated with increased risk of cardiovascular diseases (Fig. 9–1).

Cofactor for Methylmalonyl-CoA Mutase

5-Deoxyadenosylcobalamin is required by the enzyme that catalyzes the conversion of L-methylmalonyl-CoA to succinyl-CoA. This biochemical reaction plays an important role in the production of energy from fats and proteins. Succinyl-CoA is also required for the synthesis of hemoglobin, the oxygen-carrying pigment in red blood cells.[2]

Deficiency

B$_{12}$ deficiency is estimated to affect 10 to 15% of individuals over the age of 60.[3] Absorption of vitamin B$_{12}$ from food requires normal function of the stomach, pancreas, and small intestine. Stomach acid and enzymes free vitamin B$_{12}$ from food, allowing it to bind to other proteins, known as *R proteins*.[2] In the alkaline environment of the small intestine, R proteins are degraded by pancreatic enzymes, freeing vitamin B$_{12}$ to bind to intrinsic factor (IF), a protein secreted by specialized cells in the stomach. Receptors on the surface of the small intestine take up the IF-B$_{12}$ complex only in the presence of calcium, which is also supplied by the pancreas.[4] Vitamin B$_{12}$ can also be absorbed by passive diffusion, but this process is very inefficient, allowing only about 1% absorption of a vitamin B$_{12}$ dose.

Causes of Vitamin B$_{12}$ Deficiency

The most common causes of vitamin B$_{12}$ deficiency are pernicious anemia and food-bound vitamin B$_{12}$ malabsorption. Although both causes become more common with age, they are two separate conditions.[3]

Pernicious Anemia

Pernicious anemia has been estimated to be present in approximately 2% of individuals over 60.[5] Although anemia is often a symptom, the condition is actually the end stage of an autoimmune inflammation of the stomach, resulting in destruction of stomach cells by one's own antibodies. Progressive destruction of the cells that line the stomach cause decreased secretion of acid and enzymes required to release food-bound vitamin B$_{12}$. Antibodies to IF bind to IF, preventing formation of the IF-B$_{12}$ complex, further inhibiting vitamin B$_{12}$ absorption. If the body's vitamin B$_{12}$

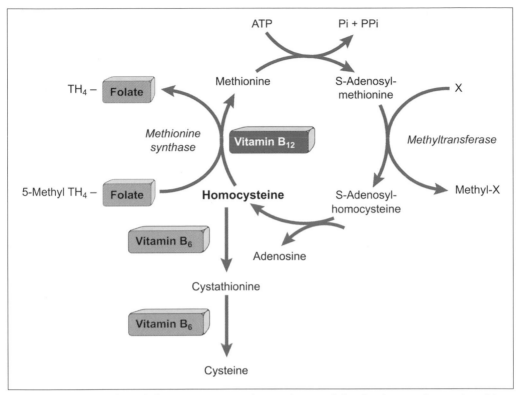

Figure 9–1. Biological methylation reactions and homocysteine metabolism. Use of S-adenosyl-methionine as the methyl donor for biological methylation reactions results in the formation of S-adenosylhomocysteine. Homocysteine is formed from the hydrolysis of S-adenosylhomocysteine. Homocysteine may be remethylated to form methionine by a folate-dependent reaction that is catalyzed by methionine synthase, a vitamin B_{12}–dependent enzyme. Alternately, homocysteine may be metabolized to cysteine in reactions catalyzed by two vitamin B_6–dependent enzymes.

stores are adequate prior to the onset of pernicious anemia, it may take years for symptoms of deficiency to develop. About 20% of the relatives of pernicious anemia patients also have pernicious anemia, suggesting a genetic predisposition. Treatment of pernicious anemia generally requires injections of vitamin B_{12}, bypassing intestinal absorption. High-dose oral supplementation is another treatment option, because consuming 1000 μg (1 mg)/d of vitamin B_{12} orally should result in the absorption of about 10 μg/d (about 1%) by passive diffusion.[3]

Food-Bound Vitamin B_{12} Malabsorption

Food-bound vitamin B_{12} malabsorption is defined as an impaired ability to absorb food or protein-bound vitamin B_{12}, although the free form is fully absorbable.[6] In the elderly, food-bound vitamin B_{12} malabsorption is thought to result mainly from atrophic gastritis, a chronic inflammation of the lining of the stomach, which ultimately results in the loss of glands in the stomach (atrophy) and decreased stomach acid production. Because stomach acid is required for the release of vitamin B_{12} from the proteins in food, vitamin B_{12} absorption is diminished. Decreased stomach acid production also provides an environment more conducive to the overgrowth of anaerobic bacteria in the stomach, interfering further with vitamin B$_{12}$ absorption.[2] Because vitamin B$_{12}$ in supplements is not bound to protein and because IF is still available, the absorption of supplemental vitamin B$_{12}$ is not reduced as it is in pernicious anemia. Thus, individuals with food-bound vitamin B$_{12}$ malabsorption do not have an increased requirement for vitamin B$_{12}$; they simply need it in the form of a supplement rather than from food.

Atrophic Gastritis

Atrophic gastritis is thought to affect 10 to 30% of people over 60 years of age and is frequently associated with infection by the bacterium *Helicobacter pylori*. *H. pylori* infection induces a chronic inflammation of the stomach, which may progress to peptic ulcer disease, atrophic gastritis, and/or gastric cancer in some individuals. The relationship of *H. pylori* infection to atrophic gastritis, gastric cancer, and vitamin B$_{12}$ deficiency is presently an area of active research.[3]

Other Causes of Vitamin B$_{12}$ Deficiency

Other causes of deficiency include surgical resection of the stomach or portions of the small intestine where receptors for the IF-B$_{12}$ complex are located. Conditions affecting the small intestine, such as malabsorption syndromes (celiac disease and tropical sprue), may also result in vitamin B$_{12}$ deficiency. Because the pancreas provides critical enzymes as well as calcium required for vitamin B$_{12}$ absorption, pancreatic insufficiency may contribute to B$_{12}$ deficiency. As vitamin B$_{12}$ is found only in foods of animal origin, a strict vegetarian (vegan) diet has resulted in cases of vitamin B$_{12}$ deficiency. In alcoholics, vitamin B$_{12}$ intake and absorption are reduced while elimination is increased.[5] Individuals with acquired immunodeficiency syndrome appear to be at increased risk of deficiency, possibly related to a failure of the IF-B$_{12}$ receptor to take up the IF-B$_{12}$ complex.[2] Long-term use of acid-reducing drugs has also been implicated in vitamin B$_{12}$ deficiency.

Symptoms of Vitamin B$_{12}$ Deficiency

Vitamin B$_{12}$ deficiency results in impairment of the activities of B$_{12}$-requiring enzymes. Impaired activity of methionine synthase may result in elevated homocysteine levels, and impaired activity of methylmalonyl-CoA mutase results in increased levels of a metabolite of L-methylmalonyl-CoA, called methylmalonic acid (MMA). Individuals with mild vitamin B$_{12}$ deficiency may not experience symptoms, although blood levels of homocysteine and/or MMA may be elevated.[7]

Megaloblastic Anemia. Diminished activity of methionine synthase in vitamin B$_{12}$ deficiency inhibits the regeneration of tetrahydrofolate and traps folate in a form that is not usable by the body (Fig. 9–2), resulting in symptoms of folate deficiency even in the presence of adequate folate levels. Thus, in both folate and vitamin B$_{12}$ deficiency, folate is unavailable to participate in DNA synthesis. This impairment of DNA synthesis affects the rapidly dividing cells of the bone marrow earlier than other cells, resulting in the production of large, immature, hemoglobin-poor red blood cells. The resulting anemia is known as *megaloblastic anemia* and is the symptom for which the disease, pernicious anemia, was named.[2] Supplementation of folic acid will provide enough usable folate to restore normal red blood cell formation. However, if vitamin B$_{12}$ deficiency was the cause, it will persist despite the resolution of the anemia. Thus, megaloblastic anemia should not be treated with folic acid until the underlying cause has been determined.[4]

Neurologic Symptoms. The neurologic symptoms of vitamin B$_{12}$ deficiency include numbness and tingling of the arms and more commonly the legs, difficulty walking, memory loss, disorientation, and dementia, with or without mood changes. Although the progression of neurologic complications is generally gradual, they are not always reversible with treatment of vitamin B$_{12}$ deficiency, especially if they have been present for a long time. Neurologic complications are not always associated with megaloblastic anemia and are the only clinical symptom of vitamin B$_{12}$ deficiency in about 25% of cases.[5] Although vi-

Table 9–1 Recommended Dietary Allowance (RDA) for Vitamin B$_{12}$

Life Stage	Age	Males, µg/d	Females, µg/d
Infants	0–6 months	0.4 (AI)	0.4 (AI)
Infants	7–12 months	0.5 (AI)	0.5 (AI)
Children	1–3 years	0.9	0.9
Children	4–8 years	1.2	1.2
Children	9–13 years	1.8	1.8
Adolescents	14–18 years	2.4	2.4
Adults	19–50 years	2.4	2.4
Adults	51 years and older	2.4*	2.4*
Pregnancy	all ages	–	2.6
Breast-feeding	all ages	–	2.8

AI, adequate intake level.
*It is advisable for this amount to be obtained by consuming foods fortified with vitamin B$_{12}$ or from a vitamin B$_{12}$–containing supplement.

tamin B$_{12}$ deficiency is known to damage the myelin sheath covering cranial, spinal, and peripheral nerves, the biochemical processes leading to neurological damage in B$_{12}$ deficiency are not well understood.[2]

Gastrointestinal Symptoms. A sore tongue, appetite loss, and constipation have also been associated with vitamin B$_{12}$ deficiency. Their origins are unclear but may be related to the stomach inflammation underlying some cases of B$_{12}$ deficiency or the increased vulnerability of the rapidly dividing cells along the gastrointestinal tract to impaired DNA synthesis.[5]

The Recommended Dietary Allowance

The current recommended dietary allowance (RDA) was revised by the Food and Nutrition Board (FNB) of the Institute of Medicine in 1998 (Table 9–1). Because of the increased risk of food-bound vitamin B$_{12}$ malabsorption in older adults, the FNB recommended that adults over 50 years of age get most of the RDA from fortified food or vitamin B$_{12}$–containing supplements.[5]

Disease Prevention

Cardiovascular Diseases

Evidence is mounting that an elevated blood homocysteine level is an independent risk factor for cardiovascular diseases (e.g., heart disease, stroke, and peripheral vascular disease). The amount of homocysteine in the blood is regulated by at least three vitamins: folate, vitamin B$_{12}$, and vitamin B$_6$ (Fig. 9–1). Analysis of the results of 12 homocysteine-lowering trials showed folic acid supplementation (0.5 to 5 mg/d) to have the greatest lowering effect on blood homocysteine levels (25%), with vitamin B$_{12}$ (0.5 mg/d or 500 µg/d) providing an additional 7% reduction.[8] The results of a sequential supplementation trial in 53 men and women indicated that after folic acid supplementation, vitamin B$_{12}$ became the major determinant of plasma homocysteine.[9]

Some evidence indicates that vitamin B$_{12}$ deficiency is a major cause of elevated homocysteine levels in people over the age of 60. Two studies found blood MMA levels to be elevated in more than 60% of elderly individuals with elevated homocysteine levels. An elevated MMA level in conjuction with elevated homocysteine suggests either a vitamin B$_{12}$ deficiency or a combined B$_{12}$ and folate deficiency, in the absence of impaired kidney function.[10] Thus, it is important to evaluate vitamin B$_{12}$ status as well as kidney function in older individuals with elevated homocysteine levels, prior to initiating homocysteine-lowering therapy. For more information regarding homocysteine and cardiovascular diseases, see Chapter 2 on folic acid.

Cancer

Folate is required for synthesis of DNA, and there is evidence that decreased availability of folate results in strands of DNA that are more susceptible to damage. Deficiency of vitamin B$_{12}$ traps folate in a form that is unusable by the body for DNA synthesis. Both vitamin B$_{12}$ and folate deficiencies result in a diminished capacity for methylation reactions (Fig. 9–2). Thus, vitamin B$_{12}$ deficiency may lead to an elevated rate of DNA damage and altered methylation of DNA, both of which are impor-

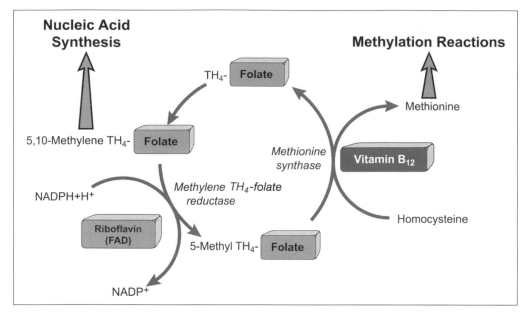

Figure 9–2. Vitamin B$_{12}$ and nucleic acid metabolism. 5,10-Methylene tetrahydrofolate (TH$_4$-folate) is required for the synthesis of nucleic acids, and 5-methyl TH$_4$-folate is required for the formation of methionine from homocysteine by the vitamin B$_{12}$–dependent enzyme methionine synthase. Methionine, in the form of S-adenosylmethionine, is required for many biological methylation reactions, including the methylation of DNA. Vitamin B$_{12}$ deficiency traps folate in a form that is unusable by the body for DNA synthesis and results in a reduced capacity for DNA methylation.

tant risk factors for cancer. A recent series of studies in young adults and older men indicated that increased levels of homocysteine and decreased levels of vitamin B$_{12}$ in the blood were associated with a biomarker of chromosome breakage in white blood cells. In a double-blind, placebo-controlled study the same biomarker of chromosome breakage was minimized in young adults who were supplemented with 700 µg of folic acid and 7 µg of vitamin B$_{12}$ daily in cereal for 2 months.[11]

A case-control study compared prediagnostic levels of serum folate, vitamin B$_6$, and vitamin B$_{12}$ in 195 women later diagnosed with breast cancer and 195 age-matched women who were not diagnosed with breast cancer.[12] Among women who were postmenopausal at the time of blood donation, the association between blood levels of vitamin B$_{12}$ and breast cancer suggested a threshold effect. The risk of breast cancer was more than doubled in those women with serum vitamin B$_{12}$ levels in the lowest quintile compared with those women in the four highest quintiles. The investigators found no relationship between breast cancer and blood levels of vitamin B$_6$, folate, or homocysteine. Because this study was observational, it cannot be determined whether decreased blood levels of vitamin B$_{12}$ were a cause or a result of breast cancer. Previously, there has been little evidence to suggest a relationship between vitamin B$_{12}$ status and breast cancer risk. However, the above studies point to a need for further investigation of the relationship between vitamin B$_{12}$ status and cancer risk.

Neural Tube Defects

Neural tube defects (NTD) may result in anencephaly or spina bifida, devastating and sometimes fatal birth defects. The defects occur between the 21st and 27th days after conception, a time when many women do not realize they are pregnant.[13] Randomized trials have demonstrated 60 to 100% reductions in NTD cases when women consumed folic acid supplements in addition to a varied diet during the month before and the month after conception. Increasing evidence indicates that the homocysteine-lowering effect of folic acid plays a critical role in lowering the risk of NTD.[14] Homocysteine may accumulate in the blood when there is inadequate folate and/or vitamin B_{12} for effective functioning of the methionine synthase enzyme. Decreased vitamin B_{12} levels in the blood and amniotic fluid of pregnant women have been associated with an increased risk of NTD, suggesting that adequate vitamin B_{12} intake in addition to folic acid may be beneficial in the prevention of NTD.

Alzheimer's Disease and Dementia

Individuals with Alzheimer's disease often have low blood levels of vitamin B_{12}. One study found lower vitamin B_{12} levels in the cerebrospinal fluid of patients with Alzheimer's disease than in patients with other types of dementia, though blood levels of vitamin B_{12} did not differ.[15] The reason for the association of low vitamin B_{12} status with Alzheimer's disease is not clear. Vitamin B_{12} deficiency, like folate deficiency, may lead to decreased synthesis of methionine and S-adenosylmethionine, adversely affecting methylation reactions essential for the metabolism of components of the myelin sheath of nerve cells, as well as neurotransmitters. Moderately increased homocysteine levels, as well as decreased folate and vitamin B_{12} levels, have also been associated with Alzheimer's disease and vascular dementia. A case-control study of 164 patients with dementia of Alzheimer's type included 76 cases in which the diagnosis of Alzheimer's disease was confirmed by examination of the brain cells after death.[16] Compared with 108 control subjects without evidence of dementia, subjects with dementia of Alzheimer's type and confirmed Alzheimer's disease had higher blood homocysteine levels and lower folate and vitamin B_{12} levels. Measures of general nutritional status indicated that the association of increased homocysteine levels and diminished vitamin B_{12} status with Alzheimer's disease was not due to dementia-related malnutrition. Low-serum vitamin B_{12} (≤ 150 pmol/L) or folate (≤ 10 nmol/L) levels were associated with a doubling of the risk of developing Alzheimer's disease in 370 elderly men and women followed over 3 years.[17] In a sample of 1092 men and women without dementia followed for an average of 10 years, those with higher plasma homocysteine levels at baseline had a significantly higher risk of developing Alzheimer's disease and other types of dementia.[18] Those with plasma homocysteine levels greater than 14 µmol/L had nearly double the risk of developing Alzheimer's disease.

Disease Treatment

Depression

Observational studies have found as many as 30% of patients hospitalized for depression to be deficient in vitamin B_{12}.[19] A recent cross-sectional study of 700 community-living, physically disabled women over the age of 65 found that vitamin B_{12}-deficient individuals were twice as likely to be severely depressed as nondeficient individuals.[20] The reasons for the relationship between vitamin B_{12} deficiency and depression are not clear. Vitamin B_{12} and folate are required for the synthesis of S-adenosylmethionine, a methyl group donor essential for the metabolism of neurotransmitters, whose bioavailability has been related to depression. Because few studies have examined the relationship of vitamin B_{12} status and the development of depression over time, it cannot yet be determined if vitamin B_{12} deficiency plays a causal role in depression. However, due to the high prevalence of vitamin B_{12} deficiency in older individuals, it may be beneficial to screen them for vitamin B_{12} deficiency as part of a medical evaluation for depression.

Sources

Food Sources

Only bacteria can synthesize vitamin B_{12}. Vitamin B_{12} is present in animal products such as meat, poultry, fish (including shellfish), and to a lesser extent milk, but it is not generally present in plant products or yeast.[1] Fresh pasteur-

Table 9–2   Food Sources of Vitamin B$_{12}$

Food	Serving	Vitamin B$_{12}$, μg
Clams, steamed	3 ounces*	84.0
Mussels, steamed	3 ounces*	20.4
Crab, steamed	3 ounces*	8.8
Salmon, baked	3 ounces*	2.4
Beef, cooked	3 ounces*	2.1
Rockfish, baked	3 ounces*	1.0
Milk	8 ounces	0.9
Brie, cheese	1 ounce	0.5
Egg, poached	1 large	0.4
Chicken, roasted	3 ounces*	0.3
Turkey, roasted	3 ounces*	0.3

*A 3-ounce serving of meat or fish is about the size of a deck of cards.

ized milk contains 0.9 μg per cup and is an important source of vitamin B$_{12}$ for some vegetarians.[5] Those vegetarians who eat no animal products need supplemental vitamin B$_{12}$ to meet their requirements. Also, individuals over the age of 50 should obtain their vitamin B$_{12}$ in supplements or fortified foods, like fortified cereal, because of the increased likelihood of food-bound vitamin B$_{12}$ malabsorption.

Most people do not have a problem obtaining the RDA of 2.4 μg/d of vitamin B$_{12}$ in food. In the United States, the average intake of vitamin B$_{12}$ is about 4.5 μg/d for young adult men and 3 μg/d for young adult women. In a sample of adults over the age of 60, men were found to have an average dietary intake of 3.4 μg/d and women 2.6 μg/d.[5] Some foods with substantial amounts of vitamin B$_{12}$ are listed in Table 9–2, along with their vitamin B$_{12}$ content in micrograms.

Supplements

Cyanocobalamin is the principal form of vitamin B$_{12}$ used in supplements, but methylcobalamin is also available. Cyanocobalalmin is available by prescription in an injectable form and as a nasal gel for the treatment of pernicious anemia. Over-the-counter preparations containing cyanocobalamin include multivitamin, vitamin B-complex, and vitamin B$_{12}$ supplements.[21]

Safety

Toxicity

No toxic or adverse effects have been associated with large intakes of vitamin B$_{12}$ from food or supplements in healthy people. Doses as high as 1 mg (1000 μg) daily by mouth or 1 mg monthly by intramuscular injection have been used to treat pernicious anemia, without significant side effects. When high doses of vitamin B$_{12}$ are given orally, only a small percentage can be absorbed, which may explain its low toxicity. Because of the low toxicity of vitamin B$_{12}$, no tolerable upper intake level was set by the Food and Nutrition Board in 1998 when the RDA was revised.[5]

Drug Interactions

A number of drugs reduce the absorption of vitamin B$_{12}$. Proton pump inhibitors (e.g., omeprazole and lansoprazole), used for therapy of Zollinger-Ellison syndrome and gastroesophageal reflux disease, markedly decrease stomach acid secretion required for the release of vitamin B$_{12}$ from food but not supplements. Long-term use of proton pump inhibitors has been found to decrease blood vitamin B$_{12}$ levels. However, vitamin B$_{12}$ deficiency does not generally develop until after at least 3 years of continuous therapy.[22] Another class of gastric acid inhibitors known as H$_2$-receptor antagonists (e.g., Tagamet, Pepsid, Zantac), often used to treat peptic ulcer disease, has also been found to decrease the absorption of vitamin B$_{12}$ from food. Because inhibition of gastric acid secretion is not as prolonged as with proton pump inhibitors, H$_2$-receptor antagonists have not been found to cause overt vitamin B$_{12}$ deficiency even after long-term use.[23] Individuals taking drugs that inhibit gastric acid secretion should consider taking vitamin B$_{12}$ in the form of a supplement because gastric acid is not required for its absorption. Other drugs found to inhibit the absorption of vitamin B$_{12}$ from food include cholestyramine (a bile acid–binding resin used in the treatment of high cholesterol), chloramphenicol, neomycin (antibiotics), and colchicine (antigout). Metformin, a medication for individuals with type II (adult onset) diabetes, decreases vitamin B_{12} absorption by tying up free calcium required for absorption of the IF-B_{12} complex. This effect is correctable by drinking milk or taking calcium carbonate tablets along with food or supplements.[4] Previous reports that megadoses of vitamin C resulted in the destruction of vitamin B_{12} have not been supported[24] and may have been an artifact of the assay used to measure vitamin B_{12} levels.[5]

Nitrous oxide, a commonly used anesthetic, both inhibits vitamin B_{12}–dependent enzymes and can produce many of the clinical features of vitamin B_{12} deficiency, such as megaloblastic anemia or neuropathy. Because nitrous oxide is commonly used for surgery in the elderly, some experts feel vitamin B_{12} deficiency should be ruled out prior to its use.[3,7]

Large doses of folic acid given to an individual with an undiagnosed vitamin B_{12} deficiency could correct megaloblastic anemia without correcting the underlying vitamin B_{12} deficiency, leaving the individual at risk of developing irreversible neurologic damage.[5] For this reason the FNB advises that all adults limit their intake of folic acid (supplements and fortification) to 1000 µg (1 mg) daily.

LPI Recommendation

A varied diet should provide enough vitamin B_{12} to prevent deficiency in most individuals 50 years of age and younger. Individuals over the age of 50, strict vegetarians, and women planning to become pregnant should take a multivitamin/multimineral supplement daily or eat a fortified breakfast cereal, which would ensure a daily intake of 6 to 30 µg of vitamin B_{12} in a form that is easily absorbed.

Older Adults

Because vitamin B_{12} malabsorption and vitamin B_{12} deficiency are more common in adults 65 years and older, some respected nutritionists recommend 100 to 400 µg/d of supplemental vitamin B_{12}, an amount provided by a number of vitamin B-complex supplements. Vitamin B_{12} injections are not necessary unless an individual has been diagnosed with pernicious anemia.

References

1. Brody T. *Nutritional Biochemistry*. 2nd ed. San Diego: Academic Press; 1999.
2. Shane B. Folic acid, vitamin B-12, and vitamin B-6. In: Stipanuk M, ed. *Biochemical and Physiological Aspects of Human Nutrition*. Philadelphia: W.B. Saunders Co.; 2000:483–518.
3. Baik HW, Russell RM. Vitamin B12 deficiency in the elderly. *Annu Rev Nutr* 1999;19:357–377.
4. Herbert V. Vitamin B-12. In: Ziegler EE, Filer LJ, eds. *Present Knowledge in Nutrition*, 7th ed. Washington, D.C.: ILSI Press; 1996:191–205.
5. Food and Nutrition Board, Institute of Medicine. Vitamin B12. *Dietary Reference Intakes: Thiamin, Riboflavin, Niacin, Vitamin B-6, Vitamin B-12, Pantothenic Acid, Biotin, and Choline*. Washington, D.C.: National Academy Press; 1998:306–356.
6. Ho C, Kauwell GP, Bailey LB. Practitioners' guide to meeting the vitamin B-12 recommended dietary allowance for people aged 51 years and older. *J Am Diet Assoc* 1999;99(6):725–727.
7. Weir DG, Scott JM. Vitamin B-12 "Cobalamin." In: Shils M, Olson JA, Shike M, Ross AC, eds. *Nutrition in Health and Disease*, 9th ed. Baltimore: Williams & Wilkins; 1999:447–458.
8. Homocysteine Lowering Trialists' Collaboration. Lowering blood homocysteine with folic acid based supplements: meta-analysis of randomised trials. Homocysteine Lowering Trialists' Collaboration. *BMJ* 1998;316(7135):894–898.
9. Quinlivan EP, McPartlin J, McNulty H, et al. Importance of both folic acid and vitamin B12 in reduction of risk of vascular disease. *Lancet* 2002;359(9302):227–228.
10. Stabler SP, Lindenbaum J, Allen RH. Vitamin B-12 deficiency in the elderly: current dilemmas. *Am J Clin Nutr* 1997;66(4):741–749.
11. Fenech M. Micronucleus frequency in human lymphocytes is related to plasma vitamin B12 and homocysteine. *Mutat Res* 1999;428(1–2):299–304.
12. Wu K, Helzlsouer KJ, Comstock GW, Hoffman SC, Nadeau MR, Selhub J. A prospective study on folate, B12, and pyridoxal 5'-phosphate (B6) and breast cancer. *Cancer Epidemiol Biomarkers Prev* 1999;8(3):209–217.
13. Eskes TK. Open or closed? A world of difference: a history of homocysteine research. *Nutr Rev* 1998;56(8):236–244.
14. Mills JL, Scott JM, Kirke PN, et al. Homocysteine and neural tube defects. *J Nutr* 1996;126(3):756S–760S.
15. Nourhashemi F, Gillette-Guyonnet S, Andrieu S, et al. Alzheimer disease: protective factors. *Am J Clin Nutr* 2000;71(2):643S–649S.
16. Clarke R, Smith AD, Jobst KA, Refsum H, Sutton L, Ueland PM. Folate, vitamin B12, and serum total homocysteine levels in confirmed Alzheimer disease. *Arch Neurol* 1998;55(11):1449–1455.
17. Wang HX, Wahlin A, Basun H, Fastbom J, Winblad B, Fratiglioni L. Vitamin B(12) and folate in relation to the development of Alzheimer's disease. *Neurology* 2001;56(9):1188–1194.
18. Seshadri S, Beiser A, Selhub J, et al. Plasma homocysteine as a risk factor for dementia and Alzheimer's disease. *N Engl J Med* 2002;346(7):476–483.

19. Hutto BR. Folate and cobalamin in psychiatric illness. *Compr Psychiatry* 1997;38(6):305–314.

20. Penninx BW, Guralnik JM, Ferrucci L, Fried LP, Allen RH, Stabler SP. Vitamin B(12) deficiency and depression in physically disabled older women: epidemiologic evidence from the Women's Health and Aging Study. *Am J Psychiatry* 2000;157(5):715–721.

21. Hendler SS, Rorvik DR, eds. *PDR for Nutritional Supplements*. Montvale, NJ: Medical Economics Company, Inc; 2001.

22. Kasper H. Vitamin absorption in the elderly. *Int J Vitam Nutr Res* 1999;69(3):169–172.

23. Termanini B, Gibril F, Sutliff VE, Yu F, Venzon DJ, Jensen RT. Effect of long-term gastric acid suppressive therapy on serum vitamin B12 levels in patients with Zollinger-Ellison syndrome. *Am J Med* 1998;104(5):422–430.

24. Simon JA, Hudes ES. Relation of serum ascorbic acid to serum vitamin B12, serum ferritin, and kidney stones in US adults. *Arch Intern Med* 1999;159(6):619–624.

10   Vitamin C

Vitamin C, also known as ascorbic acid, is a water-soluble vitamin that is essential for normal functioning of the body. Unlike most mammals, humans do not have the ability to make their own vitamin C. We must therefore obtain vitamin C through our diet.

Function

Vitamin C is required for the synthesis of collagen, an important structural component of blood vessels, tendons, ligaments, and bone. Vitamin C also plays an important role in the synthesis of the neurotransmitter norepinephrine. Neurotransmitters are critical to brain function and are known to affect mood. In addition, vitamin C is required for the synthesis of carnitine, a small molecule that is essential for the transport of fat to cellular organelles called *mitochondria*, for conversion to energy.[1] Recent research also suggests that vitamin C is involved in the metabolism of cholesterol to bile acids, which may have implications for blood cholesterol levels and the incidence of gallstones.[2]

Vitamin C is also a highly effective antioxidant. Even in small amounts vitamin C can protect indispensable molecules in the body, such as proteins, lipids (fats), carbohydrates, and nucleic acids (DNA and RNA) from damage by free radicals and reactive oxygen species that can be generated during normal metabolism as well as through exposure to toxins and pollutants (e.g., smoking). Vitamin C may also be able to regenerate other antioxidants such as vitamin E.[1]

Deficiency

Scurvy

Severe vitamin C deficiency has been known for many centuries as the potentially fatal disease scurvy. By the late 1700s the British navy was aware that scurvy could be cured by eating oranges or lemons, even though vitamin C would not be isolated until the early 1930s. Symptoms of scurvy include bleeding and bruising easily, hair and tooth loss, and joint pain and swelling. Such symptoms appear to be related to the weakening of blood vessels, connective tissue, and bone, which contain collagen. Early symptoms of scurvy-like fatigue may result from diminished levels of carnitine, needed to derive energy from fat, or decreased synthesis of the neurotransmitter norepinephrine. Scurvy is rare in developed countries because it can be prevented by as little as 10 mg of vitamin C daily.[3] However, recent cases have occurred in children and the elderly on very restricted diets.[4,5]

The Recommended Dietary Allowance

The recommended dietary allowance (RDA) for vitamin C was revised upward in 2000 from 60 mg/d for men and women to 75 mg/d for women and 90 mg/d in men (Table 10–1). The RDA continues to be based primarily on the prevention of deficiency, rather than the prevention of chronic disease and the promotion of optimum health. The recommended intake for smokers is 35 mg/d higher than for nonsmokers because smokers are under increased oxidative stress from the toxins in cigarette smoke and generally have lower blood levels of vitamin C.[6]

Disease Prevention

The amount of vitamin C required to prevent chronic disease appears to be more than that required simply for prevention of scurvy. Much of the information regarding vitamin C and the prevention of chronic disease is based on prospective studies, where vitamin C intake is

Table 10–1 Recommended Dietary Allowance (RDA) for Vitamin C

Life Stage	Age	Males, mg/d	Females, mg/d
Infants	0–6 months	40 (AI)	40 (AI)
Infants	7–12 months	50 (AI)	50 (AI)
Children	1–3 years	15	15
Children	4–8 years	25	25
Children	9–13 years	45	45
Adolescents	14–18 years	75	65
Adults	19 years and older	90	75
Smokers	19 years and older	125	110
Pregnancy	18 years and younger	–	80
Pregnancy	19 years and older	–	85
Breast-feeding	18 years and younger	–	115
Breast-feeding	19 years and older	–	120

AI, adequate intake level.

assessed in large numbers of people who are followed over time to determine whether they develop specific chronic diseases.

Cardiovascular Diseases

Seven of 12 prospective studies, which examined large numbers of people (700 to 87,000) over a number of years (3 to 20), found a significant relationship between higher levels of vitamin C intake and a lower risk of heart disease and stroke.[1] The remaining studies, which did not find a relationship between vitamin C intake and cardiovascular diseases, compared individuals who were already consuming close to 100 mg daily with those consuming higher amounts. A careful experimental study at the National Institutes of Health (NIH) demonstrated that some human tissues (leukocytes) tend to become saturated with vitamin C at a dose of 100 mg/d.[7] Thus, it is possible that once tissue saturation has been achieved, additional protective effects of vitamin C against cardiovascular diseases are small and therefore difficult to detect in prospective studies. Consistent with this possibility, at least six prospective studies have found low blood levels of vitamin C at baseline to be associated with a subsequent increase in the risk of heart disease or stroke.[1,8] In a prospective study that followed more than 2000 residents of a rural Japanese community for 20 years, the risk of stroke in those whose blood levels of vitamin C were in the highest quartile (1/4) was only 59% of those whose blood levels were in the lowest quartile.[9] Additionally, the risk of stroke in those who consumed vegetables 6 to 7 days of the week was only 58% of the risk in those who consumed vegetables 0 to 2 days of the week. The participants' blood levels of vitamin C were highly correlated with their fruit and vegetable intake. Therefore, as in many studies of vitamin C intake and cardiovascular disease risk, it is difficult to separate the effects of vitamin C on stroke risk from the effects of other components of fruits and vegetables, emphasizing the benefits of a diet rich in fruits and vegetables.

Cancer

A large number of studies have shown that increased consumption of fresh fruits and vegetables is associated with a reduced risk for most types of cancer.[10] Such studies are the basis for dietary guidelines endorsed by the U.S. Department of Agriculture and the National Cancer Institute, which recommend at least five servings of fruits and vegetables per day. A number of case-control studies have investigated the role of vitamin C in cancer prevention. Most have shown that higher intakes of vitamin C are associated with decreased incidence of cancers of the mouth, throat and vocal chords, esophagus, stomach, colon-rectum, and lung.[1] Because the possibility of bias is greater in case-control studies, prospective studies are generally given more weight in the evaluation of the effect of nutrient intake on disease. In general, prospective studies in which the lowest intake group consumed more than 86 mg of vitamin C daily have not found differences in cancer risk, while studies finding significant cancer risk reductions found them in people consuming at least 80 to 110 mg of vitamin C daily.[1]

A prospective study of 870 men over a period of 25 years found that those who consumed more than 83 mg of vitamin C daily had a striking 64% reduction in lung cancer compared with those who consumed less than 63 mg per day.[11] Although most large prospective studies found no association between breast cancer and vitamin C intake, two recent studies found dietary vitamin C intake to be inversely associated with breast cancer risk in certain subgroups. In the Nurses' Health Study, premenopausal women with a family history of breast cancer who consumed an average of 205 mg/d of vitamin C from foods had a 63% lower risk of breast cancer than those who consumed an average of 70 mg/d.[12] In the Swedish Mammography Cohort, women who were overweight and consumed an average of 110 mg/d of vitamin C had a 39% lower risk of breast cancer compared with overweight women who consumed an average of 31 mg/d.[13] A number of observational studies have found increased dietary vitamin C intake to be associated with decreased risk of stomach cancer, and laboratory experiments indicate that vitamin C inhibits the formation of carcinogenic compounds in the stomach. Infection with the bacterium *Helicobacter pylori* is known to increase the risk of stomach cancer and also appears to lower the vitamin C content of stomach secretions. Although two intervention studies did not find a decrease in the occurrence of stomach cancer with vitamin C supplementation,[6] more recent research suggests that vitamin C supplementation may be a useful addition to standard *H. pylori* eradication therapy in reducing the risk of gastric cancer.[14]

Cataracts

Cataracts are a leading cause of blindness in the United States, occurring more frequently and becoming more severe as people age. Decreased vitamin C levels in the lens of the eye have been associated with increased severity of cataracts in humans. Some, but not all, studies have observed increased dietary vitamin C intake[15] and increased blood levels of vitamin C[16] to be associated with decreased risk of cataracts. Those studies that have found a relationship suggest that vitamin C intake may have to be higher than 300 mg/d for a number of years before a protective effect can be detected.[1] Recently, a 7-year controlled intervention trial of a daily antioxidant supplement containing 500 mg of vitamin C, 400 IU of vitamin E, and 15 mg of β-carotene in 4629 men and women found no difference between the antioxidant combination and a placebo on the development and progression of age-related cataracts.[17] Therefore, the relationship between vitamin C intake and the development of cataracts requires further clarification before specific recommendations can be made.

Lead Toxicity

Although the use of lead paint and leaded gasoline has been discontinued in the United States, lead toxicity continues to be a significant health problem, especially in children living in urban areas. Abnormal growth and development have been observed in infants of women exposed to lead during pregnancy, and children who are chronically exposed to lead are more likely to develop learning disabilities and behavioral problems and to have low IQs. In adults, lead toxicity may result in kidney damage and high blood pressure. In a study of 747 older men, blood lead levels were significantly higher in those who reported total dietary vitamin C intakes averaging less than 109 mg/d compared with men who reported higher vitamin C intakes.[18] A much larger study of 19,578 people, including 4214 children from 6 to 16 years of age, found higher serum vitamin C levels to be associated with significantly lower blood lead levels.[19] An intervention trial that examined the effects of vitamin C supplementation on blood lead levels in 75 adult male smokers found that 1000 mg/d of vitamin C resulted in significantly lower blood lead levels over a 4-week treatment period compared with placebo.[20] A lower dose of 200 mg/d did not significantly affect blood lead levels, despite the finding that serum vitamin C levels were not different from those of the group that took 1000 mg/d. The mechanism for the relationship between vitamin C intake and blood lead levels is not known, although it has been postulated that vitamin C may inhibit intestinal absorption or enhance urinary excretion of lead.

Disease Treatment

Cardiovascular Diseases

Vasodilation. The ability of blood vessels to relax or dilate is compromised in individuals with atherosclerosis. The damage to the heart muscle caused by a heart attack and to the brain caused by a stroke is related, in part, to the inability of blood vessels to dilate enough to allow blood flow to the affected areas. The pain of angina pectoris is also related to insufficient dilation of the coronary arteries. Treatment with vitamin C has consistently resulted in improved dilation of blood vessels in individuals with atherosclerosis as well as those with angina pectoris, congestive heart failure, high cholesterol, and high blood pressure. Improved blood vessel dilation has been demonstrated at a dose of 500 mg of vitamin C daily.[21]

Hypertension. Individuals with high blood pressure are at increased risk of developing cardiovascular diseases. Several studies have demonstrated a blood pressure–lowering effect of vitamin C supplementation. One study of individuals with high blood pressure found that a daily supplement of 500 mg of vitamin C resulted in an average drop in systolic blood pressure of 9% after 4 weeks.[22] It should be noted that those participants who were taking antihypertensive medication continued taking it throughout the 4-week study. Because the findings regarding vitamin C and high blood pressure have not yet been replicated in larger studies, it is important for individuals with significantly high blood pressure to continue current therapy (medication, lifestyle changes, etc.) in consultation with a qualified health care provider.

Cancer

Studies in the 1970s and 1980s conducted by Linus Pauling and colleagues suggested that very large doses of vitamin C (10 g/d intravenously for 10 days followed by at least 10 g/d orally indefinitely) were helpful in increasing the survival time and improving the quality of life of terminal cancer patients.[23] However, two randomized placebo-controlled studies conducted at the Mayo clinic found no differences in outcome between terminal cancer patients receiving 10 g of vitamin C per day orally or placebo.[24] There were significant methodological differences between the Mayo Clinic and Pauling's studies, and recently, two researchers from the NIH suggested that the route of administration (intravenous versus oral) may have been the key to the discrepant results.[25] Intravenous administration can result in much higher blood levels of vitamin C than oral administration, and levels that are toxic to certain types of cancer cells in culture can be achieved with intravenous but not oral administration of vitamin C. Thus, it appears reasonable to reevaluate the use of high-dose vitamin C as cancer therapy.

Currently, there is no clinical evidence suggesting that vitamin C would adversely affect the survival of cancer patients. However, vitamin C should not be used in place of therapy that has been demonstrated effective in the treatment of a particular type of cancer, for example, chemotherapy or radiation therapy. If an individual with cancer chooses to take vitamin supplements, it is important that the clinician coordinating his or her treatment is aware of the type and dose of each supplement. Although research is under way to determine whether combinations of antioxidant vitamins might be beneficial as an adjunct to conventional cancer therapy, definitive conclusions are not yet possible.[26]

Diabetes Mellitus

Numerous observational studies have found that people with diabetes have lower plasma levels of vitamin C (approximately 30% lower) than do people without diabetes. However, a number of methodological flaws have been attributed to such studies, and it is not clear whether diabetes is the cause of lower plasma levels of vitamin C. Recently a large population-based study found no difference in blood levels of vitamin C between more than 200 individuals with newly diagnosed diabetes and 1800 individuals without diabetes, once dietary intake of vitamin C and cigarette smoking were taken into consideration.[27] Though few studies have demonstrated improved blood glucose levels upon supplementation of diabetic individuals with vitamin C, doses of between 100 and 600 mg of vitamin C daily have been found to normalize cellular sorbitol levels, which may have implications for decreasing some of the long-term complications of diabetes.[28] Cardiovascular diseases are the leading cause of death in individuals with diabetes. Vitamin C has also been found to improve blood vessel dilation, which is often impaired in diabetic individuals. The link between cardiovascular diseases and diabetes may be related to increased oxidative stress, giving credibility to the idea that the antioxidant properties of vitamin C may benefit individuals with diabetes. Although the role of vitamin C in the management of diabetes is by no means clear, maintaining an adequate intake of vitamin C may help prevent some of the complications of diabetes.

Common Cold

The work of Linus Pauling stimulated public interest in the use of large doses (greater than 1 g/d) of vitamin C to prevent infection with the viruses responsible for the common cold. Reviews of the research conducted on this issue over the past 20 years conclude that, in general, large doses of vitamin C do not have a significant effect on the incidence of the common cold.[29] However, a few studies have indicated that certain susceptible groups (e.g., individuals with low dietary intake and marathoners) may be less susceptible to the common cold when taking supplemental vitamin C. Additionally, large doses of vitamin C have been found to decrease the duration and severity of colds, an effect that may be related to the antihistamine effects found to occur with large doses (2 g) of vitamin C.[30]

Sources

Food Sources

As shown in Table 10–2, different fruits and vegetables vary in their vitamin C content, but five servings should average out to at least 200 mg of vitamin C. One fruit serving should be considered to be one medium piece of fruit, 1/2 cup of canned or cooked fruit, or 3/4 cup of fruit

Table 10–2   Food Sources of Vitamin C

Food	Serving	Vitamin C (mg)
Sweet red pepper	1/2 cup, raw chopped	141
Strawberries	1 cup, whole	82
Orange juice	3/4 cup (6 ounces)	75
Orange	1 medium	70
Grapefruit juice	3/4 cup (6 ounces)	60
Broccoli	1/2 cup, cooked	58
Grapefruit	1/2 medium	44
Potato	1 medium, baked	26
Tomato	1 medium	23

juice. One vegetable serving should be considered to be 1 cup of raw leafy vegetables, 1/2 cup of other vegetables cooked or raw, or 3/4 cup of vegetable juice.

Supplements

Vitamin C (L-ascorbic acid) is available in many forms, but there is little scientific evidence that any one form is better absorbed or more effective than another.

Natural vs. Synthetic Vitamin C. Natural and synthetic L-ascorbic acid are chemically identical and there are no known differences in their biological activities or bioavailability.[31]

Mineral Ascorbates. Mineral salts of ascorbic acid are buffered and therefore less acidic than ascorbic acid. Some people find them less irritating to the gastrointestinal tract than ascorbic acid. Sodium ascorbate and calcium ascorbate are the most common forms, although a number of other mineral ascorbates are available. Sodium ascorbate generally provides 131 mg of sodium per 1000 mg of ascorbic acid, and pure calcium ascorbate provides 114 mg of calcium per 1000 mg of ascorbic acid.

Ascorbate and Vitamin C Metabolites. One such supplement (Ester-C®) contains mainly calcium ascorbate, but also contains small amounts of the vitamin C metabolites dehydroascorbate (oxidized ascorbic acid), calcium threonate, and trace levels of xylonate and ly-xonate. Although the metabolites are supposed to increase the bioavailability of vitamin C, the only published study in humans found no difference between Ester-C® and commercially available ascorbic acid tablets with respect to the absorption and urinary excretion of vitamin C.[32]

Vitamin C with Bioflavonoids. Bioflavonoids are a class of water-soluble plant pigments that are often found in vitamin C–rich fruits and vegetables, especially citrus fruits. Although many bioflavonoids are thought to function as antioxidants, there is little evidence that the bioflavonoids in most commercial preparations increase the bioavailability or efficacy of vitamin C.[32]

Ascorbyl Palmitate. Ascorbyl palmitate is vitamin C that has been esterified to the saturated fatty acid, palmitic acid, resulting in a fat-soluble form of vitamin C. Ascorbyl palmitate has been added to a number of skin creams due to interest in its antioxidant properties as well as the important role of vitamin C in collagen synthesis.[33] Although ascorbyl palmitate is also available as an oral supplement, it is likely that most of it is hydrolyzed (broken apart) to ascorbic acid and palmitic acid in the digestive tract before it is absorbed.[34]

Safety

Toxicity

A number of possible problems with very large doses of vitamin C have been suggested, mainly based on in vitro experiments or isolated case reports, including genetic mutations, birth defects, cancer, atherosclerosis, kidney stones, "rebound scurvy," increased oxidative stress, excess iron absorption, vitamin B_{12} deficiency, and erosion of dental enamel. However, none of these adverse health effects have been confirmed, and there is no reliable scientific evidence that large amounts of vitamin C (up to 10 g/d in adults) are toxic or detrimental to health. With the latest RDA published in 2000, a tolerable upper intake level (UL) for vitamin C was set for the first time (Table 10–3). A UL of 2 g (2000 mg) daily

Table 10–3 Tolerable Upper Intake Level (UL) for Vitamin C

Life Stage	Age	UL, mg/d
Infants	0–12 months	not possible to establish*
Children	1–3 years	400
Children	4–8 years	650
Children	9–13 years	1200
Adolescents	14–18 years	1800
Adults	19 years and older	2000

*Source of intake should be from food and formula only.

was recommended to prevent most adults from experiencing diarrhea and gastrointestinal disturbances.[6] Such symptoms are not generally serious, especially if they resolve with temporary discontinuation or reduction of high-dose vitamin C supplementation.

Does Vitamin C Promote Oxidative Damage under Physiological Conditions?

Vitamin C is known to function as a highly effective antioxidant in living organisms. However, in test tube experiments, vitamin C can interact with some free metal ions to produce potentially damaging free radicals. Although free metal ions are not generally found under physiological conditions, the idea that high doses of vitamin C might be able to promote oxidative damage in vivo has received a great deal of attention. Widespread publicity has been given to a few studies suggesting a pro-oxidant effect of vitamin C,[35,36] but these studies turned out to be either flawed or of no physiological relevance.[37] A recent comprehensive review of the literature found no credible scientific evidence that supplemental vitamin C promotes oxidative damage under physiological conditions or in humans.[37] Studies that report a pro-oxidant effect for vitamin C should be evaluated carefully to determine whether the study system was physiologically relevant and to rule out the possibility of methodological and design flaws.

Drug Interactions

A number of drugs are known to lower vitamin C levels, requiring an increase in its intake. Estrogen-containing contraceptives are known to lower vitamin C levels in plasma and white blood cells. Aspirin can lower vitamin C levels if taken frequently. For example, two aspirin tablets taken every 6 hours for a week has been reported to lower white blood cell vitamin C by 50%, primarily by increasing urinary excretion of vitamin C. There is some evidence, though controversial, that vitamin C interacts with anticoagulant medications like warfarin. Large doses of vitamin C may inhibit the action of warfarin, requiring an increase in dose to maintain its effectiveness. Individuals on anticoagulants should limit their vitamin C intake to 1 g/d and have their prothrombin time monitored by the clinician following their anticoagulant therapy. Because high doses of vitamin C have been found to interfere with the interpretation of certain laboratory tests (e.g., serum bilirubin, serum creatinine, and the guaiac assay for occult blood), it is important to inform one's health care provider of any recent supplement use.[38]

LPI Recommendation

The Linus Pauling Institute recommends that generally healthy adults of all ages consume at least 200 mg of vitamin C daily. Eating five servings per day of most fruits and vegetables will provide at least 200 mg of vitamin C. Although vitamin C from supplements is easily absorbed and utilized by the body, most of the epidemiologic evidence showing decreased chronic disease risk with increased vitamin C intake is based on vitamin C consumption from fruits and vegetables, not from supplements. The amounts of vitamin C required to maintain optimum body levels in special populations, such as children, pregnant women, and older adults, have not been established. Similarly, the amounts of vitamin C required to derive therapeutic benefits in diseased individuals are not known and may be higher than 200 mg/d.

Older Adults

Although there is no conclusive evidence that generally healthy older adults (65 years and older) have a higher requirement for vitamin C than younger people, some older populations have been found to have vitamin C intakes considerably below the RDA of 75 and 90 mg/d for women and men, respectively, as well as the 200 mg/d recommended by the Linus Pauling Institute. Because older adults are at higher risk for most of the chronic diseases that adequate vitamin C intake may protect against, ensuring a daily vitamin C intake of at least 200 mg is especially important.

References

1. Carr AC, Frei B. Toward a new recommended dietary allowance for vitamin C based on antioxidant and health effects in humans. *Am J Clin Nutr* 1999;69(6): 1086–1107.
2. Simon JA, Hudes ES. Serum ascorbic acid and gallbladder disease prevalence among US adults: the Third National Health and Nutrition Examination Survey (NHANES III). *Arch Intern Med* 2000;160(7):931–936.
3. Sauberlich HE. A history of scurvy and vitamin C. In: Packer L, Fuchs J, eds. *Vitamin C in Health and Disease.* New York: Marcel Decker Inc; 1997:1–24.
4. Stephen R, Utecht T. Scurvy identified in the emergency department: a case report. *J Emerg Med* 2001; 21(3):235–237.
5. Weinstein M, Babyn P, Zlotkin S. An orange a day keeps the doctor away: scurvy in the year 2000. *Pediatrics* 2001;108(3):E55.
6. Food and Nutrition Board, Institute of Medicine. Vitamin C. *Dietary Reference Intakes for Vitamin C, Vitamin E, Selenium, and Carotenoids.* Washington, D.C.: National Academy Press; 2000:95–185.
7. Levine M, Rumsey SC, Daruwala R, Park JB, Wang Y. Criteria and recommendations for vitamin C intake. *JAMA* 1999;281(15):1415–1423.
8. Khaw KT, Bingham S, Welch A, et al. Relation between plasma ascorbic acid and mortality in men and women in EPIC-Norfolk prospective study: a prospective population study. European Prospective Investigation into Cancer and Nutrition. *Lancet* 2001;357(9257):657–663.
9. Yokoyama T, Date C, Kokubo Y, Yoshiike N, Matsumura Y, Tanaka H. Serum vitamin C concentration was inversely associated with subsequent 20-year incidence of stroke in a Japanese rural community. The Shibata study. *Stroke* 2000;31(10):2287–2294.
10. Steinmetz KA, Potter JD. Vegetables, fruit, and cancer prevention: a review. *J Am Diet Assoc* 1996;96(10): 1027–1039.
11. Kromhout D. Essential micronutrients in relation to carcinogenesis. *Am J Clin Nutr* 1987;45(5 Suppl):1361–1367.
12. Zhang S, Hunter DJ, Forman MR, et al. Dietary carotenoids and vitamins A, C, and E and risk of breast cancer. *J Natl Cancer Inst* 1999;91(6):547–556.

13. Michels KB, Holmberg L, Bergkvist L, Ljung H, Bruce A, Wolk A. Dietary antioxidant vitamins, retinol, and breast cancer incidence in a cohort of Swedish women. *Int J Cancer* 2001;91(4):563–567.
14. Feiz HR, Mobarhan S. Does vitamin C intake slow the progression of gastric cancer in *Helicobacter pylori*–infected populations? *Nutr Rev* 2002;60(1):34–36.
15. Jacques PF, Chylack LT, Jr., Hankinson SE, et al. Long-term nutrient intake and early age-related nuclear lens opacities. *Arch Ophthalmol* 2001;119(7):1009–1019.
16. Simon JA, Hudes ES. Serum ascorbic acid and other correlates of self-reported cataract among older Americans. *J Clin Epidemiol* 1999;52(12):1207–1211.
17. Age-related Eye Disease Study Research Group. A randomized, placebo-controlled, clinical trial of high-dose supplementation with vitamins C and E and beta carotene for age-related cataract and vision loss: AREDS report no. 9. *Arch Ophthalmol* 2001;119 (10):1439–1452.
18. Cheng Y, Willett WC, Schwartz J, Sparrow D, Weiss S, Hu H. Relation of nutrition to bone lead and blood lead levels in middle-aged to elderly men. The Normative Aging Study. *Am J Epidemiol* 1998;147(12): 1162–1174.
19. Simon JA, Hudes ES. Relationship of ascorbic acid to blood lead levels. *JAMA* 1999;281(24):2289–2293.
20. Dawson EB, Evans DR, Harris WA, Teter MC, McGanity WJ. The effect of ascorbic acid supplementation on the blood lead levels of smokers. *J Am Coll Nutr* 1999;18(2):166–170.
21. Gokce N, Keaney JF, Jr., Frei B, et al. Long-term ascorbic acid administration reverses endothelial vasomotor dysfunction in patients with coronary artery disease. *Circulation* 1999;99(25):3234–3240.
22. Duffy SJ, Gokce N, Holbrook M, et al. Treatment of hypertension with ascorbic acid. *Lancet* 1999;354 (9195):2048–2049.
23. Cameron E, Pauling L. Supplemental ascorbate in the supportive treatment of cancer: prolongation of survival times in terminal human cancer. *Proc Natl Acad Sci USA* 1976;73(10):3685–3689.
24. Moertel CG, Fleming TR, Creagan ET, Rubin J, O'Connell MJ, Ames MM. High-dose vitamin C versus placebo in the treatment of patients with advanced cancer who have had no prior chemotherapy: a randomized double-blind comparison. *N Engl J Med* 1985;312(3):137–141.
25. Padayatty SJ, Levine M. Reevaluation of ascorbate in cancer treatment: emerging evidence, open minds and serendipity. *J Am Coll Nutr* 2000;19(4):423–425.
26. Kaegi E. Unconventional therapies for cancer: 6. 714-X. Task Force on Alternative Therapeutic of the Canadian Breast Cancer Research Initiative. *CMAJ* 1998;158(12):1621–1624.
27. Will JC, Ford ES, Bowman BA. Serum vitamin C concentrations and diabetes: findings from the Third National Health and Nutrition Examination Survey, 1988–1994. *Am J Clin Nutr* 1999;70(1):49–52.
28. Will JC, Byers T. Does diabetes mellitus increase the requirement for vitamin C? *Nutr Rev* 1996;54(7):193–202.
29. Hemila H. Vitamin C intake and susceptibility to the common cold. *Br J Nutr* 1997;77(1):59–72.
30. Johnston CS, Martin LJ, Cai X. Antihistamine effect of supplemental ascorbic acid and neutrophil chemotaxis. *J Am Coll Nutr* 1992;11(2):172–176.
31. Gregory JF, 3rd. Ascorbic acid bioavailability in foods and supplements. *Nutr Rev* 1993;51(10):301–303.
32. Johnston CS, Luo B. Comparison of the absorption and excretion of three commercially available sources of vitamin C. *J Am Diet Assoc* 1994;94(7):779–781.
33. Austria R, Semenzato A, Bettero A. Stability of vitamin C derivatives in solution and topical formulations. *J Pharm Biomed Anal* 1997;15(6):795–801.
34. DeRitter E. Physiologic availability of dehydro-L-ascorbic acid and palmitoyl-L-ascorbic acid. *Science* 1951;113:628–631.
35. Lee SH, Oe T, Blair IA. Vitamin C-induced decomposition of lipid hydroperoxides to endogenous genotoxins. *Science* 2001;292(5524):2083–2086.
36. Podmore ID, Griffiths HR, Herbert KE, Mistry N, Mistry P, Lunec J. Vitamin C exhibits pro-oxidant properties. *Nature* 1998;392(6676):559.
37. Carr A, Frei B. Does vitamin C act as a pro-oxidant under physiological conditions? *FASEB J* 1999;13(9): 1007–1024.
38. Hendler SS, Rorvik DR, eds. *PDR for Nutritional Supplements*. Montvale, NJ: Medical Economics Company, Inc; 2001.

11 Vitamin D

Vitamin D is a fat-soluble vitamin that exists in many forms. The form utilized primarily by humans is vitamin D_3 (cholecalciferol). Animals (including humans) can convert cholesterol to 7-dehydrocholesterol, which is a precursor of vitamin D_3. Exposure to the ultraviolet light in sunlight (UVB radiation) converts 7-dehydrocholesterol in the skin to vitamin D_3. In fact, adequate exposure to sunlight can eliminate the requirement for vitamin D in the diet, making it only "conditionally essential." Vitamin D_3 is not itself biologically active, but must be modified by the body to have any physiologic effects.[1]

Function

Calcium Metabolism

Maintenance of blood calcium levels within a narrow range is vital for normal functioning of the nervous system, as well as for bone growth and maintenance of bone density. This tight regulation is accomplished through a complex system, sometimes called the *vitamin D endocrine system*, because the active form of vitamin D_3 has a mechanism of action similar to some hormones, for example, thyroid hormone.[2]

Vitamin D Endocrine System

Once vitamin D_3 enters the circulation from either the diet or the skin, it is bound to the vitamin D–binding protein and transported to the liver. In the liver, vitamin D_3 is hydroxylated on carbon number 25 to form 25-hydroxyvitamin D_3 (25-OH-D_3), also known as *calcidiol.* Though the synthesis of calcidiol is controlled in the liver, increased exposure to sunlight or increased intake of vitamin D_3 results in increased blood levels of calcidiol, making it a useful indicator of vitamin D nutritional status. Although calcidiol is the

major circulating form of vitamin D, it is not biologically active. To exert physiologic effects, calcidiol must be hydroxylated on carbon number 1 to form 1,25-dihydroxyvitamin D_3 [1,25(OH)$_2$$D_3$], also called *calcitriol.* This hydroxylation reaction is catalyzed by an enzyme in the kidneys.[2]

The parathyroid glands sense the blood calcium level and secrete parathyroid hormone (PTH) if it becomes too low, for example, when dietary calcium intake is inadequate (Fig. 11–1). PTH stimulates the activity of the 1-hydroxylase enzyme in the kidney, resulting in increased production of calcitriol, the biologically active form of vitamin D_3. Increased blood levels of calcitriol restore normal blood calcium levels in three different ways: (1) by activating the vitamin D–dependent transport system in the small intestine, increasing the absorption of dietary calcium; (2) by increasing the mobilization of calcium from bone into the circulation; and (3) by increasing the reabsorption of calcium by the kidneys. PTH is also required to increase bone calcium mobilization and calcium reabsorption by the kidneys. However, PTH is not required for the effect of calcitriol on the intestinal absorption of calcium.[1]

Vitamin D Receptor

The physiologic effects of calcitriol require proteins known as *receptors.* Calcitriol enters the cell and interacts with a vitamin D receptor (VDR) in the nucleus to form a complex. The calcitriol/VDR complex combines with another receptor, the retinoic acid X receptor (RXR), to form a heterodimer, which can then interact with small portions of DNA known as *vitamin D responsive elements* (VDRE). The interaction of a VDR/RXR heterodimer with a VDRE results in a change in the rate of transcription of a nearby gene.[2] In this manner, the activity of vitamin D–dependent calcium transporters in the small intestine, osteoblasts in bone, and

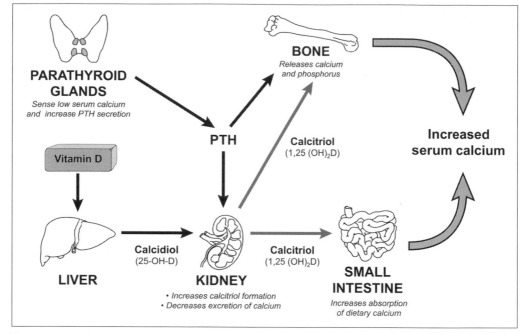

Figure 11–1. The vitamin D endocrine system. Calcium-sensing proteins in the parathyroid glands sense serum calcium levels. In response to slight declines in serum calcium, the parathyroid glands secrete parathyroid hormone (PTH). PTH stimulates the activity of the 1-hydroxylase enzyme in the kidney, resulting in increased production of calcitriol, the biologically active form of vitamin D. Calcitriol acts to restore normal serum calcium levels in three ways: (1) by activating the vitamin D–dependent transport system in the small intestine, increasing the absorption of dietary calcium; (2) by increasing the mobilization of calcium from bone into the circulation; and (3) by increasing the reabsorption of calcium by the kidneys. PTH is also required to increase bone calcium mobilization and calcium reabsorption by the kidneys.

the 1-hydroxylase enzyme in the kidneys may be increased.

Cell Differentiation

Cells that are dividing rapidly are said to be proliferating. Cell proliferation can be observed during growth and wound healing (regeneration). Differentiation results in the specialization of cells for specific functions, such as those of a nerve cell. In general, differentiation of cells leads to a decrease in proliferation. Psoriasis is a disease characterized by the proliferation of skin cells called *keratinocytes*. The identification of VDR in keratinocytes led to the use of creams containing analogs of calcitriol in the treatment of severe cases of psoriasis.[3]

Immunity

VDR have been identified in cells that play a critical role in the immune system. Specialized white blood cells, known as *T lymphocytes* or *T cells*, are involved in the recognition of foreign pathogens known as *antigens* and coordinating the immune response. Some diseases are associated with immune responses to inappropriate antigens. For example, autoimmune diseases occur when an immune response is mounted to an antigen belonging to oneself rather than a foreign antigen, and allergies occur when the antigen is an innocuous foreign substance.[4] Immune responses that are mediated by T cells can be inhibited by large doses of calcitriol. However, a deficiency of vitamin D also interferes with T-cell–mediated immunity.[3] The presence of VDR in T cells suggests that vitamin D plays a role in the function and/or the development of T cells.[5] Pharmacologic doses of calcitriol have had beneficial effects in animal models of several autoimmune diseases, mediated by T cells.[6]

Deficiency

Bone is considered a mineralized connective tissue. The matrix of bone consists mainly of connective elements known as collagen, while bone mineral consists largely of hydroxyapatite crystals, which contain large amounts of calcium and phosphorus.[1] The manifestations of severe vitamin D deficiency are seen mainly in bone.

Rickets

In infants and children, prolonged vitamin D deficiency results in a condition known as *rickets*. Rickets results in the failure of bone to mineralize. Rapidly growing bones are most severely affected by rickets. The growth plates of bones continue to enlarge, but in the absence of adequate mineralization, weight-bearing limbs (arms and legs) become bowed. In infants, rickets may result in delayed closure of the fontanelles (soft spots) in the skull, and the rib cage may become deformed due to the pulling action of the diaphragm. The treatment of rickets includes vitamin D or calcitriol supplementation, a diet that provides adequate calcium and phosphorus, and a plan for the prevention of future vitamin D deficiency. Although fortification of foods has led to complacency regarding vitamin D deficiency, nutritional rickets is still being reported in a number of U.S. cities.[7]

Osteomalacia

Although adult bones are no longer growing, they are in a constant state of turnover. Bone is a dynamic tissue that is continually remodeling in response to stress. The remodeling process involves the demineralization and remineralization of bone through the action of bone cells called *osteoclasts* and *osteoblasts*, respectively. In adults with prolonged vitamin D

deficiency, the collagenous bone matrix is preserved but bone mineral is progressively lost as a result of normal bone turnover, resulting in bone pain and osteomalacia (soft bones). Although they both result in fragile bones, osteomalacia differs from osteoporosis in several ways. Osteomalacia is relatively rare and characterized by a decreased bone mineral content in the presence of a relative increase in the collagenous bone matrix. In contrast, osteoporosis is characterized by a decrease in total bone mass, with no change in the ratio of bone mineral to collagenous bone matrix.[1] Moreover, osteoporosis is a much more common condition whose cause appears to be multifactorial.

Risk Factors for Vitamin D Deficiency

Risk factors for vitamin D deficiency include the following:

- *Infancy* Infants who have little or no sun exposure and do not consume vitamin D–fortified formula are at increased risk, especially those born just before winter in northern or southern latitudes.[7]
- *Elderly individuals with minimal sun exposure* The elderly have reduced capacity to synthesize vitamin D in response to sunlight exposure and are more likely to stay indoors or use sunscreen for the prevention of skin cancer.[8]
- *Dark skin* Those of African or Indian descent with darkly pigmented skin living in northern or southern latitudes synthesize less vitamin D on exposure to sunlight than those with light skin.[1,2]
- *Covering all exposed skin when outside* Osteomalacia has been documented in Arab women who for religious or cultural reasons cover all of their skin at all times when going outside.[1,2]
- *Fat malabsorption syndromes* Cystic fibrosis and cholestatic liver disease impair the absorption of dietary vitamin D.[1,2]
- *Inflammatory bowel disease* Patients with inflammatory bowel disease such as Crohn's disease appear to be at increased risk of vitamin D deficiency, especially those who have had small bowel resections.[9]

Table 11–1   Adequate Intake (AI) for Vitamin D

Life Stage	Age	Males, µg/d	Females, µg/d
Infants	0–6 months	5 (200 IU)	5 (200 IU)
Infants	7–12 months	5 (200 IU)	5 (200 IU)
Children	1–3 years	5 (200 IU)	5 (200 IU)
Children	4–8 years	5 (200 IU)	5 (200 IU)
Children	9–13 years	5 (200 IU)	5 (200 IU)
Adolescents	14–18 years	5 (200 IU)	5 (200 IU)
Adults	19–50 years	5 (200 IU)	5 (200 IU)
Adults	51–70 years	10(400 IU)	10 (400 IU)
Adults	71 years and older	15 (600 IU)	15 (600 IU)
Pregnancy	all ages	–	5 (200 IU)
Breastfeeding	all ages	–	5 (200 IU)

- *Kidney failure* Severe kidney disease can impair the conversion of calcidiol to the biologically active form of vitamin D, calcitriol.[1,2]
- *Genetic disease* A rare genetic disease affects the activity of the 1-hydroxylase enzyme in the kidneys that converts calcidiol to its active form, calcitriol.[1,2]
- *Seizure disorders (epilepsy)* Long-term treatment with anticonvulsant medications, such as phenytoin, can affect hepatic metabolism of vitamin D.[10]

The Adequate Intake Level

In 1997, the Food and Nutrition Board (FNB) of the Institute of Medicine felt that the issue of sunlight exposure confounded the existing data on vitamin D requirements, making it impossible to calculate a recommended dietary allowance level. Instead, the FNB set an adequate intake level that assumes that no vitamin D is synthesized in the skin through exposure to sunlight.[11] The recommendation was based on the maintenance of a healthy skeleton (Table 11–1).

Disease Prevention

Osteoporosis

Deficiency or altered metabolism of vitamin D appears to play a role in osteoporosis. Insufficient vitamin D intake results in reduced calcium absorption, increased PTH secretion, and increased resorption of bone. Increased blood levels of PTH and decreased blood levels of calcidiol, both indicators of inadequate vitamin D nutritional status, have been associated with decreased bone mineral density in older adults.[12] In temperate latitudes, for example, Boston (42 degrees north), synthesis of vitamin D by the skin does not occur from November to March. A study of postmenopausal women in Boston found that supplementation with 400 IU of vitamin D resulted in reduced bone loss from the lumbar spine in winter.[13] In a similar population of postmenopausal women, a 2-year trial of 500 mg of calcium (bringing total calcium intake to an average of 1000 mg/d) and either 100 IU or 700 IU/d of vitamin D (bringing total vitamin D intake to 200 IU or 800 IU/d, respectively) resulted in a decreased loss of bone density at the femoral neck (hip) in the group taking 700 IU of vitamin D, although there was no difference in bone loss from the spine between the two groups.[14] More recently, daily supplementation with 500 mg of calcium and 700 IU of vitamin D reduced bone loss in the femoral neck, spine, and total body in men and women over 65 years of age and reduced the frequency of nonvertebral fractures over a 3-year period.[15] When the calcium and vitamin D supplementation were discontinued, the improvements in bone density at the femoral neck and spine in both men and women were lost within 2 years. Men, but not women, retained a small improvement in total body bone density at the end of 2 years.[16] Thus, it appears that calcium and vitamin D supplementation must be maintained to provide any lasting benefit with respect to bone density.

Although the prevention of fracture is the primary goal in the prevention and treatment of osteoporosis, fewer studies have measured fracture incidence as an endpoint because the larger sample sizes and longer duration required make such studies more difficult and costly. Two large trials have examined the effect of vitamin D supplementation on the incidence of osteoporotic fractures. A French study of 3270 elderly women found a significant decrease in hip fractures after 1.5 and 3 years of supplementation with 800 IU/d of vitamin D and 1200 mg/d of calcium compared with placebo.[17] However, a Dutch study of 1916 women and 662 men found no difference in fracture incidence after 3.5 years of supplementation with 400 IU of vitamin D or placebo.[18] Overall, the evidence to date suggests that vitamin D supplements of 400 to 800 IU may be helpful in reducing bone loss and fracture rates in the elderly, especially in women living in temperate latitudes. For vitamin D supplementation to be effective in preserving bone health, adequate calcium (1000 to 1500 mg/d) must also be consumed.

Cancer

Two characteristics of cancerous cells are their lack of differentiation (specialization) and their rapid growth or proliferation. Many malignant tumors have been found to contain VDR, including breast, lung, skin (melanoma), colon, and bone. Biologically active forms of vitamin D_3, such as calcitriol and its analogs, have been found to induce differentiation and/or inhibit proliferation of a number of cancerous and noncancerous cell types.[19]

Prostate Cancer. Epidemiologic studies show correlations between risk factors for prostate cancer and conditions that can result in decreased vitamin D levels. Increased age is associated with an increased risk of prostate cancer, as well as with decreased sun exposure and decreased capacity to synthesize vitamin D_3. The incidence of prostate cancer is higher in African American men than in white American men, and the high melanin content of dark skin is known to reduce the efficiency of vitamin D_3 synthesis. Geographically, mortality from prostate cancer is inversely associated with the availability of sunlight, as it is high in the United States and northwest Europe, but low in Africa, Central America, and South America.[19]

Colorectal Cancer. The geographic distribution of colon cancer is similar to the historic geographic distribution of rickets, providing circumstantial evidence that decreased sunlight exposure and diminished vitamin D nutritional status may be related to an increased risk of colon cancer. A number of observational studies have found an association between colon cancer risk and dietary intake of vitamin D. The majority of those studies indicated that an intake of 4 µg (160 IU) of vitamin D per day or more was associated with a reduced risk of colon cancer.[20] However, two large prospective studies of women, the Nurses' Health Study[21] and the Iowa Women's Health Study,[22] did not find significant associations between vitamin D intake and the risk of colorectal cancer after statistical adjustment for other risk factors. Serum calcidiol [25(OH)D_3] levels are a marker for vitamin D nutritional status. Recently, serum calcidiol levels have been inversely associated with the risk of potentially precancerous colorectal adenomas (polyps)[23] and indices of colonic epithelial cell proliferation, which are considered biomarkers for colon cancer risk.[24]

Breast Cancer. In cell culture, the growth of some human breast cancer cell lines is inhibited by the active form of vitamin D, calcitriol. Breast cancer mortality follows a similar geographic distribution to that of colon cancer.[20,25] An examination of the data from the first National Health and Nutrition Examination Survey found that several measures of sunlight exposure and dietary vitamin D intake were associated with a reduced risk of breast cancer.[26] A case-control study of more than 300 women found blood levels of calcitriol at the time of diagnosis of breast cancer to be significantly lower in white women, but not African American women, than in comparable women without breast cancer.[27] Blood levels of calcidiol, the form of vitamin D generally used to assess vitamin D nutritional status, did not differ between women with and without breast cancer. In contrast, a case-control study of 96 white women who were subsequently diagnosed with breast cancer found that prediagnostic blood levels of calcitriol did not differ from those of a comparable group of women who did not develop breast cancer over the same period of time.[28] The average length of follow-up was 15 years. Presently, the relationship between vitamin D nutritional status and breast cancer risk in humans requires further clarification.

Disease Treatment

While reading this section it is important to remember that prolonged intake of high doses of vitamin D may result in serious side effects. The potential for vitamin D toxicity is higher if an individual is taking one of the drug formulations of calcitriol [1,25(OH)$_2$D$_3$] because it bypasses physiological control mechanisms that limit its production in the kidneys (see "Safety").

Osteoporosis

Vitamin D supplementation may be a useful adjunct to medical therapies aimed at preventing and treating osteoporosis, such as hormone replacement therapy or bisphosphonate therapy (e.g., etidronate or alendronate).[12] An uncontrolled trial in osteoporosis patients with a poor response to bisphosphonate therapy found that the addition of 25 µg (1000 IU)/d of vitamin D to the bisphosphonate regimen resulted in significantly increased bone mineral density of the lumbar spine after 1 year.[29] However, these findings require confirmation in a randomized, controlled trial.

Cancer

The active metabolite of vitamin D, calcitriol, inhibits the growth of human prostate cancer cells in culture, but the mechanism for this effect is not clear.[19] Two small nonrandomized trials have examined the effects of calcitriol on humans. Blood tests for prostate-specific antigen (PSA) measure a protein produced by prostate cells and are useful for monitoring the response of prostate cancer to treatment. In a small trial, only 2 of 13 men with prostate cancer that was unresponsive to hormone treatment showed decreased PSA levels during a course of treatment with calcitriol.[30] In another small study, six of seven prostate cancer patients had significantly decreased PSA levels after a course of treatment with calcitriol.[31] Unlike taking physiologic doses of vi-

tamin D, which must be metabolized to form calcitriol, taking pharmacologic doses of calcitriol carries with it the risk for serious side effects. Although the use of calcitriol or newly developed analogs as preventive or therapeutic agents for prostate cancer appears promising, there is presently insufficient human data to evaluate their efficacy or safety.

Autoimmune Disease

Insulin-dependent diabetes mellitus (IDDM), multiple sclerosis (MS), and rheumatoid arthritis (RA) are each examples of autoimmune disease. In IDDM, insulin-producing β cells of the pancreas are the target of the inappropriate immune response. In MS and RA, the targets are the myelin-producing cells of the central nervous system and the collagen-producing cells of the joints, respectively. The autoimmune responses are mediated by T lymphocytes (T cells). The biologically active form of vitamin D, calcitriol, has been found to modulate T-cell responses, such that the autoimmune responses are diminished. Treatment with calcitriol has had beneficial effects in animal models of IDDM, MS, and RA. In humans, increased incidence of IDDM, MS, and RA is found in geographic regions with low supplies of vitamin D (low sunlight exposure and low dietary intake). Presently, vitamin D and calcium supplementation are advocated for individuals at risk of osteoporosis from corticosteroid regimens prescribed to treat autoimmune diseases. Although the use of vitamin D and vitamin D analogs in the therapy of certain autoimmune diseases holds promise, further research is required before their safety and efficacy can be determined.[5,6]

Sources

Sunlight

Sunlight exposure provides most people with their entire vitamin D requirement. Children and young adults who spend a short time outside two or three times a week will generally synthesize all the vitamin D they need. Elderly individuals have diminished capacity to synthesize vitamin D from sunlight exposure and frequently use sunscreen or protective clothing to prevent skin cancer and sun damage. The application of sunscreen with an SPF factor of 8 reduces production of vitamin D by 95 %. In latitudes around 40 degrees north or 40 degrees south (Boston is 42 degrees north), there is insufficient UVB light available for vitamin D synthesis from November to early March. Ten degrees farther north or south (Edmonton, Canada) this "vitamin D winter" extends from mid-October to mid-March. A survey of elderly people who took a multivitamin supplement or drank three glasses of milk daily found that about 80 % of them were vitamin D–deficient by the end of winter. These findings have led some experts to recommend small amounts of regular sun exposure to elderly individuals.[2] About 15 minutes of exposure on the hands, face, and forearms three times a week in the morning or late afternoon during the spring, summer, and fall should provide adequate vitamin D and allow for storage of any excess in fat for use during the winter with minimal risk of skin damage. A sunscreen may be applied after the 15 minutes, if additional sun exposure is planned.

Food Sources

Vitamin D is found naturally in very few foods. Foods containing vitamin D include some fatty fish (herring, salmon, sardines), fish liver oils, and eggs from hens that have been fed vitamin D. In the United States, milk and infant formula are fortified with vitamin D to contain 10 μg (400 IU)/quart. However, other dairy products such as cheese and yogurt are not usually fortified with vitamin D. Some cereals and breads are also fortified with vitamin D. Accurate estimates of average dietary intakes of vitamin D are difficult because of the high variability of the vitamin D content of fortified foods.[11,32] Vitamin D contents of some vitamin D–rich foods are listed in Table 11–2, in both international units and micrograms.

Supplements

Vitamin D is available in multivitamin and single-ingredient supplements. Multivitamin supplements commonly provide 5 to 10 μg (200 to 400 IU) of vitamin D daily.[10]

Table 11–2   Food Sources of Vitamin D

Food	Serving	Vitamin D (IU)	Vitamin D (μg)
Cod liver oil	1 tablespoon	1360	34
Herring	3 ounces*	765	19.1
Salmon	3 ounces*	425	10.6
Sardines, canned	3 ounces*	255	6.4
Milk, fortified	8 ounces	100	2.5
Shrimp, canned	3 ounces*	90	2.3
Cereal, fortified	1 serving (usually 1 cup)	40 to 50	1 to 1.3
Egg yolk	1	25	0.63

*A 3-ounce serving of meat or fish is about the size of a deck of cards.

Safety

Toxicity

Vitamin D toxicity is also called *hypervitaminosis D*. Vitamin D toxicity has not been observed to result from sun exposure. Hypervitaminosis D appears to result primarily from vitamin D supplementation over many years at pharmacologic doses of 10,000 to 50,000 IU/d (250 to 1250 μg/d).[11] The adverse effects of hypervitaminosis D appear to be due mainly to the elevated blood calcium levels it induces. Symptoms include loss of appetite, nausea, vomiting, excessive thirst, excessive urination, severe itching, muscular weakness, joint pain, and ultimately disorientation, coma, and death. Blood and urinary calcium levels are elevated. If the condition persists, demineralization of bones and calcification of organs, such as the heart and kidneys, may also occur. The potential for vitamin D toxicity is higher if an individual is taking one of the drug formulations of calcitriol [1,25(OH)$_2$D$_3$] because it bypasses physiological control mechanisms that limit its production in the kidneys. Because the consequences of vitamin D toxicity are severe, the FNB of the Institute of Medicine set the tolerable upper level of intake for vitamin D at 2000 IU/d (50 μg/d) for adults, five times lower

Table 11–3 Tolerable Upper Intake Level (UL) for Vitamin D

Life Stage	Age	UL, µg/d
Infants	0–12 months	25 (1000 IU/d)
Children	1–18 years	50 (2000 IU/d)
Adults	19 years and older	50 (2000 IU/d)

than the dose generally observed to cause hypervitaminosis D in healthy individuals (Table 11–3).[11]

Drug Interactions

Anticonvulsants (phenytoin and phenobarbital) may reduce blood levels of calcidiol by affecting hepatic metabolism of vitamin D. The cholesterol-lowering medications cholestyramine and colestipol, orlistat, mineral oil, and the fat substitute olestra can decrease the intestinal absorption of vitamin D. The oral antifungal medication ketoconazole has been found to reduce blood levels of calcitriol in healthy men.[10] The induction of hypercalcemia (elevated blood calcium levels) by toxic levels of vitamin D may precipitate cardiac arrhythmia in patients on digitalis (digoxin) or verapamil, a calcium channel blocker, used to treat high blood pressure.[33]

LPI Recommendation

The Linus Pauling Institute recommends that generally healthy adults take a multivitamin/multimineral supplement that supplies 10 µg (400 IU) of vitamin D daily. If there is no reason to avoid all sun exposure, getting at least 15 minutes of sun exposure on the arms, face, and hands three times a week in the morning or late afternoon during the spring, summer, and fall may help residents of temperate latitudes (much of the United States) avoid vitamin D deficiency at the end of winter.

Older Adults

In addition to the 400 IU (10 µg) of vitamin D usually provided by a multivitamin/multimineral supplement, individuals over the age of 65 should consider taking an additional 400 IU (10 µg) of vitamin D to provide a total of 20 µg (800 IU)/d.

References

1. Brody T. *Nutritional Biochemistry*, 2nd ed. San Diego: Academic Press; 1999.
2. Holick MF. Vitamin D. In: Shils M, Olson JA, Shike M, Ross AC, eds. *Nutrition in Health and Disease*, 9th ed. Baltimore: Williams & Wilkins; 1999:329–345.
3. DeLuca HF, Zierold C. Mechanisms and functions of vitamin D. *Nutr Rev* 1998;56(2 Pt 2):S4–S10.
4. Janeway CA, Travers P. *Immunobiology: The Immune System in Health and Disease*. 3rd ed. New York: Garland Publishing Inc; 1997.
5. Cantorna MT. Vitamin D and autoimmunity: is vitamin D status an environmental factor affecting autoimmune disease prevalence? *Proc Soc Exp Biol Med* 2000;223(3):230–233.
6. Deluca HF, Cantorna MT. Vitamin D: its role and uses in immunology. *FASEB J* 2001;15(14):2579–2585.
7. Buist N. Vitamin D deficiency in Oregon: nutritional rickets resurgent. *Doernbecher Journal* 2000;6(2): 13–17.
8. Harris SS, Soteriades E, Coolidge JA, Mudgal S, Dawson-Hughes B. Vitamin D insufficiency and hyperparathyroidism in a low income, multiracial, elderly population. *J Clin Endocrinol Metab* 2000;85(11): 4125–4130.
9. Jahnsen J, Falch JA, Mowinckel P, Aadland E. Vitamin D status, parathyroid hormone and bone mineral density in patients with inflammatory bowel disease. *Scand J Gastroenterol* 2002;37(2):192–199.
10. Hendler SS, Rorvik DR, eds. *PDR for Nutritional Supplements*. Montvale, NJ: Medical Economics Company, Inc; 2001.
11. Food and Nutrition Board, Institute of Medicine. Vitamin D. *Dietary Reference Intakes: Calcium, Phosphorus, Magnesium, Vitamin D, and Fluoride*. Washington, D.C.: National Academy Press; 1997:250–287.
12. Shearer MJ. The roles of vitamins D and K in bone health and osteoporosis prevention. *Proc Nutr Soc* 1997;56(3):915–937.
13. Dawson-Hughes B, Dallal GE, Krall EA, Harris S, Sokoll LJ, Falconer G. Effect of vitamin D supplementation on wintertime and overall bone loss in healthy postmenopausal women. *Ann Intern Med* 1991;115(7): 505–512.
14. Dawson-Hughes B, Harris SS, Krall EA, Dallal GE, Falconer G, Green CL. Rates of bone loss in postmenopausal women randomly assigned to one of two dosages of vitamin D. *Am J Clin Nutr* 1995;61(5):1140–1145.
15. Dawson-Hughes B, Harris SS, Krall EA, Dallal GE. Effect of calcium and vitamin D supplementation on bone density in men and women 65 years of age or older. *N Engl J Med* 1997;337(10):670–676.
16. Dawson-Hughes B, Harris SS, Krall EA, Dallal GE. Effect of withdrawal of calcium and vitamin D supplements on bone mass in elderly men and women. *Am J Clin Nutr* 2000;72(3):745–750.
17. Chapuy MC, Arlot ME, Delmas PD, Meunier PJ. Effect of calcium and cholecalciferol treatment for three years on hip fractures in elderly women. *BMJ* 1994;308 (6936):1081–1082.
18. Lips P, Graafmans WC, Ooms ME, Bezemer PD, Bouter LM. Vitamin D supplementation and fracture incidence in elderly persons: a randomized, placebo-con-

trolled clinical trial. *Ann Intern Med* 1996;124(4):400–406.

19. Blutt SE, Weigel NL. Vitamin D and prostate cancer. *Proc Soc Exp Biol Med* 1999;221(2):89–98.

20. Garland CF, Garland FC, Gorham ED. Calcium and vitamin D: their potential roles in colon and breast cancer prevention. *Ann NY Acad Sci* 1999;889:107–119.

21. Martinez ME, Giovannucci EL, Colditz GA, et al. Calcium, vitamin D, and the occurrence of colorectal cancer among women. *J Natl Cancer Inst* 1996;88(19): 1375–1382.

22. Bostick RM, Potter JD, Sellers TA, McKenzie DR, Kushi LH, Folsom AR. Relation of calcium, vitamin D, and dairy food intake to incidence of colon cancer among older women. The Iowa Women's Health Study. *Am J Epidemiol* 1993;137(12):1302–1317.

23. Peters U, McGlynn KA, Chatterjee N, et al. Vitamin D, calcium, and vitamin D receptor polymorphism in colorectal adenomas. *Cancer Epidemiol Biomarkers Prev* 2001;10(12):1267–1274.

24. Holt PR, Arber N, Halmos B, et al. Colonic epithelial cell proliferation decreases with increasing levels of serum 25-hydroxy vitamin D. *Cancer Epidemiol Biomarkers Prev* 2002;11(1):113–119.

25. Grant WB. An ecologic study of dietary and solar ultraviolet-B links to breast carcinoma mortality rates. *Cancer* 2002;94(1):272–281.

26. John EM, Schwartz GG, Dreon DM, Koo J. Vitamin D and breast cancer risk: the NHANES I Epidemiologic follow-up study, 1971–1975 to 1992. National Health and Nutrition Examination Survey. *Cancer Epidemiol Biomarkers Prev* 1999;8(5):399–406.

27. Janowsky EC, Lester GE, Weinberg CR, et al. Association between low levels of 1,25-dihydroxyvitamin D and breast cancer risk. *Public Health Nutr* 1999;2(3):283–291.

28. Hiatt RA, Krieger N, Lobaugh B, Drezner MK, Vogelman JH, Orentreich N. Prediagnostic serum vitamin D and breast cancer. *J Natl Cancer Inst* 1998;90(6):461–463.

29. Heckman GA, Papaioannou A, Sebaldt RJ, et al. Effect of vitamin D on bone mineral density of elderly patients with osteoporosis responding poorly to bisphosphonates. *BMC Musculoskelet Disord* 2002;3(1):6.

30. Osborne JL, Schwartz GG, Smith DC, Bahnson R, Day R, Trump DL. Phase II trial of oral 1,25 dihydroxyvitamin D (calcitriol) in hormone refractory prostate cancer. *Urol Oncol* 1995;1:195.

31. Gross C, Stamey T, Hancock S, Feldman D. Treatment of early recurrent prostate cancer with 1,25-dihydroxyvitamin D3 (calcitriol). *J Urol* 1998;159(6):2035–2039.

32. Calvo MS. Dietary considerations to prevent loss of bone and renal function. *Nutrition* 2000;16(7–8):564–566.

33. Vitamins. *Drug Facts and Comparisons*. St. Louis: Facts and Comparisons; 2000:6–33.

12 Vitamin E

The term *vitamin E* describes a family of eight antioxidants, four tocopherols, alpha (α), beta (β), gamma (γ), and delta (δ), and four tocotrienols (also α, β, γ, and δ). α-Tocopherol is the only form of vitamin E that is actively maintained in the human body and is therefore the form of vitamin E found in the largest quantities in the blood and tissue.[1] Because α-tocopherol is the form of vitamin E that appears to have the greatest nutritional significance, it will be the primary topic of the following discussion. It is also the only form that meets the 2000 recommended dietary allowance (RDA) for vitamin E.

Function

α-Tocopherol

A primary function of α-tocopherol in humans appears to be that of an antioxidant. Free radicals are formed primarily in the body during normal metabolism and also upon exposure to environmental factors such as cigarette smoke or pollutants. Fats, which are an integral part of all cell membranes, are vulnerable to destruction through oxidation by free radicals. The fat-soluble vitamin α-tocopherol is uniquely suited to intercepting free radicals and preventing a chain reaction of lipid destruction. Aside from maintaining the integrity of cell membranes throughout the body, α-tocopherol also protects the fats in low-density lipoproteins (LDLs) from oxidation. Oxidized LDLs have been implicated in the development of cardiovascular diseases. When a molecule of α-tocopherol neutralizes a free radical, it is altered in such a way that its antioxidant capacity is lost. However, other antioxidants, such as vitamin C, are capable of regenerating the antioxidant capacity of α-tocopherol.[2]

Several other functions of α-tocopherol have been identified that are not likely to be related to its antioxidant capacity. α-To-copherol is known to inhibit the activity of protein kinase C, an important cell-signaling molecule, as well as to affect the expression and activity of immune and inflammatory cells. Additionally, α-tocopherol has been shown to inhibit platelet aggregation and to enhance vasodilation.[3,4]

γ-Tocopherol

The function of γ-tocopherol in humans is presently unclear. Although the most common form of vitamin E in the American diet is γ-tocopherol, blood levels of γ-tocopherol are generally 10 times lower than those of α-tocopherol. This phenomenon appears due to the action of the α-tocopherol transfer protein in the liver, which preferentially incorporates α-tocopherol into lipoproteins that are circulated in the blood and ultimately delivers α-tocopherol to different tissues in the body.[1] Because γ-tocopherol is initially absorbed in the same manner as α-tocopherol, small amounts are detectable in blood and tissue. Products of the metabolism of tocopherols, known as metabolites, can be detected in the urine. More γ-tocopherol metabolites are excreted in the urine than α-tocopherol metabolites, suggesting less γ-tocopherol is needed for use by the body.[5] Limited research in the test tube and in animals indicates that γ-tocopherol or its metabolites may play a role in the protection of the body from damage by free radicals,[6,7] but these effects have not been convincingly demonstrated in humans. In one recent prospective study, increased plasma γ-tocopherol levels were associated with a significantly reduced risk of developing prostate cancer, while significant protective associations for increased levels of plasma α-tocopherol and toenail selenium were found only when γ-tocopherol levels were also high.[8] These limited findings, in addition to the fact that taking α-tocopherol supplements lowers γ-tocopherol levels in the blood, have led some scientists to call for additional research on the effects of dietary and supplemental γ-tocopherol on health.[9]

Deficiency

Vitamin E deficiency has been observed in individuals with severe malnutrition, genetic defects of the α-tocopherol transfer protein, and fat malabsorption syndromes. For example, children with cystic fibrosis or cholestatic liver disease, who have an impaired capacity to absorb dietary fat and therefore fat-soluble vitamins, may develop symptomatic vitamin E deficiency. Severe vitamin E deficiency results mainly in neurological symptoms such as impaired balance and coordination and muscle weakness. The developing nervous system appears to be especially vulnerable to vitamin E deficiency because children with severe vitamin E deficiency from birth who are not treated with vitamin E develop neurological symptoms rapidly. In contrast, adults who develop vitamin E malabsorption may not develop neurological symptoms for 10 to 20 years. It should be noted that symptomatic vitamin E deficiency in healthy individuals who consume diets low in vitamin E has never been reported.[10]

Although true vitamin E deficiency is rare, suboptimal intake of vitamin E is relatively common in the United States. The Third National Health and Nutrition Examination Survey examined the dietary intake and serum levels of α-tocopherol in 16,295 multiethnic adults over the age of 18. Twenty-seven percent of white participants, 41% of African Americans, 28% of Mexican Americans, and 32% of the other participants were found to have serum levels of α-tocopherol less than 20 µmol/L, a value chosen because the literature suggests an increased risk for cardiovascular disease below this level.[11]

The Recommended Dietary Allowance

The RDA for vitamin E was previously 8 mg for women and 10 mg for men. The RDA was revised by the Food and Nutrition Board of the Institute of Medicine in 2000 (Table 12–1).[3]

Table 12–1 Recommended Dietary Allowance (RDA) for Vitamin E

Life Stage	Age	Males, mg/d*	Females, mg/d*
Infants	0–6 months	4 (AI)	4 (AI)
Infants	7–12 months	5 (AI)	5 (AI)
Children	1–3 years	6	6
Children	4–8 years	7	7
Children	9–13 years	11	11
Adolescents	14–18 years	15	15
Adults	19 years and older	15	15
Pregnancy	all ages	–	15
Breastfeeding	all ages	–	19

*mg of α-tocopherol.
AI, adequate intake level.

This new recommendation was based largely on the results of studies done in the 1950s in men fed vitamin E–deficient diets. In a test tube analysis, hydrogen peroxide was added to blood samples and the breakdown of red blood cells, known as hemolysis, was used to indicate vitamin E deficiency. Because hemolysis has also been reported in children with severe vitamin E deficiency, this analysis was considered to be a clinically relevant test of vitamin E status. Importantly, this means that the new RDA for vitamin E continues to be based on the prevention of deficiency symptoms rather than on health promotion and the prevention of chronic disease.

Disease Prevention

Cardiovascular Diseases

The results of at least five large observational studies suggest that increased vitamin E consumption is associated with decreased risk of myocardial infarction (heart attack) or death from heart disease in both men and women. Each study was a prospective study that measured vitamin E consumption in presumably healthy people and followed them for a number of years to determine how many of them were diagnosed with or died as a result of heart disease. In two of the studies, those individuals who consumed more than 7 mg of α-tocopherol in food were only approximately 35 % as likely to die from heart disease as those who consumed less than 3 to 5 mg of α-tocopherol.[12,13] Two other large studies found a significant reduction in the risk of heart disease only in those women and men who consumed α-tocopherol supplements of at least 100 IU (67 mg of *RRR*-α-tocopherol) daily,[14,15] with the greatest benefit observed at an intake of 800 IU (536 mg *RRR*-α-tocopherol) daily.[16] More recently, several studies have observed plasma or red blood cell levels of α-tocopherol to be inversely associated with the presence or severity of atherosclerosis detected using ultrasonography.[16–19]

In contrast, however, intervention studies with vitamin E supplements in patients with heart disease have not shown vitamin E to be effective in preventing heart attacks or death (see below).

Cancer

Many types of cancer are thought to result from oxidative damage to DNA caused by free radicals. The ability of α-tocopherol to neutralize free radicals has made it the subject of a number of cancer prevention studies. However, several large prospective studies have failed to find significant associations between α-tocopherol intake and the incidence of lung cancer or breast cancer.[3] A placebo-controlled intervention study designed to look at the effect of α-tocopherol supplementation on lung cancer in smokers found a 34 % reduction in the incidence of prostate cancer in smokers given supplements of 50 mg of synthetic α-tocopherol (equivalent to 25 mg of *RRR*-α-tocopherol) daily.[20] Because of these findings a large randomized, placebo-controlled intervention study is currently being conducted to examine the effect of α-tocopherol supplementation on prostate cancer risk.[21]

Cataracts

Cataracts appear to be formed by the oxidation of proteins in the lens of the eye, which may be prevented by antioxidants such as α-tocopherol. At least 10 observational studies have examined the association between measures of vitamin E consumption and the incidence and severity of cataracts. Of these studies, five found increased vitamin E intake to be associated with protection from cataracts, while five reported no association.[22,23] A recent intervention trial of a daily antioxidant supplement containing 500 mg of vitamin C, 400 IU of vitamin E, and 15 mg of β-carotene in 4629 men and women found that the antioxidant supplement was no different than a placebo in its effects on the development and progression of age-related cataracts over a 7-year period.[24] Another intervention trial found that a daily supplement of 50 mg of synthetic α-tocopherol (equivalent to 25 mg of *RRR*-α-tocopherol) did not alter the incidence of cataract surgery in male smokers.[25] Presently, the relationship between vitamin E intake and the development of cataracts requires further clarification before specific recommendations can be made.

Immune Function

α-Tocopherol has been shown to enhance specific aspects of the immune response that appear to decline as people age. For example, 200 mg of synthetic α-tocopherol (equivalent to 100 mg of *RRR*-α-tocopherol) daily for several months increased the formation of antibodies in response to hepatitis B vaccine and tetanus vaccine in elderly adults.[26] Whether α-tocopherol associated enhancements in the immune response actually translate to increased resistance to infections such as the flu (influenza virus) in older adults remains to be determined.[27]

Disease Treatment

Cardiovascular Diseases

Observational studies have suggested that supplemental α-tocopherol might have value in the treatment of cardiovascular disease. For example, a small observational study of men who had previously undergone a coronary artery bypass graft found a reduction in the progression of coronary artery atherosclerosis by angiography in those men who took at least 100 IU of α-tocopherol (67 mg of *RRR*-α-tocopherol) daily.[28] A randomized, placebo-controlled intervention trial in Great Britain (the CHAOS study) found that supplementing heart disease patients with either 400 or 800 IU/d of α-tocopherol (equivalent to 268 or 536 mg/d of *RRR*-α-tocopherol) for an average of 18 months resulted in a dramatic 77% reduction in nonfatal heart attacks.[29] However, total deaths from heart disease were not significantly reduced. Chronic renal dialysis patients are at much greater risk of dying from cardiovascular disease than the general population, and there is evidence that they are also under increased oxidative stress. Supplementation of renal dialysis patients with 800 IU/d of natural α-tocopherol (536 mg/d of *RRR*-α-tocopherol) for an average of 1.4 years resulted in a significantly reduced risk of heart attack compared with placebo.[30]

In contrast, three other intervention trials failed to find significant risk reductions with α-tocopherol supplementation. One study, which was designed mainly to examine cancer prevention, found that 50 mg of synthetic α-tocopherol daily (equivalent to 25 mg of *RRR*-α-tocopherol) resulted in a nonsignificant decrease in nonfatal heart attacks in those participants who had had previous heart attacks.[31] However, two other large trials found that daily supplements of 400 IU of natural α-tocopherol (equivalent to 268 mg *RRR*-α-tocopherol) and 300 mg of synthetic α-tocopherol (equivalent to 150 mg of *RRR*-α-tocopherol) in individuals with evidence of cardiovascular disease (previous heart attack, stroke, or evidence of vascular disease) did not significantly change the risk of a subsequent heart attack or stroke.[32,33] The results of several other large intervention trials, which are presently in progress, may clarify the role of α-tocopherol supplementation in the treatment of cardiovascular disease.

Diabetes Mellitus

α-Tocopherol supplementation of individuals with diabetes has been proposed because diabetes appears to increase oxidative stress and because cardiovascular complications (heart attack and stroke) are among the leading causes of death in diabetics. A number of studies have reported evidence of increased oxidative stress in diabetic individuals. Supplementation of 10 diabetic patients with 600 mg of synthetic α-tocopherol daily (equivalent to 300 mg of *RRR*-α-tocopherol) for 14 days resulted in significant reductions in urine F_2-isoprostanes, a specific marker of in vivo oxidative stress.[34] Studies of the effect of α-tocopherol supplementation on blood glucose control have been contradictory. One study reported improved control of blood glucose levels with supplementation of only 100 IU of synthetic α-tocopherol daily (equivalent to 45 mg *RRR*-α-tocopherol),[35] although studies using 900 to 1600 IU of synthetic α-tocopherol daily (equivalent to 405 to 720 mg *RRR*-α-tocopherol) found either minimal or no improvement, respectively.[36,37] Although there is reason to suspect that α-tocopherol supplementation may be beneficial for individuals with diabetes, evidence from well-controlled clinical trials is lacking.

Alzheimer's Disease and Dementia

The brain is particularly vulnerable to oxidative stress, which is thought to play a role in the pathology of neurodegenerative diseases such as Alzheimer's disease.[38] In a large, placebo-controlled intervention trial, supplementation of individuals who had moderate neurological impairment with 2000 IU of synthetic α-tocopherol daily for 2 years (equivalent to 900 mg/d of *RRR*-α-tocopherol) resulted in a significant slowing of the progression of Alzheimer's dementia.[39] After Alzheimer's disease, vascular dementia (dementia resulting from strokes) is the most common cause of dementia in the United States. A case-control study examining risk factors for vascular dementia in elderly Japanese-American men found that supplemental vitamin E and vitamin C intake was associated with a significantly decreased risk of vascular and other types of dementia but not Alzheimer's dementia.[40] Among those without dementia, vitamin E supplement use was associated with better scores on cognitive tests. Although these findings are promising, further studies are required to determine the role of α-tocopherol supplementation in the treatment of Alzheimer's disease and other types of dementia.

Sources

Food Sources

Major sources of α-tocopherol in the American diet include vegetable oils (olive, sunflower, safflower oils), nuts, whole grains, and green leafy vegetables. All eight forms of vitamin E (α-, β-, γ-, δ-tocopherols and tocotrienols) occur naturally in foods in varying amounts. The average intake of α-tocopherol from food in the United States is approximately 9 mg daily for men and 6 mg daily for women, well below the recently revised RDA of 15 mg/d of *RRR*-α-tocopherol. Many scientists believe it is difficult for an individual to consume more than 15 mg/d of α-tocopherol from food alone without also increasing fat intake above recommended levels.

Before the body's preference for α-tocopherol was clarified, the vitamin E content of food was often expressed as mg of α-tocopherol equivalents (α-TE). Presently most food composition tables and databases provide vitamin E content information only in terms of α-TE, rather than as mg of α-tocopherol. A rough approximation of the α-tocopherol content in foods can be calculated by multiplying the mg of α-TE by 0.8.[3] (*Example*: 2.0 mg α-TE × 0.8 = 1.6 mg α-tocopherol.)

The α- and γ-tocopherol values in Table 12–2 were measured in foods rather than calculated from α-TE.

Supplements

α-Tocopherol

All α-tocopherol in food is in the form of the isomer *RRR*-α-tocopherol. The same is not always true for supplements. Vitamin E supplements generally contain from 100 IU to 1000

Table 12–2 Food Sources of Vitamin E

Food	Serving	α-Tocopherol, mg	γ-Tocopherol, mg
Soy oil	1 tablespoon	1.0	10.8
Corn oil	1 tablespoon	1.5	8.2
Peanuts	1 ounce	3.2	2.4
Sunflower oil	1 tablespoon	6.6	0.7
Canola oil	1 tablespoon	2.9	0.6
Almonds	1 ounce	12.8	0.5
Olive oil	1 tablespoon	1.6	0.1
Safflower oil	1 tablespoon	4.6	0.1
Hazelnuts	1 ounce	6.1	0.03
Spinach, raw	1/2 cup, chopped	1.7	0.0
Carrots, raw	1/2 cup, chopped	0.3	0.0
Avocado (Haas)	Medium	3.3	1.2

IU of α-tocopherol. Supplements made from entirely natural sources contain only *RRR*-α-tocopherol (also labeled d-α-tocopherol). *RRR*-α-tocopherol is the isomer preferred for use by the body, making it the most bioavailable form of α-tocopherol. Synthetic α-tocopherol (also labeled dl-α-tocopherol) is correctly named *all-rac*-α-tocopherol, meaning that all eight isomers of α-tocopherol are present in the mixture. Because some isomers of α-tocopherol present in *all-rac*-α-tocopherol are not usable by the body, synthetic α-tocopherol is less bioavailable and only about half as potent. To calculate the number of mg of bioavailable α-tocopherol present in α-tocopherol supplements, use the following formulas:

Natural, RRR-, or d-α-tocopherol:
        IU × 0.67 = mg *RRR*-α-tocopherol
Example:
        100 IU = 67 mg;

Synthetic, all-rac-, or dl-α-tocopherol:
        IU × 0.45 = mg *RRR*-α-tocopherol
Example:
        100 IU = 45 mg.

γ-Tocopherol supplements and mixed tocopherol supplements are also commercially available.[41] The amounts of α- and γ-tocopherol vary in mixed tocopherol supplements, so it is important to read the label to determine the amount of each tocopherol present in the supplement.

Safety

Toxicity

Few side effects have been noted in adults taking supplements of less than 2000 mg of α-tocopherol daily (*RRR*- or *all-rac*-α-tocopherol). However, most studies of toxicity or side effects of α-tocopherol supplementation have lasted only a few weeks to a few months, and side effects occurring as a result of long-term α-tocopherol supplementation have not been adequately studied. The most worrisome possibility is that of impaired blood clotting resulting in an increased likelihood of hemorrhage in some individuals. In addition to setting the new RDA for α-tocopherol in 2000, the Food and Nutrition Board of the Institute of Medicine also set a tolerable upper intake level (UL) for α-tocopherol supplements, citing the avoidance of hemorrhage as the basis for the upper limit (Table 12–3). The Board felt that a UL of 1000 mg daily of α-tocopherol of any form (equivalent to 1500 IU of *RRR*-α-tocopherol or 1100 IU of *all-rac*-α-tocopherol) would be the highest dose unlikely to result in hemorrhage in almost all adults.[3] Although only certain isomers of α-tocopherol are retained in the circulation, all forms are absorbed and the liver must break them down and eliminate them. The rationale that any form of α-tocopherol (natural or synthetic) that can be absorbed potentially could have adverse effects is the basis for a UL that refers to all forms of α-tocopherol. Because hemorrhage is a potentially life-threatening condition, the Linus Pauling Institute also recommends that individuals do not exceed 1000 mg of α-tocopherol per day. Premature infants appear to be especially vulnerable to adverse effects of α-tocopherol supplementation, which should be used only under controlled supervision by a pediatrician. Some physicians recommend that high-dose vitamin E supplementation be discontinued 1 month before elective surgery to decrease the risk of hemorrhage.[41]

Table 12–3 Tolerable Upper Intake Level (UL) for *all rac*- and *RRR*-α-Tocopherol (*dl*- and *d*-α-Tocopherol)

Life Stage	Age	UL, mg α-Tocopherol/d
Infants	0–12 months	not possible to establish*
Children	1–3 years	200
Children	4–8 years	300
Children	9–13 years	600
Adolescents	14–18 years	800
Adults	19 years and older	1000

*Source of intake should be from food and formula only.

Drug Interactions

Individuals on anticoagulant therapy (blood thinners) or antiplatelet drugs (e.g., dipyramidole) as well as individuals who are vitamin K–deficient should not take α-tocopherol supplements without close medical supervision because of the increased risk of hemorrhage. A number of medications may decrease the absorption of vitamin E, including cholestyramine, colestipol, isoniazid, mineral oil, orlistat, sucralfate, and the fat substitute olestra. Anticonvulsant drugs such as phenobarbital, phenytoin, or carbamazepine may decrease plasma levels of vitamin E.[3,41]

LPI Recommendation

Researchers at the Linus Pauling Institute feel there exists credible evidence that a dose of 200 mg of natural source *d*- or *RRR*-α-tocopherol daily for adults may help protect against chronic diseases like heart disease, stroke, and some types of cancer. The amount of α-tocopherol required for such beneficial effects appears to be much greater than that which could be achieved through diet alone. A supplement containing the equivalent of 200 mg/d of *RRR*-α-tocopherol is well below the upper level of 1000 mg considered safe for most adults, but high enough to saturate plasma levels and systematically increase α-tocopherol levels in tissues. α-Tocopherol supplements are unlikely to be absorbed unless taken with food.

Older Adults
The Linus Pauling Institute's recommendation of 200 mg/d of natural source *d-* or *RRR*-α-tocopherol is also appropriate for generally healthy adults 65 years and older, who are at higher risk for chronic diseases like heart disease, stroke, cataracts, and cancer.

References

1. Traber MG. Utilization of vitamin E. *Biofactors* 1999;10(2–3):115–120.
2. Traber MG. Vitamin E. In: Shils M, Olson JA, Shike M, Ross AC, eds. *Nutrition in Health and Disease*, 9th ed. Baltimore: Williams & Wilkins; 1999:347–362.
3. Food and Nutrition Board, Institute of Medicine. Vitamin E. *Dietary Reference Intakes for Vitamin C, Vitamin E, Selenium, and Carotenoids*. Washington, D.C.: National Academy Press; 2000:95–185.
4. Traber MG. Does vitamin E decrease heart attack risk? Summary and implications with respect to dietary recommendations. *J Nutr* 2001;131(2):395S–397S.
5. Traber MG, Elsner A, Brigelius-Flohe R. Synthetic as compared with natural vitamin E is preferentially excreted as alpha-CEHC in human urine: studies using deuterated alpha-tocopheryl acetates. *FEBS Lett* 1998;437(1–2):145–148.
6. Christen S, Woodall AA, Shigenaga MK, Southwell-Keely PT, Duncan MW, Ames BN. Gamma-tocopherol traps mutagenic electrophiles such as NO(X) and complements alpha-tocopherol: physiological implications. *Proc Natl Acad Sci USA* 1997;94(7):3217–3222.
7. Li D, Saldeen T, Mehta JL. Gamma-tocopherol decreases ox-LDL-mediated activation of nuclear factor-kappaB and apoptosis in human coronary artery endothelial cells. *Biochem Biophys Res Commun* 1999;259(1):157–161.
8. Helzlsouer KJ, Huang HY, Alberg AJ, et al. Association between alpha-tocopherol, gamma-tocopherol, selenium, and subsequent prostate cancer. *J Natl Cancer Inst* 2000;92(24):2018–2023.
9. Jiang Q, Christen S, Shigenaga MK, Ames BN. Gamma-tocopherol, the major form of vitamin E in the US diet, deserves more attention. *Am J Clin Nutr* 2001;74(6):714–722.
10. Sokol R. Vitamin E. In: Ziegler EE, Filer LJ, eds. *Present Knowledge in Nutrition*, 7th ed: ILSI Press; 1996:130–136.
11. Ford ES, Sowell A. Serum alpha-tocopherol status in the United States population: findings from the Third National Health and Nutrition Examination Survey. *Am J Epidemiol* 1999;150(3):290–300.
12. Knekt P, Reunanen A, Jarvinen R, Seppanen R, Heliovaara M, Aromaa A. Antioxidant vitamin intake and coronary mortality in a longitudinal population study. *Am J Epidemiol* 1994;139(12):1180–1189.
13. Kushi LH, Folsom AR, Prineas RJ, Mink PJ, Wu Y, Bostick RM. Dietary antioxidant vitamins and death from coronary heart disease in postmenopausal women. *N Engl J Med* 1996;334(18):1156–1162.
14. Rimm EB, Stampfer MJ, Ascherio A, Giovannucci E, Colditz GA, Willett WC. Vitamin E consumption and the risk of coronary heart disease in men. *N Engl J Med* 1993;328(20):1450–1456.
15. Stampfer MJ, Hennekens CH, Manson JE, Colditz GA, Rosner B, Willett WC. Vitamin E consumption and the risk of coronary disease in women. *N Engl J Med* 1993;328(20):1444–1449.
16. Cherubini A, Zuliani G, Costantini F, et al. High vitamin E plasma levels and low low-density lipoprotein oxidation are associated with the absence of atherosclerosis in octogenarians. *J Am Geriatr Soc* 2001;49(5):651–654.
17. Gale CR, Ashurst HE, Powers HJ, Martyn CN. Antioxidant vitamin status and carotid atherosclerosis in the elderly. *Am J Clin Nutr* 2001;74(3):402–408.
18. McQuillan BM, Hung J, Beilby JP, Nidorf M, Thompson PL. Antioxidant vitamins and the risk of carotid atherosclerosis. The Perth Carotid Ultrasound Disease Assessment study (CUDAS). *J Am Coll Cardiol* 2001;38(7):1788–1794.
19. Simon E, Gariepy J, Cogny A, Moatti N, Simon A, Paul JL. Erythrocyte, but not plasma, vitamin E concentration is associated with carotid intima-media thickening in asymptomatic men at risk for cardiovascular disease. *Atherosclerosis* 2001;159(1):193–200.
20. Heinonen OP, Albanes D, Virtamo J, et al. Prostate cancer and supplementation with alpha-tocopherol and beta-carotene: incidence and mortality in a controlled trial. *J Natl Cancer Inst* 1998;90(6):440–446.
21. Klein EA, Thompson IM, Lippman SM, et al. SELECT: the next prostate cancer prevention trial. Selenium and Vitamin E Cancer Prevention Trial. *J Urol* 2001;166(4):1311–1315.
22. Jacques PF. The potential preventive effects of vitamins for cataract and age-related macular degeneration. *Int J Vitam Nutr Res* 1999;69(3):198–205.
23. Gale CR, Hall NF, Phillips DI, Martyn CN. Plasma antioxidant vitamins and carotenoids and age-related cataract. *Ophthalmology* 2001;108(11):1992–1998.
24. AREDS report no. 9. A randomized, placebo-controlled, clinical trial of high-dose supplementation with vitamins C and E and beta carotene for age-related cataract and vision loss: report no. 9. *Arch Ophthalmol* 2001;119(10):1439–1452.
25. Teikari JM, Rautalahti M, Haukka J, et al. Incidence of cataract operations in Finnish male smokers unaffected by alpha tocopherol or beta carotene supplements. *J Epidemiol Community Health* 1998;52(7):468–472.
26. Meydani SN, Meydani M, Blumberg JB, et al. Vitamin E supplementation and in vivo immune response in healthy elderly subjects: a randomized controlled trial. *JAMA* 1997;277(17):1380–1386.
27. Han SN, Meydani SN. Vitamin E and infectious diseases in the aged. *Proc Nutr Soc* 1999;58(3):697–705.
28. Azen SP, Qian D, Mack WJ, et al. Effect of supplementary antioxidant vitamin intake on carotid arterial wall intima-media thickness in a controlled clinical trial of cholesterol lowering. *Circulation* 1996;94(10):2369–2372.
29. Stephens NG, Parsons A, Schofield PM, Kelly F, Cheeseman K, Mitchinson MJ. Randomised controlled trial of vitamin E in patients with coronary disease: Cambridge Heart Antioxidant Study (CHAOS). *Lancet* 1996;347(9004):781–786.

30. Boaz M, Smetana S, Weinstein T, et al. Secondary prevention with antioxidants of cardiovascular disease in endstage renal disease (SPACE): randomised placebo-controlled trial. *Lancet* 2000;356(9237):1213–1218.

31. Rapola JM, Virtamo J, Ripatti S, et al. Randomised trial of alpha-tocopherol and beta-carotene supplements on incidence of major coronary events in men with previous myocardial infarction. *Lancet* 1997;349 (9067):1715–1720.

32. Yusuf S, Dagenais G, Pogue J, Bosch J, Sleight P. Vitamin E supplementation and cardiovascular events in high-risk patients. The Heart Outcomes Prevention Evaluation Study Investigators. *N Engl J Med* 2000;342(3):154–160.

33. Gruppo Italiano per lo Studio della Sopravvivenza nell'Infarto miocardico. Dietary supplementation with n-3 polyunsaturated fatty acids and vitamin E after myocardial infarction: results of the GISSI-Prevenzione trial. Gruppo Italiano per lo Studio della Sopravvivenza nell'Infarto miocardico. *Lancet* 1999; 354(9177):447–455.

34. Davi G, Ciabattoni G, Consoli A, et al. In vivo formation of 8-iso-prostaglandin f2alpha and platelet activation in diabetes mellitus: effects of improved metabolic control and vitamin E supplementation. *Circulation* 1999;99(2):224–229.

35. Jain SK, McVie R, Jaramillo JJ, Palmer M, Smith T. Effect of modest vitamin E supplementation on blood gly-cated hemoglobin and triglyceride levels and red cell indices in type I diabetic patients. *J Am Coll Nutr* 1996;15(5):458–461.

36. Paolisso G, D'Amore A, Galzerano D, et al. Daily vitamin E supplements improve metabolic control but not insulin secretion in elderly type II diabetic patients. *Diabetes Care* 1993;16(11):1433–1437.

37. Reaven PD, Herold DA, Barnett J, Edelman S. Effects of Vitamin E on susceptibility of low-density lipoprotein and low-density lipoprotein subfractions to oxidation and on protein glycation in NIDDM. *Diabetes Care* 1995;18(6):807–816.

38. Meydani M. Antioxidants and cognitive function. *Nutr Rev* 2001;59(8 Pt 2):S75–80.

39. Sano M, Ernesto C, Thomas RG, et al. A controlled trial of selegiline, alpha-tocopherol, or both as treatment for Alzheimer's disease. The Alzheimer's Disease Cooperative Study. *N Engl J Med* 1997;336(17):1216–1222.

40. Masaki KH, Losonczy KG, Izmirlian G, et al. Association of vitamin E and C supplement use with cognitive function and dementia in elderly men. *Neurology* 2000;54(6):1265–1272.

41. Hendler SS, Rorvik DR, eds. *PDR for Nutritional Supplements*. Montvale, NJ: Medical Economics Company, Inc; 2001.

13 Vitamin K

Vitamin K is a fat-soluble vitamin. The "K" is derived from the German word *koagulation.* Coagulation refers to blood clotting, because vitamin K is essential for the functioning of several proteins involved in blood clotting.[1] There are two naturally occurring forms of vitamin K. Plants synthesize phylloquinone, also known as vitamin K_1. Bacteria synthesize a range of vitamin K forms, using repeating five-carbon units in the side chain of the molecule. These forms of vitamin K are designated menaquinone-n (MK-n), where *n* stands for the number of five-carbon units. MK-n are collectively referred to as vitamin K_2.[2] MK-4 is not produced in significant amounts by bacteria, but appears to be synthesized by animals (including humans) from phylloquinone. MK-4 is found in a number of organs other than the liver at higher concentrations than phylloquinone. This fact, along with the existence of a unique pathway for its synthesis, suggests there is some unique function of MK-4 that is yet to be discovered.[3]

Function

The only known biological role of vitamin K is that of the required coenzyme for a vitamin K–dependent carboxylase that catalyzes the carboxylation of the amino acid glutamic acid, resulting in its conversion to gamma (γ)-carboxyglutamic acid (Gla).[4] Although vitamin K–dependent carboxylation occurs only on specific glutamic acid residues in a small number of proteins, it is critical to the calcium-binding function of those proteins.[5,6]

Coagulation

The ability to bind calcium ions (Ca^{2+}) is required for the activation of the seven vitamin K–dependent clotting factors in the coagulation cascade. The term *coagulation cascade* refers to a series of events, each dependent on the other, that stops bleeding through clot formation. Vitamin K–dependent γ-carboxylation of specific glutamic acid residues in those proteins makes it possible for them to bind calcium. Factors II (prothrombin), VII, IX, and X make up the core of the coagulation cascade. Protein Z appears to enhance the action of thrombin (the activated form of prothrombin) by promoting its association with phospholipids in cell membranes. Protein C and protein S are anticoagulant proteins that provide control and balance in the coagulation cascade. Because uncontrolled clotting may be as life-threatening as uncontrolled bleeding, control mechanisms are built in to the coagulation cascade. Vitamin K–dependent coagulation factors are synthesized in the liver. Consequently, severe liver disease results in lower blood levels of vitamin K–dependent clotting factors and an increased risk of uncontrolled bleeding (hemorrhage).[7]

Some people are at risk of forming clots, which could block the flow of blood in arteries of the heart, brain, or lungs, resulting in heart attack, stroke, or pulmonary embolism, respectively. Some oral anticoagulants, such as warfarin, inhibit coagulation through antagonism of the action of vitamin K. Although vitamin K is a fat-soluble vitamin, the body stores very little of it, and its stores are rapidly depleted without regular dietary intake. Perhaps because of its limited ability to store vitamin K, the body recycles it through a process called the *vitamin K cycle.* The vitamin K cycle allows a small amount of vitamin K to function in the γ-carboxylation of proteins many times, decreasing the dietary requirement. Warfarin prevents the recycling of vitamin K by inhibiting two important reactions and creating a functional vitamin K deficiency (Fig. 13–1). Inadequate γ-carboxylation of vitamin K–dependent coagulation proteins interferes with the coagulation cascade and inhibits blood clot formation. Large quantities of dietary or supplemental vitamin K can overcome the anti-

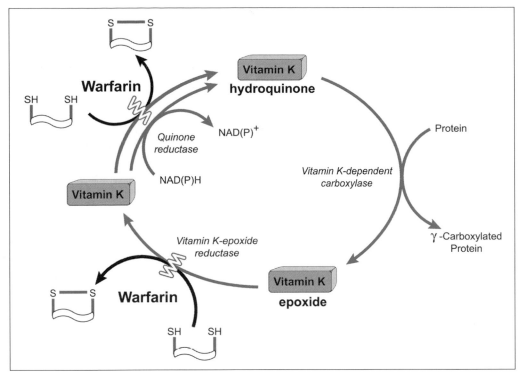

Figure 13–1. The vitamin K cycle. Warfarin is a vitamin K antagonist that inhibits the recycling of vitamin K at two dithiol-dependent steps.

coagulant effect of vitamin K antagonists, so patients taking these drugs are cautioned against consuming very large or highly variable quantities of vitamin K in their diets. Experts now advise a reasonably constant dietary intake of vitamin K that meets current dietary recommendations (90 to 120 μg/d) for patients on vitamin K antagonists like warfarin.[8]

Bone Mineralization

Three vitamin K–dependent proteins have been isolated in bone. Osteocalcin is a protein synthesized by osteoblasts (bone-forming cells). The synthesis of osteocalcin by osteoblasts is regulated by the active form of vitamin D, $1,25(OH)_2D_3$ or calcitriol. The mineral-binding capacity of osteocalcin requires vitamin K–dependent γ-carboxylation of three glutamic acid residues. The function of osteocalcin is unclear but is thought to be related to bone mineralization. Matrix Gla protein (MGP) has been found in bone, cartilage,

and soft tissue, including blood vessels. The results of animal studies suggest MGP prevents the calcification of soft tissue and cartilage while facilitating normal bone growth and development. The vitamin K–dependent anticoagulant protein S is also synthesized by osteoblasts, but its role in bone metabolism is unclear. Children with inherited protein S deficiency suffer complications related to increased blood clotting as well as to decreased bone density.[6,7,9]

Cell Proliferation

Gas6 is a vitamin K–dependent protein that was identified in 1993. It has been found throughout the nervous system, as well in the heart, lungs, stomach, kidneys, and cartilage. Although the exact mechanism of its action has not been determined, Gas6 appears to be a cellular growth regulation factor with cell-signaling activities. It may also play important roles in the developing and aging nervous system.[10,11]

Deficiency

Overt vitamin K deficiency results in impaired blood clotting, usually demonstrated by laboratory tests that measure clotting time. Symptoms include easy bruising and bleeding that may be manifested as nosebleeds, bleeding gums, blood in the urine, blood in the stool, tarry black stools, or extremely heavy menstrual bleeding. In infants, vitamin K deficiency may result in life-threatening bleeding within the skull (intracranial hemorrhage).[7]

Adults

Vitamin K deficiency is uncommon in healthy adults for a number of reasons: (1) vitamin K is widespread in foods, (2) the vitamin K cycle conserves vitamin K, and (3) bacteria that normally inhabit the large intestine synthesize menaquinones (vitamin K_2), though it is unclear whether a significant amount is absorbed and utilized. Adults at risk of vitamin K deficiency include those taking vitamin K antagonist anticoagulant drugs and individuals with significant liver damage or disease.[7]

Infants

Newborn babies that are exclusively breast-fed are at increased risk of vitamin K deficiency for the following reasons: (1) human milk is relatively low in vitamin K compared with formula, (2) the newborn's intestines are not yet colonized with bacteria that synthesize menaquinones, and (3) the vitamin K cycle may not be fully functional in newborns, especially premature infants. Infants whose mothers are on anticonvulsant medication to prevent seizures are also at risk of vitamin K deficiency. Vitamin K deficiency in newborns may result in a bleeding disorder called *hemorrhagic disease of the newborn* (HDN). Because HDN is life-threatening and easily prevented, the American Academy of Pediatrics and a number of similar international organizations recommend that an injection of phylloquinone (vitamin K_1) be administered to all newborns.[12]

Table 13–1 Adequate Intake (AI) for Vitamin K

Life Stage	Age	Males, µg/d	Females, µg/d
Infants	0–6 months	2.0	2.0
Infants	7–12 months	2.5	2.5
Children	1–3 years	30	30
Children	4–8 years	55	55
Children	9–13 years	60	60
Adolescents	14–18 years	75	75
Adults	19 years and older	120	90
Pregnancy	18 years and younger	–	75
Pregnancy	19 years and older	–	90
Breastfeeding	18 years and younger	–	75
Breastfeeding	19 years and older	–	90

Controversy Surrounding Vitamin K Administration and the Newborn

Controversy arose regarding the routine use of vitamin K injections for newborns in the early 1990s when two retrospective studies were published that suggested the possibility of an association between vitamin K injections in newborns and the development of childhood leukemia and other forms of childhood cancer. However, two large retrospective studies in the United States and Sweden that reviewed the medical records of 54,000 and 1.3 million children, respectively, found no evidence of a relationship between childhood cancers and vitamin K injections at birth.[13,14] Moreover, a pooled analysis of six case-control studies including 2431 children diagnosed with childhood cancer and 6338 control children found no evidence that vitamin K injections for newborns increased the risk of childhood leukemia.[15] In a policy statement, the American Academy of Pediatrics recommended that routine vitamin K prophylaxis for newborns be continued because HDN is life-threatening and the risks of cancer are unproven and unlikely.[16]

The Adequate Intake Level

In January 2001, the Food and Nutrition Board of the Institute of Medicine established the adequate intake (AI) level for vitamin K in the United States based on consumption levels of healthy individuals (Table 13–1).[17]

Disease Prevention

Osteoporosis

The discovery of vitamin K–dependent proteins in bone has led to research on the role of vitamin K in maintaining bone health.

Dietary Vitamin K and Osteoporotic Fracture. Epidemiologic studies have demonstrated a relationship between vitamin K and age-related bone loss (osteoporosis). The Nurses Health Study followed more than 72,000 women for 10 years. Investigators found that women whose vitamin K intake was in the lowest quintile (1/5) had a 30% higher risk of hip fracture than women with vitamin K intakes in the highest four quintiles.[18] A study of over 800 elderly men and women followed in the Framingham Heart Study for 7 years found that men and women with dietary intakes in the highest quartile (1/4) had only 35% of the risk of hip fracture experienced by those with dietary vitamin K intakes in the lowest quartile (approximately 250 μg vs. 50 μg of vitamin K). However, the investigators found no association between dietary vitamin K intake and bone mineral density in the Framingham subjects.[19] Because the primary dietary source of vitamin K is generally green leafy vegetables, high vitamin K intake could just be a marker for a healthy diet that is high in fruits and vegetables.[20]

Vitamin K–Dependent Carboxylation of Osteocalcin and Osteoporotic Fracture. Osteocalcin, a bone-related protein that circulates in the blood, has been shown to be a sensitive marker of bone formation. Vitamin K is required for the γ-carboxylation of osteocalcin. Undercarboxylation of osteocalcin adversely affects its capacity to bind to bone mineral, and the degree of osteocalcin γ-carboxylation has been found to be a sensitive indicator of vitamin K nutritional status.[3] Blood levels of undercarboxylated osteocalcin (ucOC) were found to be higher in postmenopausal women than premenopausal women and markedly higher in women over the age of 70. In a study of 195 institutionalized elderly women, the relative risk of hip fracture was six times higher in those who had elevated ucOC levels at the beginning of the study.[21] In a much larger sample of 7500 elderly women living independently, blood ucOC was also predictive of fracture risk. Although vitamin K deficiency would seem the most likely cause of elevated blood ucOC, investigators have also documented an inverse relationship between measures of vitamin D nutritional status and ucOC levels, as well as a significant lowering of ucOC by vitamin D supplementation.[6] It is also possible that an increased ucOC level is a marker for poor vitamin D or protein nutritional status.

Vitamin K Antagonists and Osteoporotic Fracture. Certain oral anticoagulants, such as warfarin, are known to be antagonists of vitamin K. Two recent studies examined the chronic use of warfarin and the risk of fracture in older women. One study reported no association between long-term warfarin treatment and fracture risk,[22] although the other found a significantly higher risk of rib and vertebral fractures in warfarin users compared to nonusers.[23] A meta-analysis of the results of 11 published studies found that oral anticoagulation therapy was associated with a very modest reduction in bone density at the wrist and no change in bone density at the hip or spine.[24]

Vitamin K Supplementation Studies and Osteoporosis. Vitamin K supplementation of 1000 μg (1 mg)/d of phylloquinone (vitamin K_1) for 2 weeks (more than 10 times the AI for vitamin K) resulted in a decrease of ucOC levels in postmenopausal women, as well as increases in several biochemical markers of bone formation. In Japan, intervention trials in hemodialysis patients and osteoporotic women using very high pharmacologic doses (45 mg/d) of menatetranone (MK-4) have reported significant reductions in the rate of bone loss.[25,26] MK-4 is not found in significant amounts in the diet but can be synthesized in

small amounts by humans from phylloquinone. The dose used in the Japanese studies is about 50 times higher than the AI for
vitamin K. Experts are not sure whether the
effects of such high doses of MK-4 represent a
true vitamin K effect. Nutritional supplements in the United States do not contain
MK-4.

In the absence of long-term interventional
studies using nutritionally optimal doses of vitamin K, evidence of a relationship between vitamin K nutritional status and bone health in
adults is considered weak. Further investigation is required to determine the physiological
function of vitamin K–dependent proteins in
bone and the mechanisms by which vitamin K
affects bone health and osteoporotic fracture
risk.[6]

Vascular Calcification and Cardiovascular Disease

One of the hallmarks of cardiovascular disease
is the formation of atherosclerotic plaques in
arterial walls. Calcification of atherosclerotic
plaques occurs as the condition progresses, resulting in decreased elasticity of the affected
vessels and increased risk of clot formation,
the usual cause of a heart attack or stroke. One
study of postmenopausal women found low
dietary vitamin K intake to be associated with
increased risk of aortic calcification, as visualized by chest X-ray.[27] Additionally, laboratory
tests examining the vitamin K–dependent γ-
carboxylation of osteocalcin indicated that elevated blood levels of ucOC were also associated with increased aortic calcification.
The mechanism by which vitamin K may promote mineralization of bone, while inhibiting
mineralization (calcification) of vessels, is not
entirely clear. One hypothesis is based on the
function of two different bone proteins,
osteocalcin and MGP. MGP has been found to
inhibit the calcification of cartilage and bone
during early embryonic development.
Osteocalcin appears later during bone
development and appears to promote bone
mineralization. Some investigators have hypothesized that high levels of MGP found in
calcified vessels may represent a defense
against vessel calcification but that inadequate
vitamin K nutritional status results in inadequate carboxylation, and presumably inactive
MGP. Thus, insufficient dietary vitamin K may
increase the risk of vascular calcification.[28] It
should be noted that this line of reasoning is
based on animal research and only one epidemiologic study in humans. Further investigations are necessary to establish the nature
of the role of bone proteins in human atherosclerotic plaque calcification.

Disease Treatment

Presently, there is insufficient evidence to support the use of vitamin K to treat diseases or
health conditions other than vitamin K deficiency, which should be treated under medical
supervision.

Sources

Food Sources

Phylloquinone (vitamin K_1) is the major dietary form of vitamin K. Green leafy vegetables
and some vegetable oils (soybean, cottonseed,
canola, and olive) are major contributors of dietary vitamin K. Hydrogenation of vegetable
oils may decrease the absorption and biological effect of dietary vitamin K.[29] Early analyses
of the vitamin K content of foods tended to be
overestimates, and older nutritional texts and
tables report higher values.[3] More accurate
analyses have been used in the compilation of
a new table of the vitamin K content of foods. A
number of good sources of vitamin K are listed
in Table 13–2 along with their vitamin K content in micrograms.

Intestinal Bacteria

Bacteria that normally colonize the large intestine synthesize menaquinones (vitamin K_2),
an active form of vitamin K. Until recently it
was thought that up to 50 % of the human vitamin K requirement might be met by bacterial
synthesis. Recent research indicates that the
contribution of bacterial synthesis is much less
than previously thought, although the exact
contribution remains unclear.[30]

Table 13–2 Food Sources of Vitamin K

Food	Serving	Vitamin K, μg
Kale, raw	1 cup, chopped	547
Broccoli, cooked	1 cup, chopped	420
Parsley, raw	1 cup, chopped	324
Swiss chard, raw	1 cup, chopped	299
Spinach, raw	1 cup, chopped	120
Leaf lettuce, raw	1 cup, shredded	118
Watercress, raw	1 cup, chopped	85
Soybean oil	1 tablespoon	26.1
Canola oil	1 tablespoon	19.7
Mayonnaise	1 tablespoon	11.9
Olive oil	1 tablespoon	6.6

Supplements

In the United States vitamin K is available over the counter in multivitamin and other supplements in doses that generally range from 10 to 120 μg/dose.[31] Menatetranone (MK-4) is used to treat osteoporosis in Japan but is not available as a supplement in the United States.

Safety

Toxicity

Although allergic reaction is possible, there is no known toxicity associated with high doses of phylloquinone (vitamin K_1) or menaquinone (vitamin K_2) forms of vitamin K.[17] The same is not true for menadione (vitamin K_3) and its derivatives. Menadione can interfere with the function of glutathione, one of the body's natural antioxidants, resulting in oxidative damage to cell membranes. Menadione given by injection has induced liver toxicity, jaundice, and hemolytic anemia (due to the rupture of red blood cells) in infants and is no longer used for treatment of vitamin K deficiency.[5,7] No tolerable upper intake level has been established for vitamin K.

Drug Interactions

The anticoagulant effect of vitamin K antagonists (e.g., warfarin) may be inhibited by very high dietary or supplemental vitamin K intake. It is generally recommended that individuals using warfarin try to consume the AI for vitamin K (90 to 120 μg) while avoiding large fluctuations in vitamin K intake that might interfere with the adjustment of their anticoagulant dose.[8] Large doses of vitamin A and vitamin E have been found to antagonize vitamin K. Excess vitamin A appears to interfere with vitamin K absorption, while a form of vitamin E (tocopherol quinone) may inhibit vitamin K–dependent carboxylase enzymes. Bleeding was reported in a man taking 5 mg of warfarin and 1200 IU of vitamin E daily.[7] When given to pregnant women, warfarin, anticonvulsants, rifampin, and isoniazid can interfere with fetal vitamin K synthesis and place the newborn at increased risk of vitamin K deficiency.[12]

Prolonged use of broad-spectrum antibiotics may decrease vitamin K synthesis by intestinal bacteria. Cephalosporins and salicylates may decrease vitamin K recycling by inhibiting vitamin K epoxide reductase. Cholestyramine, cholestipol, orlistat, mineral oil, and the fat substitute olestra may decrease vitamin K absorption.[31]

LPI Recommendation

Although the AI for vitamin K was recently increased, it is not clear if it will be enough to optimize the γ-carboxylation of vitamin K–dependent proteins in bone. Multivitamins generally contain 10 to 25 μg of vitamin K, and vitamin K or "bone" supplements may contain 100 to 120 μg of vitamin K. To consume the amount of vitamin K associated with a decreased risk of hip fracture in the Framingham Heart Study (about 250 μg/d), an individual would need to eat a little more than $^1/_2$ cup of chopped broccoli or a large salad of mixed greens every day. Though the dietary intake of vitamin K required for optimal function of all vitamin K–dependent proteins is not yet known, the Linus Pauling Institute recommends taking a multivitamin/mineral supplement and eating at least 1 cup of dark green leafy vegetables daily. Replacing dietary saturated fats like butter and cheese with monounsaturated fats found in olive oil and canola oil will also increase dietary vitamin K intake and may also decrease the risk of cardiovascular diseases.

> **Older Adults**
> Because adults 65 years and older are at increased risk of osteoporosis and hip fracture, the above recommendation for a multivitamin/mineral supplement and at least 1 cup of dark green leafy vegetables per day is especially relevant.

References

1. Brody T. *Nutritional Biochemistry*, 2nd ed. San Diego: Academic Press; 1999.
2. Shearer MJ. Vitamin K. *Lancet* 1995;345(8944):229–234.
3. Booth SL, Suttie JW. Dietary intake and adequacy of vitamin K. *J Nutr* 1998;128(5):785–788.
4. Furie B, Bouchard BA, Furie BC. Vitamin K-dependent biosynthesis of gamma-carboxyglutamic acid. *Blood* 1999;93(6):1798–1808.
5. Suttie JW. Vitamin K. In: Ziegler EE, Filer LJ, eds. *Present Knowledge in Nutrition*, 7th ed. Washington, D.C.: ILSI Press; 1996:137–145.
6. Shearer MJ. The roles of vitamins D and K in bone health and osteoporosis prevention. *Proc Nutr Soc* 1997;56(3):915–937.
7. Olson RE. Vitamin K. In: Shils M, Olson JA, Shike M, Ross AC, eds. *Nutrition in Health and Disease*, 9th ed. Baltimore: Williams & Wilkins; 1999:363–380.
8. Booth SL, Centurelli MA. Vitamin K: a practical guide to the dietary management of patients on warfarin. *Nutr Rev* 1999;57(9 Pt 1):288–296.
9. Booth SL. Skeletal functions of vitamin K-dependent proteins: not just for clotting anymore. *Nutr Rev* 1997;55(7):282–284.
10. Ferland G. The vitamin K–dependent proteins: an update. *Nutr Rev* 1998;56(8):223–230.
11. Tsaioun KI. Vitamin K-dependent proteins in the developing and aging nervous system. *Nutr Rev* 1999;57(8):231–240.
12. Thorp JA, Gaston L, Caspers DR, Pal ML. Current concepts and controversies in the use of vitamin K. *Drugs* 1995;49(3):376–387.
13. Klebanoff MA, Read JS, Mills JL, Shiono PH. The risk of childhood cancer after neonatal exposure to vitamin K. *N Engl J Med* 1993;329(13):905–908.
14. Ekelund H, Finnstrom O, Gunnarskog J, Kallen B, Larsson Y. Administration of vitamin K to newborn infants and childhood cancer. *BMJ* 1993;307(6896):89–91.
15. Roman E, Fear NT, Ansell P, et al. Vitamin K and childhood cancer: analysis of individual patient data from six case-control studies. *Br J Cancer* 2002;86(1):63–69.
16. American Academy of Pediatrics Vitamin K Ad Hoc Task Force. Controversies concerning vitamin K and the newborn. *Pediatrics* 1993;91(5):1001–1003.
17. Food and Nutrition Board, Institute of Medicine. Vitamin K. *Dietary Reference Intakes for Vitamin A, Vitamin K, Arsenic, Boron, Chromium, Copper, Iodine, Iron, Manganese, Molybdenum, Nickel, Silicon, Vanadium, and Zinc*. Washington, D.C.: National Academy Press; 2001:162–196.
18. Feskanich D, Weber P, Willett WC, Rockett H, Booth SL, Colditz GA. Vitamin K intake and hip fractures in women: a prospective study. *Am J Clin Nutr* 1999;69(1):74–79.
19. Booth SL, Tucker KL, Chen H, et al. Dietary vitamin K intakes are associated with hip fracture but not with bone mineral density in elderly men and women. *Am J Clin Nutr* 2000;71(5):1201–1208.
20. Booth SL, Mayer J. Warfarin use and fracture risk. *Nutr Rev* 2000;58(1):20–22.
21. Szulc P, Chapuy MC, Meunier PJ, Delmas PD. Serum undercarboxylated osteocalcin is a marker of the risk of hip fracture in elderly women. *J Clin Invest* 1993;91(4):1769–1774.
22. Jamal SA, Browner WS, Bauer DC, Cummings SR. Warfarin use and risk for osteoporosis in elderly women. Study of Osteoporotic Fractures Research Group. *Ann Intern Med* 1998;128(10):829–832.
23. Caraballo PJ, Heit JA, Atkinson EJ, et al. Long-term use of oral anticoagulants and the risk of fracture. *Arch Intern Med* 1999;159(15):1750–1756.
24. Caraballo PJ, Gabriel SE, Castro MR, Atkinson EJ, Melton LJ, 3rd. Changes in bone density after exposure to oral anticoagulants: a meta-analysis. *Osteoporos Int* 1999;9(5):441–448.
25. Iwamoto J, Takeda T, Ichimura S. Effect of menatetrenone on bone mineral density and incidence of vertebral fractures in postmenopausal women with osteoporosis: a comparison with the effect of etidronate. *J Orthop Sci* 2001;6(6):487–492.
26. Vermeer C, Jie KS, Knapen MH. Role of vitamin K in bone metabolism. *Annu Rev Nutr* 1995;15:1–22.
27. Jie KS, Bots ML, Vermeer C, Witteman JC, Grobbee DE. Vitamin K intake and osteocalcin levels in women with and without aortic atherosclerosis: a population-based study. *Atherosclerosis* 1995;116(1):117–123.
28. Schurgers LJ, Dissel PE, Spronk HM, et al. Role of vitamin K and vitamin K-dependent proteins in vascular calcification. *Z Kardiol* 2001;90(Suppl 3):57–63.
29. Booth SL, Lichtenstein AH, O'Brien-Morse M, et al. Effects of a hydrogenated form of vitamin K on bone formation and resorption. *Am J Clin Nutr* 2001;74(6):783–790.
30. Suttie JW. The importance of menaquinones in human nutrition. *Annu Rev Nutr* 1995;15:399–417.
31. Hendler SS, Rorvik DR, eds. *PDR for Nutritional Supplements*. Montvale, NJ: Medical Economics Company, Inc; 2001.

14 Calcium

Calcium is the most common mineral in the human body. About 99% of the calcium in the body is found in bones and teeth, and the other 1% is found in the blood and soft tissue. Calcium levels in the blood and fluid surrounding the cells (extracellular fluid) must be maintained within a very narrow concentration range for normal physiological functioning. The physiological functions of calcium are so vital to survival that the body will demineralize bone to maintain normal blood calcium levels when calcium intake is inadequate. Thus, adequate dietary calcium is a critical factor in maintaining a healthy skeleton.[1]

Function

Structure

Calcium is a major structural element in bones and teeth. The mineral component of bone consists mainly of hydroxyapatite crystals, which contain large amounts of calcium and phosphorus (about 40% calcium and 60% phosphorus).[2] Bone is a dynamic tissue that is remodeled throughout life. Bone cells called *osteoclasts* begin the process of remodeling by dissolving or resorbing bone. Bone-forming cells called *osteoblasts* then synthesize new bone to replace the bone that was resorbed. During normal growth, bone formation exceeds bone resorption. Osteoporosis may result when bone resorption exceeds formation.[1]

Cell Signaling

Calcium plays a role in mediating the constriction and relaxation of blood vessels (vasoconstriction and vasodilation), nerve impulse transmission, muscle contraction, and the secretion of hormones, such as insulin.[3] Excitable cells, such as skeletal muscle and nerve cells, contain voltage-dependent calcium channels in their cell membranes that allow for rapid changes in calcium concentrations. For example, when a muscle fiber receives a nerve impulse that stimulates it to contract, calcium channels in the cell membrane open to allow a few calcium ions into the muscle cell. These calcium ions bind to activator proteins within the cell that release a flood of calcium ions from storage vesicles inside the cell. The binding of calcium to the protein troponin-c initiates a series of steps that lead to muscle contraction. The binding of calcium to the protein calmodulin activates enzymes that break down muscle glycogen to provide energy for muscle contraction.[1]

Cofactor for Enzymes and Proteins

Calcium is necessary to stabilize or allow for optimal activity of a number of proteins and enzymes. The binding of calcium ions is required for the activation of the seven "vitamin K–dependent" clotting factors in the coagulation cascade. The term *coagulation cascade* refers to a series of events, each dependent on the other that stops bleeding through clot formation.[4]

Regulation of Calcium Levels

Calcium concentrations in the blood and fluid that surrounds cells are tightly controlled to preserve normal physiological functioning (Fig. 14–1). When blood calcium decreases (e.g., in the case of inadequate calcium intake), calcium-sensing proteins in the parathyroid glands send signals resulting in the secretion of parathyroid hormone (PTH).[5] PTH stimulates the conversion of vitamin D to its active form, calcitriol, in the kidneys. Calcitriol increases the absorption of calcium from the small intestine. Together with PTH, calcitriol stimulates the release of calcium from bone by activating osteoclasts (bone-resorbing cells) and decreases the urinary excretion of calcium by increasing its reabsorption in the kidneys.

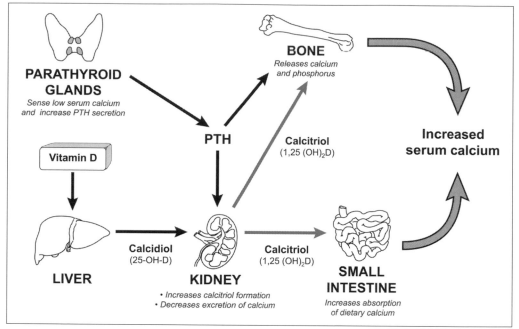

Figure 14–1. Regulation of serum calcium. Calcium-sensing proteins in the parathyroid glands sense serum calcium levels. In response to slight declines in serum calcium, the parathyroid glands secrete para-thyroid hormone (PTH). PTH stimulates the activity of the 1-hydroxylase enzyme in the kidney, resulting in increased production of calcitriol, the biologically active form of vitamin D. Calcitriol acts to restore normal serum calcium levels in three ways: (1) by activating the vitamin D–dependent transport system in the small intestine, increasing the absorption of dietary calcium; (2) by increasing the mobilization of calcium from bone into the circulation; and (3) by increasing the reabsorption of calcium by the kidneys. PTH is also required to increase bone calcium mobilization and calcium reabsorption by the kidneys.

When blood calcium rises to normal levels, the parathyroid glands stop secreting PTH and the kidneys begin to excrete any excess calcium in the urine. Although this complex system allows for rapid and tight control of blood calcium levels, it does so at the expense of the skeleton.[1]

Deficiency

A low blood calcium level usually implies abnormal parathyroid function and is rarely due to low dietary calcium intake as the skeleton provides a large reserve of calcium for maintaining normal blood levels. Other causes of abnormally low blood calcium levels include chronic kidney failure, vitamin D deficiency, and low blood magnesium levels that occur mainly in cases of severe alcoholism. Magne-sium deficiency results in a decrease in the responsiveness of osteoclasts to PTH. A chronically low calcium intake in growing individuals may prevent the attainment of optimal peak bone mass. Once peak bone mass is achieved, inadequate calcium intake may contribute to accelerated bone loss and ultimately the development of osteoporosis.[1]

Nutrient Interactions

Vitamin D is required for optimal calcium absorption. Several other nutrients (and non-nutrients) influence the retention of calcium by the body and may affect calcium nutritional status.

Sodium. Increased sodium intake results in increased loss of calcium in the urine, possibly due to competition between sodium and calcium for reabsorption in the kidney or by an effect of sodium on PTH secretion. Each 2.3-g increment of sodium (5.8 g of salt; NaCl) excreted by the kidney has been found to draw about 24 to 40 mg of calcium into the urine. Because urinary losses account for about half of the difference in calcium retention among individuals, dietary sodium has a large potential to influence bone loss. In adult women, each extra gram of sodium consumed per day is projected to produce an additional rate of bone loss of 1% per year if all of the calcium loss comes from the skeleton. Although animal studies have shown bone loss to be greater with high salt intakes, no controlled clinical trials have been conducted to confirm the relationship between salt intake and bone loss in humans.[1,6] However, a 2-year study of postmenopausal women found increased urinary sodium excretion (an indicator of increased sodium intake) to be associated with decreased bone mineral density at the hip.[7]

Protein. As dietary protein intake increases, the urinary excretion of calcium also increases. Recommended calcium intakes for the U.S. population are higher than those for populations of less industrialized nations because protein intake in the United States is generally higher. The U.S. recommended dietary allowance (RDA) for protein is 46 to 50 g/d for adult women and 58 to 63 g/d for adult men. However, the average intake of protein in the United States tends to be higher (65 to 70 g/d in adult women and 90 to 110 g/d in adult men).[3] Weaver and colleagues have calculated that each additional gram of protein results in an additional loss of 1.75 mg of calcium per day. Because only 30% of dietary calcium is generally absorbed, each 1-g increase in protein intake per day would require an additional 5.8 mg of calcium per day to offset the calcium loss.[8] At the other end of the spectrum of protein intake, the effect of dietary protein insufficiency on bone health has received much less attention. Inadequate protein intakes have been associated with poor recovery from osteoporotic fractures, and serum albumin values (an indicator of protein nutritional status) have been found to be inversely related to hip fracture risk.[3]

Phosphorus. Phosphorus, which is typically found in protein-rich foods, tends to decrease the excretion of calcium in the urine. However, phosphorus-rich foods also tend to increase the calcium content of digestive secretions, resulting in increased calcium loss in the feces. Thus, phosphorus does not offset the net loss of calcium associated with increased protein intake.[1] Increasing intakes of phosphates from soft drinks and food additives have caused concern among some researchers regarding the implications for bone health. Diets high in phosphorus and low in calcium have been found to increase PTH secretion, as have diets low in calcium.[3,6] Although the effect of high phosphorus intakes on calcium balance and bone health are presently unclear, the substitution of large quantities of soft drinks for milk or other sources of dietary calcium is cause for concern with respect to bone health in adolescents and adults.

Caffeine. Caffeine in large amounts increases urinary calcium for a short time. However, caffeine intakes of 400 mg/d did not significantly change urinary calcium excretion over 24 hours in premenopausal women when compared with a placebo.[9] Although one observational study found accelerated bone loss in postmenopausal women who consumed less than 744 mg of calcium per day and reported that they drank 2 to 3 cups of coffee per day,[10] a more recent study that measured caffeine intake found no association between caffeine intake and bone loss in postmenopausal women.[11] On average, one 8-ounce cup of coffee decreases calcium retention by only 2 to 3 mg.[1]

The Adequate Intake Level

Updated recommendations for calcium intake based on the optimization of bone health were released by the Food and Nutrition Board (FNB) of the Institute of Medicine in 1997 (Table 14–1). The setting of an adequate intake level (AI) rather than an RDA for calcium reflects the difficulty of estimating the intake of dietary calcium that will result in optimal accumulation and retention of calcium in the skeleton when other factors such as genetics, hormones, and physical activity also interact to affect bone health.[3]

Table 14–1   Adequate Intake (AI) for Calcium

Life Stage	Age	Males, mg/d	Females, mg/d
Infants	0–6 months	210	210
Infants	7–12 months	270	270
Children	1–3 years	500	500
Children	4–8 years	800	800
Children	9–13 years	1300	1300
Adolescents	14–18 years	1300	1300
Adults	19–50 years	1000	1000
Adults	51 years and older	1200	1200
Pregnancy	18 years and younger	–	1300
Pregnancy	19 years and older	–	1000
Breast-feeding	18 years and younger	–	1300
Breast-feeding	19 years and older	–	1000

Disease Prevention

Colorectal Cancer

Colorectal cancer is the most common gastrointestinal cancer and the second leading cause of cancer deaths in the United States. Colorectal cancer is caused by a combination of genetic and environmental factors, but the degree to which these two factors influence the risk of colon cancer in individuals varies widely. In individuals with familial adenomatous polyposis, the cause of colon cancer is thought to be almost entirely genetic, although dietary factors appear to influence the risk of colon cancer in others. Animal studies are strongly supportive of a protective role for calcium in intestinal cancers.[12] In humans, controlled clinical trials have found modest decreases in the recurrence of colorectal adenomas (precancerous polyps) with calcium supplementation of 1200 to 2000 mg/d.[13,14] However, most large prospective studies have found increased calcium intake to be only weakly associated with a decreased risk of colorectal cancer. These weak associations might be explained by the presence of groups within the population that differ in their response to calcium. A recent case-control study of 511 men found that increased calcium intake was more strongly associated with decreased colorectal cancer risk in those men with higher circulating levels of a growth factor known as insulin-like growth factor–1 (IGF-1).[15] There is some evidence that individuals with increased circulating levels of IGF-1 are at increased risk of colorectal cancer, and increased calcium intake may benefit this subgroup more than others. Before conclusions can be drawn, more research is needed to clarify whether specific subgroups in the larger population have different calcium requirements with respect to decreasing the risk of colorectal cancer.

Osteoporosis

Osteoporosis is a skeletal disorder in which bone strength is compromised, resulting in an increased risk of fracture. Sustaining a hip fracture is one of the most serious consequences of osteoporosis. Nearly one third of those who sustain osteoporotic hip fractures enter nursing homes within the year following the fracture, and one person in five dies within 1 year of sustaining an osteoporotic hip fracture. Although osteoporosis is most commonly diagnosed in white postmenopausal women, women of other racial groups and ages, men, and children may also develop osteoporosis.[16]

Osteoporosis is a multifactorial disorder, and nutrition is only one factor contributing to its development and progression.[2] Other factors that increase the risk of developing osteoporosis include, but are not limited to, increased age, female gender, estrogen deficiency, smoking, metabolic disease (e.g., hyperthyroidism), and the use of certain medications (e.g., corticosteroids and anticonvulsants). A predisposition to osteoporotic fracture is related to one's peak bone mass and to the rate of bone loss after peak bone mass has been attained. After adult height has been reached, the skeleton continues to accumulate bone until the third decade of life. Genetic factors exert a strong influence on peak bone mass, but lifestyle factors can also play a significant role. Strategies for reducing the risk of osteoporotic fracture include the attainment of maximal peak bone mass and the reduction of bone loss later in life. Although, calcium is the nutrient consistently found to be most important for attaining peak bone mass and preventing osteoporosis, adequate vitamin D intake is also required for optimal calcium absorption.[16]

Physical exercise is another lifestyle factor of benefit in the prevention of osteoporosis and osteoporotic fracture. There is evidence to suggest that physical activity early in life contributes to the attainment of higher peak bone mass. Exercise in the presence of adequate calcium and vitamin D intake probably has a modest effect on slowing the rate of bone loss later in life. One compilation of published calcium trials indicated that the beneficial skeletal effect of increased physical activity was achievable only at calcium intakes above 1000 mg/d.[17] High-impact exercise and resistance exercise (weights) are likely the most beneficial for reducing bone loss. Lower-impact exercises like walking, swimming, and cycling have beneficial effects on other aspects of health and function, but their effects on bone loss have been minimal. However, exercise later in life, even beyond 90 years of age, can still increase strength and reduce the likelihood of a fall, another important risk factor for hip fracture.[16]

Supplemental calcium alone cannot usually restore lost bone in individuals with osteoporosis. However, optimal treatment of osteoporosis with any drug therapy also requires adequate intake of calcium (1200 mg/d) and vitamin D (600 IU/d).[2,16]

Kidney Stones

Approximately 12% of the U.S. population will have a kidney stone at some time. Most kidney stones are composed of calcium oxalate or calcium phosphate. Although their cause is usually unknown, abnormally elevated urinary calcium (hypercalciuria) increases the risk of developing calcium stones. Increasing dietary calcium increases urinary calcium slightly, and the rise is more pronounced in those with hypercalciuria. However, other dietary factors such as sodium and protein are also known to increase urinary calcium.[18,19] A large prospec-

tive epidemiologic study that followed men over a period of 12 years found the incidence of symptomatic kidney stones to be 44% lower in men in the highest quintile (1/5) of calcium intake, averaging 1326 mg/d, compared with men in the lowest quintile of calcium intake, averaging 516 mg/d.[20] Similar results were observed in a large prospective study of women over 4 years.[21] The authors of the two epidemiologic studies suggested that increased dietary calcium might inhibit the absorption of dietary oxalate and reduce urinary oxalate, a risk factor for calcium oxalate stones. Support for this idea comes from a study in which people ingested oxalic acid with or without supplemental calcium.[22] Providing 200 mg of elemental calcium along with the oxalic acid significantly reduced its absorption and urinary oxalate excretion.

Although calcium stone formers have been advised to restrict calcium intake in the past, a cross-sectional study of 282 patients with calcium oxalate stones found that dietary salt, as measured by urinary sodium excretion, was the dietary factor most strongly associated with urinary calcium excretion.[23] A study of 85 calcium stone–forming patients found that those with low bone mineral density were significantly more likely to have higher salt intake and higher urinary sodium excretion, leading the authors to suggest that reduced salt intake should be recommended for calcium stone–forming patients.[24] Findings that calcium stone–forming patients with lower calcium intakes are more likely to have decreased bone mineral density also call into question the therapeutic use of dietary calcium restriction. At present, the only dietary change proven effective in reducing kidney stone recurrence is increasing fluid intake, although no controlled clinical trials of calcium supplementation or restriction have been reported in the literature.[1,18]

Pregnancy-Induced Hypertension

Pregnancy-induced hypertension (PIH) occurs in 10% of pregnancies and is a major health risk for pregnant women and their unborn children. PIH is a term that includes gestational hypertension, preeclampsia, and eclampsia. Gestational hypertension is defined as an abnormally high blood pressure that usually develops after the 20th week of pregnancy. In addition to gestational hypertension, preeclampsia includes the development of edema (severe swelling) and proteinuria (protein in the urine). Preeclampsia may progress to eclampsia (also called toxemia) in which life-threatening convulsions and coma may occur.[25] Although the cause of PIH is not entirely understood, calcium metabolism appears to play a role. Risk factors for PIH include first pregnancies, multiple gestations (e.g., twins or triplets), chronic high blood pressure, diabetes, and some autoimmune diseases. Data from epidemiologic studies suggest an inverse relationship between calcium intake and the incidence of PIH, but the results of experimental research on calcium supplementation and PIH have been less clear. A systematic review of randomized placebo-controlled studies found that calcium supplementation reduced the incidence of high blood pressure in pregnant women at high risk of PIH, as well as in pregnant women with low dietary calcium intake. However, in women at low risk of PIH and with adequate calcium intake the benefit of calcium supplementation was judged small and unlikely to be clinically significant.[26] A large multicenter clinical trial of Calcium for Preeclampsia Prevention in over 4500 pregnant women found no effect of 2000 mg/d of supplemental calcium on PIH. However, women in the placebo group had a mean intake of 980 mg/d, while those in the supplemental group had a mean intake of 2300 mg/d.[27] For the general population, meeting current recommendations for calcium intake during pregnancy may also help prevent PIH. Further research is required to determine whether women at high risk for PIH would benefit from calcium supplementation above the current recommendations.

Lead Toxicity

Children who are chronically exposed to lead, even in small amounts, are more likely to develop learning disabilities and behavioral problems and to have low IQs. Abnormal growth and neurological development may occur in the infants of women exposed to lead during pregnancy. In adults, lead toxicity may

result in kidney damage and high blood pressure. Although the use of lead paint and leaded gasoline has been discontinued in the United States, lead toxicity continues to be a significant health problem, especially in children living in urban areas. A study of over 300 children aged 1 through 8 years in an urban neighborhood found that 49% had blood lead levels above current guidelines, indicating excessive lead exposure, and only 59% of children ages 1 to 3 years and 41% of children ages 4 to 8 years had calcium intakes meeting the recommended levels.[28] Adequate calcium intake appears to be protective against lead toxicity in at least two ways. Increased dietary intake of calcium is known to decrease the gastrointestinal absorption of lead. Once lead enters the body it tends to accumulate in the skeleton, where its may remain for more than 20 years. Adequate calcium intake also prevents exposure to lead mobilized from the skeleton during bone demineralization. A recent study of blood lead levels during pregnancy found that women with inadequate calcium intake during the second half of pregnancy were more likely to have elevated blood lead levels, probably related to increased bone demineralization with the release of accumulated lead into the blood.[29] Lead in the blood of a pregnant woman is readily transported across the placenta resulting in fetal lead exposure at a time when the developing nervous system is highly vulnerable. In postmenopausal women, increased calcium intake was associated with decreased blood lead levels, along with other factors known to decrease bone demineralization, for example, estrogen replacement therapy and physical activity.[30]

Disease Treatment

Hypertension

The relationship between calcium intake and blood pressure has been investigated extensively over the past two decades. An analysis of 23 large observational studies found a reduction in systolic blood pressure of 0.34 mm of mercury (mm Hg) per 100 mg of calcium consumed daily and a reduction in diastolic blood pressure of 0.15 mm Hg per 100 mg calcium.[31]

A large systematic review of 42 randomized clinical trials examining the effect of calcium supplementation on blood pressure compared with placebo found an overall reduction of 1.44 mm Hg in systolic blood pressure and a reduction of 0.84 mm Hg in diastolic blood pressure.[32] Calcium supplementation in these randomized clinical trials ranged from 500 to 2000 mg/d, with 1000 to 1500 mg/d being the most common dose. In the Dietary Approaches to Stop Hypertension (DASH) study, 549 people were randomized to one of three diets for 8 weeks: (1) a control diet that was low in fruit, vegetables, and dairy products; (2) a diet rich in fruits (approximately five servings per day) and vegetables (approximately three servings per day); and (3) a combination diet rich in fruits and vegetables and low-fat dairy products (approximately three servings per day).[33] The combination diet represented an increase of about 800 mg of calcium per day over the control and fruit/vegetable-rich diets for a total of about 1200 mg of calcium per day. The combination diet reduced systolic blood pressure 5.5 mm Hg and diastolic blood pressure 3 mm Hg more than the control diet, and the fruit/vegetable diet reduced systolic blood pressure 2.8 mm Hg and diastolic blood pressure 1.1 mm Hg more than the control diet. Among those participants diagnosed with hypertension, the combination diet reduced systolic blood pressure by 11.4 mm Hg and diastolic pressure by 5.5 mm Hg more than the control diet, and the reduction for the fruit/vegetable diet was 7.2 mm Hg systolic and 2.8 mm Hg diastolic compared with the control diet.[34] This research indicates that a calcium intake at the recommended level (1000 to 1200 mg/d) may be helpful in preventing and treating moderate hypertension.[35]

Sources

Food Sources

Average dietary intakes of calcium in the United States are well below the levels recommended by the FNB for every age and gender group, especially in females. Only about 25% of boys and 10% of girls ages 9 to 17 are estimated to meet the FNB recommendations. Dairy foods provide 75% of the calcium in the American diet. However, it is typically during the most critical period for peak bone mass development that adolescents tend to replace milk with soft drinks.[1,3]

Although dairy products represent a rich and absorbable source of calcium, certain vegetables and grains also provide calcium. However, the bioavailability of that calcium must be taken into consideration. Although the calcium-rich plants in the kale family (broccoli, bok choy, cabbage, mustard, and turnip greens) contain calcium that is as bioavailable as milk, some food components have been found to inhibit the absorption of calcium. Oxalic acid, also known as *oxalate*, is the most potent inhibitor of calcium absorption and is found in high concentrations in spinach and rhubarb and somewhat lower concentrations in sweet potato and dried beans. Phytic acid is a less potent inhibitor of calcium absorption than oxalic acid. Yeast possess an enzyme (phytase) that breaks down phytic acid in grains during fermentation, lowering the phytic acid content of breads and other fermented foods. Only concentrated sources of phytate such as wheat bran or dried beans substantially reduce calcium absorption.[1] Table 14–2 lists a number of calcium-rich foods, along with their calcium content, the percent of that calcium that is generally absorbed, the estimated absorbable calcium from that food, and the number of servings of that food required to equal the absorbable calcium from one glass of milk.[8]

Supplements

Most experts recommend obtaining as much calcium as possible from foods, because calcium in foods is accompanied by other important nutrients that assist the body in utilizing calcium. However, calcium supplements may be necessary for those who have difficulty consuming enough calcium from foods. No multivitamin/multimineral tablet contains 100% of the recommended daily value for calcium because it is too bulky and the resulting pill would be too large to swallow. Calcium supplements come in several forms (calcium salts), but only part of the calcium salt is elemental calcium. All supplement labels in the United

Table 14–2   Food Sources and Relative Absorbability of Calcium[8]

Food	Serving	Elemental Calcium, mg	% Calcium Absorbed	Estimated Absorbable Calcium, mg	Servings Needed to Equal 8 Ounces of Milk*
Milk	8 ounces	300	32	96	1.0
Cheddar cheese	1.5 ounces	303	32	97	1.0
Yogurt	8 ounces	300	32	96	1.0
Tofu, calcium set	1/2 cup	258	31	80	1.2
Cheese food	1.5 ounces	241	32	77	1.2
Chinese cabbage	1/2 cup, cooked	239	40	95	1.0
Rhubarb	1/2 cup, cooked	174	9	10	9.5
Spinach	1/2 cup, cooked	115	5	6	16.3
White beans	1/2 cup, cooked	113	22	25	3.9
Bok choy	1/2 cup, cooked	79	54	43	2.3
Kale	1/2 cup, cooked	61	49	30	3.2
Pinto beans	1/2 cup, cooked	45	27	12	8.1
Red beans	1/2 cup, cooked	41	24	10	9.7
Broccoli	1/2 cup, cooked	35	61	22	4.5

Reproduced with permission by the *American Journal of Clinical Nutrition*. © Am J Clin Nutr. American Society for Clinical Nutrition.
*All other foods are compared with milk in terms of calcium availability.

States list the elemental calcium content in milligrams and refer to it as calcium. Some also list the calcium salt content (e.g., calcium carbonate) in milligrams. The formulas below may be used to calculate the amount of elemental calcium in a supplement from its calcium salt content.[36]

- *Calcium carbonate* (40% elemental calcium) multiply mg of calcium carbonate by 0.40 (*Example*: 500 mg calcium carbonate × 0.40 = 200 mg elemental calcium)
- *Calcium citrate* (21% elemental calcium) multiply by 0.21 (*Example*: 950 mg of calcium citrate × 0.21 = 200 mg elemental calcium)
- *Calcium lactate* (13% elemental calcium) multiply by 0.13 (*Example*: 1550 mg of calcium lactate × 0.13 = 200 mg elemental calcium)
- *Calcium gluconate* (9% elemental calcium) multiply by 0.09 (*Example*: 2200 mg of cal-

cium gluconate × 0.09 = 200 mg of elemental calcium)

To maximize absorption, take no more than 500 mg of elemental calcium at one time. Most calcium supplements should be taken with meals, although calcium citrate can be taken anytime.

Lead in Calcium Supplements

Several years ago concern was raised regarding the lead levels in calcium supplements obtained from natural sources (oyster shell, bone meal, dolomite). In 1993 investigators found measurable quantities of lead in most of the 70 different preparations they tested.[37] Since then manufacturers have made an effort to reduce the amount of lead in calcium supplements to less than 0.5 μg/1000 mg of elemental calcium. The federal limit is 7.5 μg/1000 mg elemental calcium. Because lead is so widespread and long lasting on earth, no one can guarantee entirely lead-free food or supplements. A recent study found measurable lead in 8 of 21 supplements, in amounts averaging between 1 and 2 μg/1000 mg of elemental calcium.[38] Calcium inhibits intestinal absorption of lead, and adequate calcium intake is protective against lead toxicity, so trace amounts of lead in calcium supplementation may pose less of a risk of excessive lead exposure than inadequate calcium consumption. Although most calcium sources today are relatively safe, looking for supplements that are labeled "lead-free" and avoiding large doses of supplemental calcium (more than 1500 mg/d) are ways to avoid incidental lead exposure.

Safety

Toxicity

Abnormally elevated blood calcium (hypercalcemia) resulting from the over consumption of calcium has never been documented to occur from foods, only from calcium supplements. Mild hypercalcemia may be without symptoms, or may result in loss of appetite, nausea, vomiting, constipation, abdominal pain, dry mouth, thirst, and frequent urination. More severe hypercalcemia may result in confusion, delirium, coma, and, if not treated, death. Hypercalcemia has been reported only with the consumption of large quantities of calcium supplements usually in combination with antacids, particularly in the days when peptic ulcers were treated with large quantities of milk, calcium carbonate (antacid), and sodium bicarbonate (absorbable alkalai).[1] This condition was termed *milk alkalai syndrome* and has been reported at calcium supplement levels from 1.5 to 16.5 g/d for 2 days to 30 years. Since the treatment for peptic ulcers has changed, the incidence of this syndrome has decreased considerably.[3]

Although the risk of forming kidney stones is increased in individuals with abnormally elevated urinary calcium (hypercalciuria), this condition is not usually related to calcium intake but rather to increased excretion of calcium by the kidneys. Overall, increased dietary

Table 14–3 Tolerable Upper Intake Level (UL) for Calcium

Life Stage	Age	UL, mg/d
Infants	0–12 months	Not possible to establish*
Children	1–18 years	2500
Adults	19 years and older	2500

*Source of intake should be from food and formula only.

calcium has been associated with a decreased risk of kidney stones. However, in a large prospective study, the risk of developing kidney stones in women taking supplemental calcium was 20% higher than in those who did not.[21] This effect may be related to the fact that calcium supplements can be taken without food, eliminating their beneficial effect of decreasing intestinal oxalate absorption. Based on the adverse effects above, as well as the potential for decreased absorption of other essential minerals (see below), the FNB of the Institute of Medicine set the tolerable upper level of intake for calcium in adults at 2500 mg of calcium per day (Table 14–3).[3]

Do High Calcium Intakes Increase the Risk of Prostate Cancer?

Recent epidemiologic studies have raised concern that high calcium intakes are associated with increased risk of prostate cancer. A large prospective cohort study in the United States followed more than 50,000 male health professionals for 8 years and found that men whose calcium intake was 2000 mg/d or more had a risk of developing advanced prostate cancer that was three times higher than men whose calcium intake was less than 500 mg/d and a risk of developing metastasized prostate cancer that was more than four times greater.[39] The results of a case-control study in Sweden that compared the calcium consumption of 526 men diagnosed with prostate cancer with that of 536 controls were similar.[40] Neither study found calcium intake to be associated with an increased risk of total prostate cancer or nonadvanced prostate cancer. More recently, another prospective study of U.S. physicians found that increased intake of calcium from dairy foods was associated with an increased risk of prostate cancer.[41] Although this study did not examine supplement use, each 500 mg/d increase in calcium from dairy foods was associated with a 16% increase in the risk of prostate cancer (advanced and nonadvanced).

The physiologic mechanisms underlying the relationship between calcium intake and prostate cancer are not yet clear. High levels of dietary calcium may lead to decreased circulating levels of calcitriol, the active form of vitamin D. In experimental studies conducted in prostate cancer cell lines and animal models, calcitriol has been found to have protective effects. However, the findings of studies conducted in humans on serum calcitriol levels and prostate cancer risk have been much less consistent.

Not all epidemiologic studies have demonstrated an association between calcium intake and prostate cancer. In total, 7 of 14 case-control studies and five of nine prospective cohort studies have reported statistically significant positive associations between prostate cancer and some measure of dairy product consumption. Of those studies that have examined calcium intake, three of six case-control studies and two of four cohort studies reported statistically significant associations between prostate cancer and calcium intake.[42] One Serbian case-control study found increased calcium intake to be associated with a decreased risk of prostate cancer.[43] The lack of agreement among these studies suggests complex interactions among risk factors for prostate cancer. Until the relationship between calcium and prostate cancer is clarified, it is reasonable for men to consume a total of 1000 to 1200 mg/d of calcium (diet and supplements combined), which is the intake level recommended by the FNB.[3]

Drug Interactions

Taking calcium supplements in combination with thiazide diuretics (e.g., hydrochlorthiazide) increases the risk of developing hypercalcemia due to increased reabsorption of calcium in the kidneys. High doses of supplemental calcium could increase the likelihood of abnormal heart rhythms in people taking digitalis (digoxin) for heart failure. Calcium supplements may also decrease the efficacy of calcium channel blockers. Calcium may decrease the absorption of tetracycline- and quinolone-class antibiotics, bisphosphonates, and levothyroxine, so it is advisable to separate doses of these medications and calcium-rich foods or supplements by 2 hours. Use of H_2 blockers (e.g., cimetidine) and proton pump inhibitors (e.g., omeprazole) may decrease the absorption of calcium carbonate and calcium phosphate.[36,44]

Nutrient Interactions

The presence of calcium decreases iron absorption from nonheme sources (i.e., most supplements and food sources other than meat). However, up to 12 weeks of calcium supplementation has not been found to change iron nutritional status, probably due to a compensatory increase in iron absorption. Individuals taking iron supplements should take them 2 hours apart from calcium-rich foods or supplements to maximize iron absorption. High calcium intakes in rats have produced relative magnesium deficiencies, but calcium intake was not found to affect magnesium retention in humans.[1] Although a number of studies did not find high calcium intakes to affect zinc absorption or zinc nutritional status, a recent study in 10 men and women indicated that 600 mg of calcium consumed with a meal decreased the absorption of zinc from that meal by 50%.[45]

LPI Recommendation

The Linus Pauling Institute supports the AI recommended by the FNB. Following these recommendations should provide adequate calcium to promote skeletal health and may also decrease the risks of some chronic diseases.

Children and Adolescents

To promote the attainment of maximal peak bone mass, children and adolescents (9 to 18 years) should consume a total (diet plus supplements) of 1300 mg/d of calcium.

Adults
After adult height has been reached, the skeleton continues to accumulate bone until the third decade of life when peak bone mass is attained. To promote the attainment of maximal peak bone mass and to minimize bone loss later in life, adult men and women, 50 years of age and younger, should consume a total (diet plus supplements) of 1000 mg/d of calcium.

Older Adults
To minimize bone loss, men older than 51 years and postmenopausal women should consume a total (diet plus supplements) of 1200 mg/d of calcium. Taking a multivitamin/multimineral supplement containing at least 10 μg (400 IU)/d of vitamin D will help to ensure adequate calcium absorption (see Chapter 11, "Vitamin D").

Pregnant and Breast-Feeding Women
Pregnant and breast-feeding adolescents (under 19 years of age) should consume a total of 1300 mg/d of calcium, and pregnant and breast-feeding adults (19 to 50 years) should consume a total of 1000 mg/d of calcium.

References

1. Weaver CM, Heaney RP. Calcium. In: Shils M, Olson JA, Shike M, Ross AC, eds. Nutrition in Health and Disease, 9th ed. Baltimore: Williams & Wilkins; 1999:141–155.
2. Heaney RP. Calcium, dairy products and osteoporosis. J Am Coll Nutr 2000;19(2 Suppl):83S–99S.
3. Food and Nutrition Board, Institute of Medicine. Calcium. Dietary Reference Intakes: Calcium, Phosphorus, Magnesium, Vitamin D, and Fluoride. Washington, D.C.: National Academy Press; 1997:71–145.
4. Brody T. Nutritional Biochemistry, 2nd ed. San Diego: Academic Press; 1999.
5. Pearce SH, Thakker RV. The calcium-sensing receptor: insights into extracellular calcium homeostasis in health and disease. J Endocrinol 1997;154(3):371–378.
6. Calvo MS. Dietary considerations to prevent loss of bone and renal function. Nutrition 2000;16(7–8):564–566.
7. Devine A, Criddle RA, Dick IM, Kerr DA, Prince RL. A longitudinal study of the effect of sodium and calcium intakes on regional bone density in postmenopausal women. Am J Clin Nutr 1995;62(4):740–745.
8. Weaver CM, Proulx WR, Heaney R. Choices for achieving adequate dietary calcium with a vegetarian diet. Am J Clin Nutr 1999;70(3 Suppl):543S–548S.
9. Barger-Lux MJ, Heaney RP, Stegman MR. Effects of moderate caffeine intake on the calcium economy of premenopausal women. Am J Clin Nutr 1990;52(4):722–725.
10. Harris SS, Dawson-Hughes B. Caffeine and bone loss in healthy postmenopausal women. Am J Clin Nutr 1994;60(4):573–578.
11. Lloyd T, Johnson-Rollings N, Eggli DF, Kieselhorst K, Mauger EA, Cusatis DC. Bone status among postmenopausal women with different habitual caffeine intakes: a longitudinal investigation. J Am Coll Nutr 2000;19(2):256–261.
12. Bostick R. Diet and nutrition in the prevention of colon cancer. In: Bendich A, Deckelbaum RJ, eds. Preventive Nutrition: The Comprehensive Guide for Health Professionals, 2nd ed. Totowa: Humana Press, Inc; 2001:57–95.
13. Baron JA, Beach M, Mandel JS, et al. Calcium supplements and colorectal adenomas. Polyp Prevention Study Group. Ann NY Acad Sci 1999;889:138–145.
14. Bonithon-Kopp C, Kronborg O, Giacosa A, Rath U, Faivre J. Calcium and fibre supplementation in prevention of colorectal adenoma recurrence: a randomised intervention trial. European Cancer Prevention Organisation Study Group. Lancet 2000;356 (9238):1300–1306.
15. Ma J, Giovannucci E, Pollak M, et al. Milk intake, circulating levels of insulin-like growth factor-I, and risk of colorectal cancer in men. J Natl Cancer Inst 2001;93(17):1330–1336.
16. National Institutes of Health. Osteoporosis Prevention, Diagnosis, and Therapy. NIH Consensus Statement 2000;17(1):1–36.
17. Specker BL. Evidence for an interaction between calcium intake and physical activity on changes in bone mineral density. J Bone Miner Res 1996;11(10):1539–1544.
18. Martini LA, Wood RJ. Should dietary calcium and protein be restricted in patients with nephrolithiasis? Nutr Rev 2000;58(4):111–117.
19. Heller HJ. The role of calcium in the prevention of kidney stones. J Am Coll Nutr 1999;18(5 Suppl):373S–378S.
20. Curhan GC, Willett WC, Rimm EB, Stampfer MJ. A prospective study of dietary calcium and other nutrients and the risk of symptomatic kidney stones. N Engl J Med 1993;328(12):833–838.
21. Curhan GC, Willett WC, Speizer FE, Spiegelman D, Stampfer MJ. Comparison of dietary calcium with supplemental calcium and other nutrients as factors affecting the risk for kidney stones in women. Ann Intern Med 1997;126(7):497–504.
22. Liebman M, Chai W. Effect of dietary calcium on urinary oxalate excretion after oxalate loads. Am J Clin Nutr 1997;65(5):1453–1459.
23. Burtis WJ, Gay L, Insogna KL, Ellison A, Broadus AE. Dietary hypercalciuria in patients with calcium oxalate kidney stones. Am J Clin Nutr 1994;60(3):424–429.
24. Martini LA, Cuppari L, Colugnati FA, et al. High sodium chloride intake is associated with low bone density in calcium stone-forming patients. Clin Nephrol 2000;54(2):85–93.
25. Ritchie LD, King JC. Dietary calcium and pregnancy-induced hypertension: is there a relation? Am J Clin Nutr 2000;71(5 Suppl):1371S–1374S.
26. Kulier R, de Onis M, Gulmezoglu AM, Villar J. Nutritional interventions for the prevention of mater-

nal morbidity. *Int J Gynaecol Obstet* 1998;63(3):231–246.

27. Levine RJ, Hauth JC, Curet LB, et al. Trial of calcium to prevent preeclampsia. *N Engl J Med* 1997;337(2):69–76.

28. Bruening K, Kemp FW, Simone N, Holding Y, Louria DB, Bogden JD. Dietary calcium intakes of urban children at risk of lead poisoning. *Environ Health Perspect* 1999;107(6):431–435.

29. Hertz-Picciotto I, Schramm M, Watt-Morse M, Chantala K, Anderson J, Osterloh J. Patterns and determinants of blood lead during pregnancy. *Am J Epidemiol* 2000;152(9):829–837.

30. Muldoon SB, Cauley JA, Kuller LH, Scott J, Rohay J. Lifestyle and sociodemographic factors as determinants of blood lead levels in elderly women. *Am J Epidemiol* 1994;139(6):599–608.

31. Birkett NJ. Comments on a meta-analysis of the relation between dietary calcium intake and blood pressure. *Am J Epidemiol* 1998;148(3):223–228; discussion 232–223.

32. Griffith LE, Guyatt GH, Cook RJ, Bucher HC, Cook DJ. The influence of dietary and nondietary calcium supplementation on blood pressure: an updated metaanalysis of randomized controlled trials. *Am J Hypertens* 1999;12(1 Pt 1):84–92.

33. Appel LJ, Moore TJ, Obarzanek E, et al. A clinical trial of the effects of dietary patterns on blood pressure. DASH Collaborative Research Group. *N Engl J Med* 1997;336(16):1117–1124.

34. Conlin PR, Chow D, Miller ER, 3rd, et al. The effect of dietary patterns on blood pressure control in hypertensive patients: results from the Dietary Approaches to Stop Hypertension (DASH) trial. *Am J Hypertens* 2000;13(9):949–955.

35. Miller GD, DiRienzo DD, Reusser ME, McCarron DA. Benefits of dairy product consumption on blood pressure in humans: a summary of the biomedical literature. *J Am Coll Nutr* 2000;19(2 Suppl):147S–164S.

36. Hendler SS, Rorvik DR, eds. *PDR for Nutritional Supplements*. Montvale, NJ: Medical Economics Company, Inc; 2001.

37. Bourgoin BP, Evans DR, Cornett JR, Lingard SM, Quattrone AJ. Lead content in 70 brands of dietary calcium supplements. *Am J Public Health* 1993;83(8):1155–1160.

38. Ross EA, Szabo NJ, Tebbett IR. Lead content of calcium supplements. *JAMA* 2000;284(11):1425–1429.

39. Giovannucci E, Rimm EB, Wolk A, et al. Calcium and fructose intake in relation to risk of prostate cancer. *Cancer Res* 1998;58(3):442–447.

40. Chan JM, Giovannucci E, Andersson SO, Yuen J, Adami HO, Wolk A. Dairy products, calcium, phosphorous, vitamin D, and risk of prostate cancer (Sweden). *Cancer Causes Control* 1998;9(6):559–566.

41. Chan JM, Stampfer MJ, Ma J, Gann PH, Gaziano JM, Giovannucci EL. Dairy products, calcium, and prostate cancer risk in the Physicians' Health Study. *Am J Clin Nutr* 2001;74(4):549–554.

42. Chan JM, Giovannucci EL. Dairy products, calcium, and vitamin D and risk of prostate cancer. *Epidemiol Rev* 2001;23(1):87–92.

43. Vlajinac HD, Marinkovic JM, Ilic MD, Kocev NI. Diet and prostate cancer: a case-control study. *Eur J Cancer* 1997;33(1):101–107.

44. Minerals. *Drug Facts and Comparisons*. St. Louis: Facts and Comparisons; 2000:27–51.

45. Wood RJ, Zheng JJ. High dietary calcium intakes reduce zinc absorption and balance in humans. *Am J Clin Nutr* 1997;65(6):1803–1809.

15 Chromium

Although trivalent chromium is recognized as a nutritionally essential mineral, scientists are not yet certain exactly how it functions in the body. The two most common forms of chromium are trivalent chromium (III) and hexavalent chromium (VI). Chromium (III) is the principal form in foods, as well as the form utilized by the body. Chromium (VI) is derived from chromium (III) by heating at alkaline pH and is used as a source of chromium for industrial purposes. It is a strong irritant and is recognized as a carcinogen when inhaled. At low levels, chromium (VI) is readily reduced to chromium (III) by reducing substances in foods and the acidic environment of the stomach that serve to prevent the ingestion of chromium (VI).[1-3]

Function

A biologically active form of chromium participates in glucose metabolism by enhancing the effects of insulin. Insulin is secreted by specialized cells in the pancreas in response to increased blood glucose levels, for example, after a meal. Insulin binds to insulin receptors on the surface of cells, activating those receptors and stimulating glucose uptake by cells. Through its interaction with insulin receptors, insulin provides cells with glucose for energy and prevents blood glucose levels from becoming elevated. In addition to its effects on carbohydrate (glucose) metabolism, insulin also influences the metabolism of fat and protein. A decreased response to insulin or decreased insulin sensitivity may result in impaired glucose tolerance or type 2 diabetes, also known as non-insulin–dependent diabetes mellitus. Type 2 diabetes is characterized by elevated blood glucose levels and insulin resistance.[3]

The precise structure of the biologically active form of chromium is not known. Recent research suggests that a low-molecular-weight chromium-binding substance (LMWCr) may enhance the response of the insulin receptor to insulin. The following is a proposed model for the effect of chromium on insulin action (Fig. 15–1). First, the inactive form of the insulin receptor is converted to the active form by binding insulin. The binding of insulin by the insulin receptor stimulates the movement of chromium into the cell and results in binding of chromium to apoLMWCr, a form of the LMWCr that lacks chromium. Once it binds chromium the LMWCr binds to the insulin receptor and enhances its activity. The ability of the LMWCr to activate the insulin receptor is dependent on its chromium content. When insulin levels drop due to normalization of blood glucose levels, the LMWCr may be released from the cell to terminate its effects.[4]

Nutrient Interactions

Iron. Chromium competes for one of the binding sites on the iron transport protein, transferrin. However, supplementation of older men with 925 µg of chromium per day for 12 weeks did not significantly affect measures of iron nutritional status.[5] A study of younger men found an insignificant decrease in transferrin saturation with iron after supplementation of 200 µg of chromium per day for 8 weeks, but no long-term studies have addressed this issue.[6] Iron overload in hereditary hemochromatosis may interfere with chromium transport by competing for transferrin binding. This has led to the hypothesis that decreased chromium transport might contribute to the diabetes associated with hereditary hemochromatosis.[3]

Vitamin C. Chromium uptake is enhanced in animals when given at the same time as vitamin C.[1] In a study of three women, administration of 100 mg of vitamin C together with 1 mg of chromium resulted in higher plasma levels of chromium than 1 mg of chromium without vitamin C.[3]

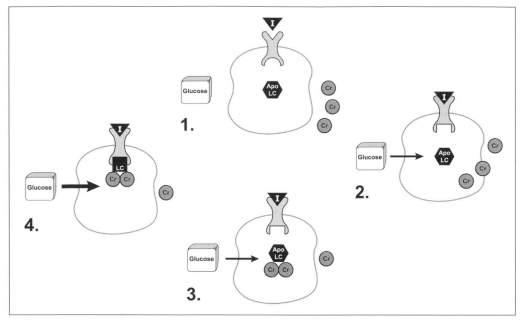

Figure 15–1. A proposed model for the enhancing effects of chromium on insulin activity. (1) Insulin binds to and activates the insulin receptor. (2) Insulin receptor activation stimulates the movement of chromium into the cell. (3) Chromium binds to a peptide known as Apo-LMWCr (Apo-LC). (4) Functional LMWCr (LC) binds to the insulin receptor and enhances its activity.

Carbohydrates. Diets high in simple sugars (e.g., sucrose), compared with diets high in complex carbohydrates (e.g., whole grains), increase urinary chromium excretion in adults. This effect may be related to increased insulin secretion in response to the consumption of simple sugars compared with complex carbohydrates.[3]

Deficiency

Chromium deficiency was reported in three patients on long-term intravenous feeding who did not receive supplemental chromium in their intravenous solutions. These patients developed evidence of abnormal glucose utilization and increased insulin requirements that responded to chromium supplementation. Additionally, impaired glucose tolerance in malnourished infants responded to an oral dose of chromium chloride. Because chromium appears to enhance the action of insulin and chromium deficiency has resulted in impaired glucose tolerance, chromium insufficiency has been hypothesized to be a contributing factor to the development of type 2 diabetes.[3,7]

Several studies of male runners indicated that urinary chromium loss was increased by endurance exercise, suggesting that chromium needs may be greater in individuals who exercise regularly.[8] In a more recent study, resistive exercise (weight lifting) was found to increase urinary excretion of chromium in older men. However, chromium absorption was also increased, leading to little or no net loss of chromium as a result of resistive exercise.[9]

At present, research on the effects of inadequate chromium intake and risk factors for chromium insufficiency are limited by the lack of sensitive and accurate tests for determining chromium nutritional status.[1,3]

The Adequate Intake Level

Because there was not enough information on chromium requirements to set a recommended dietary allowance, the Food and

Table 15–1   Adequate Intake (AI) for Chromium

Life Stage	Age	Males, μg/d	Females, μg/d
Infants	0–6 months	0.2	0.2
Infants	7–12 months	5.5	5.5
Children	1–3 years	11	11
Children	4–8 years	15	15
Children	9–13 years	25	21
Adolescents	14–18 years	35	24
Adults	19–50 years	35	25
Adults	51 years and older	30	20
Pregnancy	18 years and younger	–	29
Pregnancy	19 years and older	–	30
Breastfeeding	18 years and younger	–	44
Breastfeeding	19 years and older	–	45

Nutrition Board (FNB) set an adequate intake level based on the chromium content in normal diets (Table 15–1).[3]

Disease Prevention

Impaired Glucose Tolerance and Type 2 Diabetes Mellitus

In 12 of 15 controlled studies of people with impaired glucose tolerance, chromium supplementation was found to improve some measure of glucose utilization or to have beneficial effects on blood lipid profiles.[10] Impaired glucose tolerance refers to a metabolic state between normal glucose regulation and overt diabetes. Generally, blood glucose levels are higher than normal but lower than those accepted as diagnostic for diabetes. Impaired glucose tolerance is associated with increased risk for cardiovascular diseases but is not associated with the other classic complications of

diabetes. About 25 to 30% of individuals with impaired glucose tolerance eventually develop type 2 diabetes.[11] Generally, chromium supplementation at doses of about 200 μg/d, in a variety of forms for 2 to 3 months, were found to be beneficial. The reasons for the variation or lack of effect in some studies are not clear, but chromium depletion is not the only known cause of impaired glucose tolerance. Additionally, the lack of an accurate measure of chromium nutritional status prevents researchers from identifying those individuals who are most likely to benefit from chromium supplementation.[1,12]

Cardiovascular Diseases

Impaired glucose tolerance and type 2 diabetes are associated with adverse changes in lipid profiles and increased risk of cardiovascular diseases. Studies examining the effects of chromium supplementation on lipid profiles have been notable for their inconsistent results. Although some studies have observed reductions in total cholesterol, low-density lipoprotein cholesterol, and triglyceride levels or increases in high-density lipoprotein cholesterol levels, others have observed no effect. Such inconsistent responses of lipid and lipoprotein levels to chromium supplementation may reflect differences in chromium nutritional status. It is possible that only those individuals with insufficient chromium will experience beneficial effects on lipid profiles due to chromium supplementation.[1,2,10]

Health Claims

Increases Muscle Mass. Claims that chromium supplementation increases lean body mass and decreases body fat are based on the relationship between chromium and insulin action. In addition to affecting glucose metabolism, insulin is known to affect fat and protein metabolism. At least 12 placebo-controlled studies have compared the effect of chromium supplementation (200 to 1000 μg as chromium picolinate per day) with or without an exercise program on lean body mass and measures of body fat. In general, those studies that have used the most sensitive and accurate methods of measuring body fat and lean mass (dual-energy X-ray absorbtiometry and hydrodensitometry or underwater weighing) do not indicate a beneficial effect of chromium supplementation on body composition.[2,10]

Promotes Weight Loss. Controlled studies of chromium supplementation (200 to 400 µg as chromium picolinate per day) have demonstrated little if any beneficial effect on weight or fat loss,[13] and claims of weight loss in humans appear to be exaggerated. In 1997 the U.S. Federal Trade Commission ruled that there is no basis for claims that chromium picolinate promotes weight loss and fat loss in humans.[2,10,12]

Disease Treatment

Type 2 Diabetes Mellitus

Type 2 diabetes is characterized by elevated blood glucose levels and insulin resistance. Although insulin levels in type 2 diabetics may be higher than in healthy individuals, the physiological effects of insulin are reduced. Because chromium is known to enhance the action of insulin, the relationship between chromium nutritional status and type 2 diabetes has generated considerable scientific interest. Individuals with type 2 diabetes have been found to have higher rates of urinary chromium loss than healthy individuals, especially those with diabetes of more than 2 years' duration.[14] Prior to 1997, well-designed studies of chromium supplementation in individuals with type 2 diabetes showed no improvement in blood glucose control, though they provided some evidence of reduced insulin levels and improved blood lipid profiles.[15] In 1997, the results of a large placebo-controlled trial conducted in China indicated that chromium supplementation might be beneficial in the treatment of type 2 diabetes.[16] One hundred eighty participants took either a placebo, 200 µg/d, or 1000 µg/d of chromium in the form of chromium picolinate. At the end of 4 months, blood glucose levels were 15 to 19% lower in those who took 1000 µg/d compared with those who took a placebo. Blood glucose levels in those who took 200 µg/d did not differ signif-

icantly from those who took a placebo. Insulin levels were lower in those who took either 200 µg/d or 1000 µg/d. Glycosylated hemoglobin levels, a measure of long-term control of blood glucose, were also lower in both chromium-supplemented groups, but they were lowest in the group taking 1000 µg/d. Because the chromium nutritional status of the Chinese participants was not evaluated, and the prevalence of obesity was much lower than is typically associated with type 2 diabetics in the United States, extrapolation of these results to a U.S. population is difficult. However, the findings in the Chinese population emphasize the need for large-scale randomized controlled trials of chromium supplementation for type 2 diabetes in the United States.[15]

Gestational Diabetes

Few studies have examined the effects of chromium supplementation on gestational diabetes. Gestational diabetes occurs in about 2% of pregnant women and usually appears in the second or third trimester of pregnancy. Blood glucose levels must be tightly controlled to prevent adverse effects on the developing fetus. After delivery, glucose tolerance generally reverts to normal. However, 30 to 40% of women who have had gestational diabetes develop type 2 diabetes within 5 to 10 years. An observational study in pregnant women did not find serum chromium levels to be associated with measures of glucose tolerance or insulin resistance in late pregnancy, although serum chromium levels may not reflect tissue chromium levels.[17] Women with gestational diabetes whose diets were supplemented with 4 µg of chromium per kilogram of body weight daily as chromium picolinate for 8 weeks had decreased fasting blood glucose and insulin levels compared with those who took a placebo. However, insulin therapy rather than chromium picolinate was required to normalize severely elevated blood glucose levels.[2,18]

Table 15–2   Food Sources of Chromium

Food	Serving	Chromium, μg
Broccoli	1/2 cup	11.0
Turkey ham (processed)	3 ounces*	10.4
Grape juice	8 fluid ounces	7.5
Waffle	1 (~2.5 ounces)	6.7
English muffin	1	3.6
Potatoes	1 cup, mashed	2.7
Bagel	1	2.5
Orange juice	8 fluid ounces	2.2
Beef	3 ounces*	2.0
Turkey breast	3 ounces*	1.7
Apple w/peel	1 medium	1.4
Green beans	1/2 cup	1.1
Banana	1 medium	1.0

*A 3-ounce serving of meat or fish is about the size of a deck of cards.

Sources

Food Sources

The amount of chromium in foods is variable, and it has been measured accurately in relatively few foods. Presently, there is no large database for the chromium content of foods. Processed meats, whole grain products, ready-to-eat bran cereals, green beans, broccoli, and spices are relatively rich in chromium. Foods high in simple sugars, such as sucrose and fructose, are not only low in chromium but have been found to promote chromium loss.[2] Estimated average chromium intakes in the United States range from 23 to 29 μg/d for adult women and 39 to 54 μg/d for adult men.[3] The chromium content of some foods is listed in Table 15–2 in micrograms (μg).[19] Because chromium content in different batches of the same food has been found to vary significantly, the information in the Table 15–2 should serve only as a guide to the chromium content of foods.

Supplements

Chromium (III) is available as a supplement in several forms: chromium chloride, chromium nicotinate, chromium picolinate, and high-chromium yeast. They are available as stand-alone supplements or in combination products. Doses typically range from 50 to 200 μg of elemental chromium.[20] Chromium nicotinate and chromium picolinate may be more bioavailable than chromium chloride.[10] In much of the research on impaired glucose tolerance and type 2 diabetes, chromium picolinate was the source of chromium. However, some concerns have been raised over the long-term safety of chromium picolinate supplementation.

Safety

Toxicity

Hexavalent chromium or chromium (VI) is a recognized carcinogen. Exposure to chromium (VI) in dust is associated with increased incidence of lung cancer and is known to cause inflammation of the skin (dermatitis). In contrast, there is little evidence that trivalent chromium or chromium (III) is toxic to humans. Because no adverse effects have been convincingly associated with excess intake of chromium (III) from food or supplements, the FNB of the Institute of Medicine did not set a tolerable upper level of intake for chromium. Because information is limited, the FNB acknowledged a potential for adverse effects of high intakes of supplemental chromium (III) and advised caution.[3]

Most of the concerns regarding the long-term safety of chromium (III) supplementation arise from several studies in cell culture, suggesting chromium (III), especially in the form of chromium picolinate, may increase DNA damage.[21-23] Presently, there is no evidence that chromium (III) increases DNA damage in living organisms,[3] and a study in 10 women taking 400 μg/d of chromium as chromium picolinate found no evidence of increased oxidative damage to DNA as measured by antibodies to an oxidized DNA base.[24]

Several studies have demonstrated the safety of daily doses of up to 1000 μg of chromium for several months.[16,25] However, there have been a few isolated reports of serious adverse reactions to chromium picolinate. Kidney failure was reported 5 months after a 6-week course of 600 µg of chromium per day in the form of chromium picolinate,[26] and kidney failure and impaired liver function were reported after the use of 1200 to 2400 µg/d of chromium in the form of chromium picolinate over a period of 4 to 5 months.[27] Individuals with preexisting kidney or liver disease may be at increased risk of adverse effects and should limit supplemental chromium intake.[3]

Drug Interactions

Little is known about drug interactions with chromium in humans. Large doses of calcium carbonate or magnesium hydroxide-containing antacids decreased chromium absorption in rats. Aspirin and indomethacin (a nonsteroidal anti-inflammatory drug) increased chromium absorption in rats.[1]

LPI Recommendation

The lack of sensitive indicators of chromium nutritional status in humans makes it difficult to determine the level of chromium intake most likely to promote optimum health. Following the Linus Pauling Institute recommendation to take a multivitamin/multimineral supplement containing 100 % of the daily values (DV) of most nutrients will generally provide 60 to 120 µg/d of chromium, well above the adequate intake level of 20 to 25 µg/d for adult women and 30 to 35 µg/d for adult men.

Because impaired glucose tolerance and type 2 diabetes are associated with potentially serious health problems, individuals considering high-dose chromium supplementation to treat either condition should do so in collaboration with a qualified health care provider.

Older Adults

Although the requirement for chromium is not known to be higher for adults 65 years and older, one study found that chromium concentrations in hair, sweat, and urine decreased with age.[28] Following the Linus Pauling Institute recommendation to take a multivitamin/multimineral supplement containing 100 % of the DV of most nutrients should provide sufficient chromium for most older adults.

References

1. Stoecker BJ. Chromium. In: Shils M, Olson JA, Shike M, Ross AC, eds. *Nutrition in Health and Disease*, 9th ed. Baltimore: Williams & Wilkins; 1999:277–282.
2. Lukaski HC. Chromium as a supplement. *Annu Rev Nutr* 1999;19:279–302.
3. Food and Nutrition Board, Institute of Medicine. Chromium. *Dietary Reference Intakes for Vitamin A, Vitamin K, Boron, Chromium, Copper, Iodine, Iron, Manganese, Molybdenum, Nickel, Silicon, Vanadium, and Zinc*. Washington, D.C.: National Academy Press; 2001:6:197–223.
4. Vincent JB. Elucidating a biological role for chromium at a molecular level. *Acc Chem Res* 2000;33(7):503–510.
5. Campbell WW, Beard JL, Joseph LJ, Davey SL, Evans WJ. Chromium picolinate supplementation and resistive training by older men: effects on iron-status and hematologic indexes. *Am J Clin Nutr* 1997;66(4):944–949.
6. Lukaski HC, Bolonchuk WW, Siders WA, Milne DB. Chromium supplementation and resistance training: effects on body composition, strength, and trace element status of men. *Am J Clin Nutr* 1996;63(6):954–965.
7. Jeejeebhoy KN. The role of chromium in nutrition and therapeutics and as a potential toxin. *Nutr Rev* 1999;57(11):329–335.
8. Lukaski HC. Magnesium, zinc, and chromium nutriture and physical activity. *Am J Clin Nutr* 2000;72(2 Suppl):585S–593S.
9. Rubin MA, Miller JP, Ryan AS, et al. Acute and chronic resistive exercise increase urinary chromium excretion in men as measured with an enriched chromium stable isotope. *J Nutr* 1998;128(1):73–78.
10. Kobla HV, Volpe SL. Chromium, exercise, and body composition. *Crit Rev Food Sci Nutr* 2000;40(4):291–308.
11. Goldman L, Bennett JC. *Cecil Textbook of Medicine*, 21st ed. Philadelphia: W.B. Saunders Co.; 2000.
12. Anderson RA. Effects of chromium on body composition and weight loss. *Nutr Rev* 1998;56(9):266–270.
13. Volpe SL, Huang HW, Larpadisorn K, Lesser II. Effect of chromium supplementation and exercise on body composition, resting metabolic rate and selected biochemical parameters in moderately obese women following an exercise program. *J Am Coll Nutr* 2001; 20(4):293–306.
14. Morris BW, MacNeil S, Hardisty CA, Heller S, Burgin C, Gray TA. Chromium homeostasis in patients with type II (NIDDM) diabetes. *J Trace Elem Med Biol* 1999; 13(1–2):57–61.
15. Hellerstein MK. Is chromium supplementation effective in managing type II diabetes? *Nutr Rev* 1998;56(10):302–306.
16. Anderson RA, Cheng N, Bryden NA, Polansky MM, Chi J, Feng J. Elevated intakes of supplemental chromium improve glucose and insulin variables in individuals with type II diabetes. *Diabetes* 1997;46(11):1786–1791.
17. Gunton JE, Hams G, Hitchman R, McElduff A. Serum chromium does not predict glucose tolerance in late pregnancy. *Am J Clin Nutr* 2001;73(1):99–104.

18. Jovanovic-Peterson L, Peterson CM. Vitamin and mineral deficiencies which may predispose to glucose intolerance of pregnancy. *J Am Coll Nutr* 1996;15(1):14–20.

19. Anderson RA, Bryden NA, Polansky MM. Dietary chromium intake. Freely chosen diets, institutional diet, and individual foods. *Biol Trace Elem Res* 1992;32:117–121.

20. Hendler SS, Rorvik DR, eds. *PDR for Nutritional Supplements*. Montvale, NJ: Medical Economics Company, Inc; 2001.

21. Stearns DM, Wise JP, Sr., Patierno SR, Wetterhahn KE. Chromium(III) picolinate produces chromosome damage in Chinese hamster ovary cells. *Faseb J* 1995;9(15):1643–1648.

22. Speetjens JK, Collins RA, Vincent JB, Woski SA. The nutritional supplement chromium(III) tris(picolinate) cleaves DNA. *Chem Res Toxicol* 1999;12(6):483–487.

23. Blasiak J, Kowalik J. A comparison of the in vitro genotoxicity of tri- and hexavalent chromium. *Mutat Res* 2000;469(1):135–145.

24. Kato I, Vogelman JH, Dilman V, et al. Effect of supplementation with chromium picolinate on antibody titers to 5-hydroxymethyl uracil. *Eur J Epidemiol* 1998;14(6):621–626.

25. Hathcock JN. Vitamins and minerals: efficacy and safety. *Am J Clin Nutr* 1997;66(2):427–437.

26. Wasser WG, Feldman NS, D'Agati VD. Chronic renal failure after ingestion of over-the-counter chromium picolinate. *Ann Intern Med* 1997;126(5):410.

27. Cerulli J, Grabe DW, Gauthier I, Malone M, McGoldrick MD. Chromium picolinate toxicity. *Ann Pharmacother* 1998;32(4):428–431.

28. Davies S, McLaren Howard J, Hunnisett A, Howard M. Age-related decreases in chromium levels in 51,665 hair, sweat, and serum samples from 40,872 patients—implications for the prevention of cardiovascular disease and type II diabetes mellitus. *Metabolism* 1997;46(5):469–473.

16 Copper

Copper (Cu) is an essential trace element for humans and animals. In the body, copper shifts between the cuprous (Cu$^+$) and the cupric (Cu^{2+}) forms, though the majority of the body's copper is in the Cu^{2+} form. The ability of copper to easily accept and donate electrons explains its important role in oxidation-reduction (redox) reactions and the scavenging of free radicals.[1] Although Hippocrates is said to have prescribed copper compounds to treat diseases as early as 400 B.C.,[2] scientists are still uncovering new information regarding the functions of copper in the human body.

Function

Copper is a critical functional component of a number of essential enzymes, known as *cuproenzymes*. Some of the physiologic functions known to be copper-dependent are discussed below.

Energy Production

The copper-dependent enzyme cytochrome c oxidase plays a critical role in cellular energy production. By catalyzing the reduction of molecular oxygen (O$_2$) to water (H$_2$O), cytochrome c oxidase generates an electrical gradient used by the mitochondria to create the vital energy-storing molecule adenosine triphosphate.[3]

Connective Tissue Formation

Another cuproenzyme, lysyl oxidase, is required for the cross-linking of collagen and elastin, which are essential for the formation of strong and flexible connective tissue. The action of lysyl oxidase helps maintain the integrity of connective tissue in the heart and blood vessels and plays a role in bone formation.[2]

Iron Metabolism

Two copper-containing enzymes, ceruloplasmin (ferroxidase I) and ferroxidase II, have the capacity to oxidize ferrous iron (Fe^{2+}) to ferric iron (Fe^{3+}), the form of iron that can be loaded onto the protein transferrin for transport to the site of red blood cell formation. Although the ferroxidase activity of these two cuproenzymes has not yet been proven to be physiologically significant, the fact that iron mobilization from storage sites is impaired in copper deficiency supports their role in iron metabolism.[2,4]

Central Nervous System

A number of reactions essential to normal function of the brain and nervous system are catalyzed by cuproenzymes.
- *Neurotransmitter synthesis* Dopamine-β-mono-oxygenase catalyzes the conversion of dopamine to the neurotransmitter norepinephrine.[4]
- *Metabolism of neurotransmitters* Mono-amine oxidase (MAO) plays a role in the metabolism of the neurotransmitters norepinephrine, epinephrine, and dopamine. MAO also functions in the degradation of the neurotransmitter serotonin, which is the basis for the use of MAO inhibitors as antidepressants.[5]
- *Formation and maintenance of myelin* The myelin sheath is made of phospholipids whose synthesis depends on cytochrome c oxidase activity.[2]

Melanin Formation

The cuproenzyme tyrosinase is required for the formation of the pigment melanin. Melanin is formed in cells called *melanocytes* and plays a role in the pigmentation of the hair, skin, and eyes.[2]

Antioxidant Functions

Superoxide dismutase (SOD) functions as an antioxidant by catalyzing the conversion of superoxide radicals (free radicals) to hydrogen peroxide, which can subsequently be reduced to water by other antioxidant enzymes.[6] Two forms of SOD contain copper: (1) copper/zinc SOD is found within most cells of the body, including red blood cells, and (2) extracellular SOD is a copper-containing enzyme found in high levels in the lungs and low levels in blood plasma.[2]

Ceruloplasmin may function as an antioxidant in two different ways. Free copper and iron ions are powerful catalysts of free radical damage. By binding copper, ceruloplasmin prevents free copper ions from catalyzing oxidative damage. The ferroxidase activity of ceruloplasmin (oxidation of ferrous iron) facilitates iron loading onto its transport protein, transferrin, and may prevent free ferrous ions (Fe^{2+}) from participating in harmful free radical–generating reactions.[6]

Regulation of Gene Expression

Copper-dependent transcription factors regulate transcription of specific genes. Thus, cellular copper levels may affect the synthesis of proteins by enhancing or inhibiting the transcription of specific genes. Genes regulated by copper-dependent transcription factors include genes for copper/zinc superoxide dismutase (Cu/Zn SOD), catalase (another antioxidant enzyme), and proteins related to the cellular storage of copper.[3]

Nutrient Interactions

Iron. Adequate copper nutritional status appears to be necessary for normal iron metabolism and red blood cell formation. Anemia is a clinical sign of copper deficiency, and iron has been found to accumulate in the livers of copper-deficient animals, indicating that copper (probably in the form of ceruloplasmin) is required for iron transport to the bone marrow for red blood cell formation.[2] Infants fed a high iron formula absorbed less copper than infants fed a low iron formula, suggesting that high iron intakes may interfere with copper absorption in infants.[5]

Zinc. High supplemental zinc intakes of 50 mg/d or more for extended periods of time may result in copper deficiency. High dietary zinc increases the synthesis of an intestinal cell protein called *metallothionein*, which binds certain metals and prevents their absorption by trapping them in intestinal cells. Metallothionein has a stronger affinity for copper than zinc, so high levels of metallothionein induced by excess zinc cause a decrease in intestinal copper absorption. High copper intakes have not been found to affect zinc nutritional status.[2,5]

Fructose. High fructose diets have exacerbated copper deficiency in rats but not in pigs, whose gastrointestinal systems are more like those of humans. Very high levels of dietary fructose (20% of total calories) did not result in copper depletion in humans, suggesting that fructose intake does not result in copper depletion at levels relevant to normal diets.[2,5]

Vitamin C. Although vitamin C supplements have produced copper deficiency in laboratory animals, the effect of vitamin C supplements on copper nutritional status in humans is less clear. Two small studies in healthy young adult men indicate that the oxidase activity of ceruloplasmin may be impaired by relatively high doses of supplemental vitamin C. In one study, vitamin C supplementation of 1500 mg/d for 2 months resulted in a significant decline in ceruloplasmin oxidase activity.[7] In the other study, supplements of 605 mg of vitamin C/d for 3 weeks resulted in decreased ceruloplasmin oxidase activity, although copper absorption did not decline.[8] Neither of these studies found vitamin C supplementation to adversely affect copper nutritional status.

Deficiency

Clinically evident or frank copper deficiency is relatively uncommon. Serum copper levels and ceruloplasmin levels may fall to 30% of normal in cases of severe copper deficiency. One of the most common clinical signs of copper defi-

Table 16–1 Recommended Dietary Allowance (RDA) for Copper

Life Stage	Age	Males, µg/d	Females, µg/d
Infants	0–6 months	200 (AI)	200 (AI)
Infants	7–12 months	220 (AI)	220 (AI)
Children	1–3 years	340	340
Children	4–8 years	440	440
Children	9–13 years	700	700
Adolescents	14–18 years	890	890
Adults	19 years and older	900	900
Pregnancy	all ages	–	1000
Breastfeeding	all ages	–	1300

AI, adequate intake level.

ciency is an anemia that is unresponsive to iron therapy but is corrected by copper supplementation. The anemia is thought to result from defective iron mobilization due to decreased ceruloplasmin activity. Copper deficiency may also result in abnormally low numbers of white blood cells known as *neutrophils* (neutropenia), a condition that may be accompanied by increased susceptibility to infection. Osteoporosis and other abnormalities of bone development related to copper deficiency are most common in copper-deficient low birth weight infants and young children. Less common features of copper deficiency may include loss of pigmentation, neurological symptoms, and impaired growth.[2,3]

Individuals at Risk of Deficiency

Cow's milk is relatively low in copper, and cases of copper deficiency have been reported in high-risk infants and children fed only cow's milk formula. High-risk individuals include: premature infants, especially those with low birth weight; infants with prolonged diarrhea; infants and children recovering from malnutrition; and individuals with malabsorption syndromes including celiac disease, sprue, and short bowel syndrome due to surgical removal of a large portion of the intestine. Individuals

receiving intravenous total parenteral nutrition or other restricted diets may also require supplementation with copper and other trace elements.[2,3] Cystic fibrosis patients may also be at increased risk of copper insufficiency.[9]

The Recommended Dietary Allowance

A variety of indicators were used to establish the recommended dietary allowance (RDA) for copper, including plasma copper concentration, serum ceruloplasmin activity, superoxide dismutase activity in red blood cells, and platelet copper concentration.[5] The RDA for copper reflects the results of depletion–repletion studies and is based on the prevention of deficiency (Table 16–1).

Disease Prevention

Cardiovascular Diseases

Although it is clear that severe copper deficiency results in heart abnormalities and damage (cardiomyopathy) in some animal species, the pathology differs from atherosclerotic cardiovascular diseases prevalent in humans.[5] Studies in humans have produced inconsistent results, and their interpretation is hindered by the lack of a reliable marker of copper nutritional status. Outside the body, free copper is known to be a pro-oxidant and is frequently used to produce oxidation of low-density lipoprotein (LDL) in the test tube. Recently, ceruloplasmin has been found to stimulate LDL oxidation in the test tube,[10] leading some scientists to propose that increased copper levels could increase the risk of atherosclerosis by promoting the oxidation of LDL. However, there is little evidence that copper or ceruloplasmin promotes LDL oxidation in the human body. Additionally, the cuproenzymes, superoxide dismutase and ceruloplasmin, are known to have antioxidant properties, leading some experts to propose that copper deficiency rather than excess copper increases the risk of cardiovascular diseases.[11]

Epidemiologic Studies. Several epidemiologic studies have found increased serum copper levels to be associated with increased risk of cardiovascular disease. A recent prospective study in the United States examined serum copper levels in more than 4400 men and women 30 years of age and older.[12] During the following 16 years, 151 participants died from coronary heart disease (CHD). After adjusting for other risk factors of heart disease, those with serum copper levels in the two highest quartiles had a significantly greater risk of dying from CHD. Three other case-control studies conducted in Europe had similar findings. Serum copper largely reflects serum ceruloplasmin and is not a sensitive indicator of copper nutritional status. Serum ceruloplasmin levels are known to increase by 50 % or more under certain conditions of physical stress, such as trauma, inflammation, or disease. Because over 90 % of serum copper is carried in ceruloplasmin, elevated serum copper may simply be a marker of the inflammation that accompanies atherosclerosis. In contrast to the serum copper findings, two autopsy studies found copper levels in heart muscle to be lower in patients who died of CHD than those who died of other causes.[13] Additionally, the copper content of white blood cells has been positively correlated with the degree of patency of coronary arteries in CHD patients,[14,15] and patients with a history of myocardial infarction (heart attack) had lower concentrations of extracellular superoxide dismutase than those without a history of myocardial infarction.[16]

Experimental Studies. Although studies in very small numbers of adults fed experimental diets low in copper have demonstrated adverse changes in blood cholesterol levels, including increased total and LDL cholesterol levels and decreased high-density lipoprotein cholesterol levels,[17] other studies have not confirmed those results.[18] Copper supplementation of 2 to 3 mg/d for 4 to 6 weeks did not result in clinically significant changes in cholesterol levels.[11,19] Recent research has also failed to find evidence that increased copper intake increases oxidative stress. In a multicenter placebo-controlled study, copper supplementation of 3 and 6 mg/d for 6 weeks did not result in increased susceptibility of LDL to oxidation induced outside the body (ex vivo)

by copper or peroxynitrite (a reactive nitrogen species).[20] Moreover, supplementation with 3 and 6 mg/d of copper decreased the ex vivo oxidizability of red blood cells,[21] indicating that relatively high intakes of copper do not increase the susceptibility of LDL or red blood cells to oxidation.

Summary. Although free copper and ceruloplasmin can promote LDL oxidation in the test tube, there is little evidence that increased dietary copper increases oxidative stress in humans. Increased serum copper levels have been associated with increased cardiovascular disease risk, but the significance of these findings is unclear due to the association between serum ceruloplasmin levels and inflammatory conditions. Clarification of the relationships between copper nutritional status, ceruloplasmin levels, and cardiovascular disease risk requires further research.

Immune System Function

Copper is known to play an important role in the development and maintenance of immune system function, but the exact mechanism of its action is not yet known. Neutropenia (abnormally low numbers of white blood cells called *neutrophils*) is a clinical sign of copper deficiency in humans. Adverse effects of insufficient copper on immune function appear most pronounced in infants. Infants with Menkes disease, a genetic disorder that results in severe copper deficiency, suffer from frequent and severe infections.[22,23] In a study of 11 malnourished infants with evidence of copper deficiency, the ability of certain white blood cells to engulf pathogens increased significantly after 1 month of copper supplementation.[24] More recently, 11 men on a low-copper diet (0.66 mg/d for 24 days and 0.38 mg/d for another 40 days) showed a decreased proliferation response when white blood cells called *mononuclear cells* isolated from their blood were presented with an immune challenge in cell culture.[25] Although severe copper deficiency has adverse effects on immune function, the effects of marginal copper insufficiency in humans are not yet clear.

Osteoporosis

The copper-dependent enzyme lysyl oxidase is required for the maturation (cross-linking) of collagen, a key element in the organic matrix of bone. Osteoporosis has been observed in infants and adults with severe copper deficiency, but it is not clear whether marginal copper deficiency contributes to osteoporosis. Research regarding the role of copper nutritional status in age-related osteoporosis is limited. Serum copper levels of 46 elderly patients with hip fractures were reported to be significantly lower than matched controls.[26] A small study in perimenopausal women, who consumed an average of 1 mg of dietary copper daily, reported decreased loss of bone mineral density from the lumbar spine after copper supplementation of 3 mg/d for 2 years.[27] Marginal copper intake of 0.7 mg/d for 6 weeks significantly increased a measurement of bone resorption (breakdown) in healthy adult males.[28] However, copper supplementation of 3 to 6 mg/d for 6 weeks had no effect on biochemical markers of bone resorption or bone formation in a study of healthy adult men and women.[29] Although severe copper deficiency is known to adversely affect bone health, the effects of marginal copper deficiency and copper supplementation on bone metabolism and age-related osteoporosis require further research before conclusions can be drawn.

Disease Treatment

Presently, there is insufficient evidence to support the use of copper to treat diseases or health conditions other than frank copper deficiency.

Sources

Food Sources

Copper is found in a wide variety of foods and is most plentiful in organ meats, shellfish, nuts, and seeds. Wheat bran cereals and whole grain products are also good sources of copper. According to national surveys, the average dietary intake of copper in the United States is approximately 1.0 to 1.1 mg (1000 to

Table 16–2   Food Sources of Copper

Food	Serving	Copper, µg
Liver (beef), cooked	1 ounce	1265
Oysters, cooked	1 medium oyster	670
Cashews	1 ounce	629
Crab meat, cooked	3 ounces	624
Clams, cooked	3 ounces	585
Sunflower seeds	1 ounce	519
Lentils, cooked	1 cup	497
Hazelnuts	1 ounce	496
Mushrooms, raw	1 cup (sliced)	344
Almonds	1 ounce	332
Chocolate (semi-sweet)	1 ounce	198
Hot cocoa mix	1 ounce (1 packet)	169
Peanut butter (chunky)	2 tablespoons	165
Shredded wheat cereal	2 biscuits	143

1100 µg)/d for adult women and 1.2 to 1.6 mg (1200 to 1600 µg)/d for adult men.[5] The copper content of some foods that are relatively rich in copper is listed in micrograms in Table 16–2.

Supplements

Copper supplements are available as cupric oxide, copper gluconate, copper sulfate, and copper amino acid chelates.[30]

Safety

Toxicity

Copper toxicity is rare in the general population. Acute copper poisoning has occurred through the contamination of beverages by storage in copper-containing containers as well as from contaminated water supplies.[31] In the United States, the health-based guideline for a maximum water copper concentration of 1.3 mg/L is enforced by the Environmental Protection Agency.[32] Symptoms of acute copper toxicity include abdominal pain, nausea,

Table 16–3 Tolerable Upper Intake Level (UL) for Copper

Life Stage	Age	UL, µg/d
Infants	0–12 months	not possible to establish*
Children	1–3 years	1000
Children	4–8 years	3000
Children	9–13 years	5000
Adolescents	14–18 years	8000
Adults	19 years and older	10,000

*Source of intake should be from food and formula only.

vomiting, and diarrhea, which help prevent additional ingestion and absorption of copper. More serious signs of acute copper toxicity include severe liver damage, kidney failure, coma, and death. Of more concern from a nutritional standpoint is the possibility of liver damage resulting from long-term exposure to lower doses of copper. In generally healthy individuals, doses of up to 10 mg (10,000 µg) daily have not resulted in liver damage. For this reason, the U.S. Food and Nutrition Board recently set the tolerable upper level of intake for copper at 10 mg/d from food and supplements (Table 16–3). It should be noted that individuals with genetic disorders affecting copper metabolism (Wilson's disease, Indian childhood cirrhosis, and idiopathic copper toxicosis) may be at risk of adverse effects of chronic copper toxicity at significantly lower intake levels.[5]

Drug Interactions

Relatively little is known about the interaction of copper with drugs. Penicillamine is used to bind copper and enhance its elimination in Wilson's disease, a genetic disorder resulting in copper overload. Because it dramatically increases the urinary excretion of copper, individuals taking penicillamine for reasons other than copper overload may have an increased requirement for copper. Antacids may interfere with copper absorption when used in very high amounts.[2]

LPI Recommendation

The RDA for copper (900 µg/d for adults) is sufficient to prevent deficiency, but the lack of clear indicators of copper nutritional status in humans makes it difficult to determine the level of copper intake most likely to promote optimum health or prevent chronic disease. A varied diet should provide enough copper for most people. For those who are concerned that their diet may not provide adequate copper, a multivitamin/multimineral supplement will generally provide at least the RDA for copper.

Older Adults
Because aging has not been associated with significant changes in the requirement for copper, our recommendation for copper is the same for adults over the age of 65.[33]

References

1. Linder MC, Hazegh-Azam M. Copper biochemistry and molecular biology. *Am J Clin Nutr* 1996;63(5):797S–811S.
2. Turnlund JR. Copper. In: Shils M, Olson JA, Shike M, Ross AC, eds. *Nutrition in Health and Disease*, 9th ed. Baltimore: Williams & Wilkins; 1999:241–252.
3. Uauy R, Olivares M, Gonzalez M. Essentiality of copper in humans. *Am J Clin Nutr* 1998;67(5 Suppl):952S–959S.
4. Harris ED. Copper. In: O'Dell BL, Sunde RA, eds. *Handbook of Nutritionally Essential Minerals*. New York: Marcel Dekker, Inc.; 1997:231–273.
5. Food and Nutrition Board, Institute of Medicine. Copper. *Dietary Reference Intakes for Vitamin A, Vitamin K, Boron, Chromium, Copper, Iodine, Iron, Manganese, Molybdenum, Nickel, Silicon, Vanadium, and Zinc*. Washington, D.C.: National Academy Press; 2001:224–257.
6. Johnson MA, Fischer JG, Kays SE. Is copper an antioxidant nutrient? *Crit Rev Food Sci Nutr* 1992;32(1):1–31.
7. Finley EB, Cerklewski FL. Influence of ascorbic acid supplementation on copper status in young adult men. *Am J Clin Nutr* 1983;37(4):553–556.
8. Jacob RA, Skala JH, Omaye ST, Turnlund JR. Effect of varying ascorbic acid intakes on copper absorption and ceruloplasmin levels of young men. *J Nutr* 1987;117(12):2109–2115.
9. Percival SS, Kauwell GP, Bowser E, Wagner M. Altered copper status in adult men with cystic fibrosis. *J Am Coll Nutr* 1999;18(6):614–619.
10. Fox PL, Mazumder B, Ehrenwald E, Mukhopadhyay CK. Ceruloplasmin and cardiovascular disease. *Free Radic Biol Med* 2000;28(12):1735–1744.

11. Jones AA, DiSilvestro RA, Coleman M, Wagner TL. Copper supplementation of adult men: effects on blood copper enzyme activities and indicators of cardiovascular disease risk. *Metabolism* 1997;46(12):1380–1383.

12. Ford ES. Serum copper concentration and coronary heart disease among US adults. *Am J Epidemiol* 2000;151(12):1182–1188.

13. Klevay LM. Cardiovascular disease from copper deficiency—a history. *J Nutr* 2000;130(2S Suppl):489S–92S.

14. Kinsman GD, Howard AN, Stone DL, Mullins PA. Studies in copper status and atherosclerosis. *Biochem Soc Trans* 1990;18(6):1186–1188.

15. Mielcarz G, Howard AN, Mielcarz B, et al. Leucocyte copper, a marker of copper body status is low in coronary artery disease. *J Trace Elem Med Biol* 2001;15(1):31–35.

16. Wang XL, Adachi T, Sim AS, Wilcken DE. Plasma extracellular superoxide dismutase levels in an Australian population with coronary artery disease. *Arterioscler Thromb Vasc Biol* 1998;18(12):1915–1921.

17. Klevay LM. Lack of a recommended dietary allowance for copper may be hazardous to your health. *J Am Coll Nutr* 1998;17(4):322–326.

18. Milne DB, Nielsen FH. Effects of a diet low in copper on copper-status indicators in postmenopausal women. *Am J Clin Nutr* 1996;63(3):358–364.

19. Medeiros DM, Milton A, Brunett E, Stacy L. Copper supplementation effects on indicators of copper status and serum cholesterol in adult males. *Biol Trace Elem Res* 1991;30(1):19–35.

20. Turley E, McKeown A, Bonham MP, et al. Copper supplementation in humans does not affect the susceptibility of low density lipoprotein to in vitro induced oxidation (FOODCUE project). *Free Radic Biol Med* 2000;29(11):1129–1134.

21. Rock E, Mazur A, O'Connor J M, Bonham MP, Rayssiguier Y, Strain JJ. The effect of copper supplementation on red blood cell oxidizability and plasma antioxidants in middle-aged healthy volunteers. *Free Radic Biol Med* 2000;28(3):324–329.

22. Percival SS. Copper and immunity. *Am J Clin Nutr* 1998;67(5 Suppl):1064S–1068S.

23. Failla ML, Hopkins RG. Is low copper status immunosuppressive? *Nutr Rev* 1998;56(1 Pt 2):S59–S64.

24. Heresi G, Castillo-Duran C, Munoz C, Arevalo M, Schlesinger L. Phagocytosis and immunoglobulin levels in hypocupremic children. *Nutr Res* 1985;5:1327–1334.

25. Kelley DS, Daudu PA, Taylor PC, Mackey BE, Turnlund JR. Effects of low-copper diets on human immune response. *Am J Clin Nutr* 1995;62(2):412–416.

26. Conlan D, Korula R, Tallentire D. Serum copper levels in elderly patients with femoral-neck fractures. *Age Ageing* 1990;19(3):212–214.

27. Eaton-Evans J, Mellwrath EM, Jackson WE, McCartney H, Strain JJ. Copper supplementation and the maintenance of bone mineral density in middle-aged women. *J Trace Elem Exp Med* 1996;9:87–94.

28. Baker A, Harvey L, Majask-Newman G, Fairweather-Tait S, Flynn A, Cashman K. Effect of dietary copper intakes on biochemical markers of bone metabolism in healthy adult males. *Eur J Clin Nutr* 1999;53(5):408–412.

29. Baker A, Turley E, Bonham MP, et al. No effect of copper supplementation on biochemical markers of bone metabolism in healthy adults. *Br J Nutr* 1999;82(4):283–290.

30. Hendler SS, Rorvik DR, eds. *PDR for Nutritional Supplements*. Montvale, NJ: Medical Economics Company, Inc; 2001.

31. Bremner I. Manifestations of copper excess. *Am J Clin Nutr* 1998;67(5 Suppl):1069S–1073S.

32. Fitzgerald DJ. Safety guidelines for copper in water. *Am J Clin Nutr* 1998;67(5 Suppl):1098S–1102S.

33. Wood RJ, Suter PM, Russell RM. Mineral requirements of elderly people. *Am J Clin Nutr* 1995;62(3):493–505.

17 Fluoride (Fluorine)

Fluorine occurs naturally in the Earth's crust, water, and food as the negatively charged ion, fluoride (F⁻). Fluoride is considered a trace element because only small amounts are present in the body (about 2.6 g in adults), and because the daily requirement for maintaining dental health is only a few milligrams a day. About 95% of the total body fluoride is found in bones and teeth.[1] Although its role in the prevention of dental caries (tooth decay) is well established, fluoride is not generally considered an essential mineral element because humans do not require it for growth or to sustain life.[2] However, if one considers the prevention of chronic disease (dental caries) an important criterion in determining essentiality, then fluoride might well be considered an essential trace element.[3]

Function

Fluoride is absorbed in the stomach and small intestine. Once in the circulation it rapidly enters mineralized tissue (bones and developing teeth). At usual intake levels, fluoride does not accumulate in soft tissue. The predominant mineral elements in bone are crystals of calcium and phosphate, known as *hydroxyapatite crystals*. Fluoride's high chemical reactivity and small radius allow it to either displace the larger hydroxyl ion in the hydroxyapatite crystal, forming fluoroapatite, or to increase crystal density by entering spaces within the hydroxyapatite crystal. Fluoroapatite hardens tooth enamel and stabilizes bone mineral.[4]

Nutrient Interactions

Both calcium and magnesium form insoluble complexes with fluoride and are capable of significantly decreasing fluoride absorption when present in the same meal. However, the absorption of fluoride in the form of monofluorophosphate, unlike sodium fluoride, is unaffected by calcium. A diet low in chloride (i.e., salt) has been found to increase fluoride retention by reducing urinary excretion of fluoride.[1]

Deficiency

In humans, the only clear effect of inadequate fluoride intake is an increased risk of dental caries (tooth decay) for individuals of all ages. Epidemiologic investigations of patterns of water consumption and the prevalence of dental caries across different climates and geographic regions with different water fluoride concentrations in the United States led to the development of a recommended optimum range of fluoride concentration of 0.7 to 1.2 mg/L or parts per million (ppm), with the lower concentration recommended for warmer climates where water consumption is higher and the higher concentration for colder climates. A number of studies conducted prior to the introduction of fluoride-containing toothpastes demonstrated that the prevalence of dental caries was 40 to 60% lower in communities with optimal water fluoride concentrations than in communities with low water fluoride concentrations.[5]

The Adequate Intake Level

The Food and Nutrition Board (FNB) of the Institute of Medicine updated its recommendations for fluoride intake in 1997 (Table 17–1). The FNB felt there was inadequate data to set a recommended dietary allowance; instead adequate intake levels were based on estimated intakes (0.05 mg/kg of body weight) that have been shown to reduce the occurrence of dental caries most effectively without causing the unwanted side effect of tooth enamel mottling known as dental fluorosis.[5] See the section below on safety for a discussion of dental fluorosis.

Table 17–1   Adequate Intake (AI) for Fluoride

Life Stage	Age	Males, mg/d	Females, mg/d
Infants	0–6 months	0.01	0.01
Infants	7–12 months	0.5	0.5
Children	1–3 years	0.7	0.7
Children	4–8 years	1.0	1.0
Children	9–13 years	2.0	2.0
Adolescents	14–18 years	3.0	3.0
Adults	19 years and older	4.0	3.0
Pregnancy	all ages	–	3.0
Breastfeeding	all ages	–	3.0

Disease Prevention

Dental Caries

Specific cariogenic (cavity-causing) bacteria found in dental plaque are capable of metabolizing certain carbohydrates (sugars) and converting them to organic acids, which can dissolve susceptible tooth enamel. If unchecked, the bacteria may penetrate deeper layers of the tooth and progress into the soft pulp tissue at the center. Untreated caries can lead to severe pain, local infection, tooth loss or extraction, nutritional problems, and serious systemic infections in susceptible individuals.[6] Increased fluoride intake, most commonly through water fluoridation, has been found to decrease dental caries in children and adults. Fluoride consumed in water appears to have a systemic effect in children before teeth erupt, as well as a topical (surface) effect in adults and children after teeth have erupted. Between 1950 and 1980 clinical studies in 20 different countries demonstrated that adding fluoride to community water supplies (0.7 to 1.2 ppm) reduced caries by 40 to 50 % in primary (baby) teeth and 50 to 60 % in permanent teeth.[7]

Although the role of fluoride in preventing dental caries is well established, the mechanisms for its effects are not entirely understood. Originally, it was believed that fluoride incorporated into the enamel during tooth development resulted in a more acid-resistant enamel. More recent research indicates that the primary action of fluoride occurs topically after the teeth erupt into the mouth. When enamel is partially demineralized by organic acids, fluoride in the saliva can enhance the remineralization of enamel through its interactions with calcium and phosphate. In the presence of fluoride, remineralized enamel contains more fluoride and is more resistant to demineralization. In salivary concentrations associated with optimum fluoride intake, fluoride has been found to inhibit bacterial enzymes, resulting in reduced acid production by cariogenic bacteria.[6,7]

Osteoporosis

Although fluoride in pharmacologic doses has been shown to be a potent therapeutic agent for increasing spinal bone mass, there is little evidence that water fluoridation at optimum levels for the prevention of dental caries is helpful in the prevention of osteoporosis. The majority of studies conducted to date have failed to find clinically significant differences in bone mineral density or fracture incidence between residents of areas with fluoridated water supplies and residents in areas without fluoridated water supplies.[8] Two relatively recent studies found drinking water fluoridation to be associated with decreased incidence of hip fracture in the elderly. One study in Italy found a significantly greater risk of femoral (hip) fractures in men and women residing in an area with low water fluoridation (0.05 ppm) compared with the risk in a similar population whose water supply was naturally fluoridated (1.45 ppm) at higher than optimum levels for prevention of dental caries.[9] Another study in Germany found no significant difference in bone mineral density between residents of a community whose water supply had been optimally fluoridated for 30 years (1 ppm) compared with those who resided in a community without fluoridated water.[10] However, the incidence of hip fracture was significantly lower in women over the age of 85 who resided in the community with fluoridated water compared with women of the same age who resided in the area without fluoridated water, despite higher calcium levels in the nonfluoridated water supply.

Disease Treatment

Osteoporosis

Osteoporosis is characterized by decreased bone mineral density (BMD) and increased bone fragility and susceptibility to fracture. In general, decreased BMD is associated with increased risk of fracture. However, the usual relationship between BMD and fracture risk does not always hold true when very high (pharmacologic) doses of fluoride are used to treat osteoporosis. Most available therapies for osteoporosis (e.g., estrogen, calcitonin, and bisphosphonates) decrease bone loss (resorption), resulting in very small increases in BMD. Pharmacologic doses of fluoride are capable of producing large increases in the BMD of the lumbar spine. Despite dramatic increases in lumbar spine BMD, therapeutic trials of fluoride in patients with osteoporosis have not consistently demonstrated significant decreases in the occurrence of vertebral fracture.[11] A meta-analysis of 11 controlled studies that included 1429 participants found that fluoride treatment resulted in increased BMD at the lumbar spine but did not substantially decrease the risk of vertebral fractures.[12] This meta-analysis also found that increasing doses of fluoride increased the risk of nonvertebral fractures without lowering the risk of vertebral fractures.

Early studies using high doses of sodium fluoride (75 mg/d) may have induced rapid bone mineralization in the absence of adequate calcium and vitamin D, resulting in denser bones that were not mechanically stronger.[13] Some controlled studies using lower doses, intermittent dosage schedules, or slow release formulations (enteric-coated sodium fluoride) have demonstrated a decreased incidence of vertebral fracture along with increased bone density of the lumbar spine.[14–16] Analysis of bone architecture has also shed some light on the inconsistent effect of fluoride therapy in reducing vertebral fractures. Recent research indicates that osteo-

porosis may be associated with an irreversible change in the architecture of bone known as *decreased trabecular connectivity*. Normal bone consists of a series of plates interconnected by thick rods. Severely osteoporotic bone has fewer plates, and the rods may be fractured or disconnected (decreased trabecular connectivity). Despite the increase in bone density it stimulates, fluoride therapy probably cannot restore connectivity in patients with severe bone loss. Thus, fluoride therapy may be less effective in osteoporotic individuals who have already lost substantial trabecular connectivity.[11,17]

Serious side effects have been associated with the high doses of fluoride used to treat osteoporosis. They include gastrointestinal irritation, joint pain in the lower extremities, the development of calcium deficiency, and the development of stress fractures. The reasons for the occurrence of lower extremity joint pain and stress fractures in patients taking fluoride for osteoporosis remain unclear but may be related to rapid increases in bone formation without sufficient calcium to support such an increase.[11] Presently, enteric-coated sodium fluoride or monofluorophosphate preparations offer a lower side effect profile than the high-dose sodium fluoride used in earlier trials. Additionally, sufficient calcium and vitamin D must be provided to support fluoride-induced bone formation. Although fluoride therapy may be beneficial for the treatment of osteoporosis in appropriately selected and closely monitored individuals, uncertainty about its safety and benefit in reducing fractures has kept the Food and Drug Administration from approving fluoride therapy for osteoporosis.[18] Combinations of lower doses of fluoride with antiresorptive agents, such as estrogen or bisphosphonates, may also improve therapeutic results while minimizing side effects and are considered worthy of further study.[19,20]

Table 17–2   Food Sources of Fluoride

Food	Serving	Fluoride, mg
Canned sardines, with bones	100 g (3.5 ounces)	0.2–0.4
Tea	100 mL (3.5 fluid ounces)	0.1–0.6
Fish, without bones	100 g (3.5 ounces)	0.01–0.17
Chicken	100 g (3.5 ounces)	0.06–0.10

Table 17–3   Fluoride Supplement Schedule Recommended by the American Dental Association, the American Academy of Pediatric Dentistry, and the American Academy of Pediatrics

Age	Fluoride Ion Level in Drinking Water, ppm*		
	< 0.3 ppm	0.3–0.6 ppm	> 0.6 ppm
Birth– 6 months	None	None	None
6 months– 3 years	0.25 mg/d**	None	None
3 years– 6 years	0.50 mg/d	0.25 mg/d	None
6 years– 16 years	1.0 mg/d	0.50 mg/d	None

*1.0 part per million (ppm) = 1 mg/L.
**2.2 mg sodium fluoride contains 1 mg fluoride ion.

Sources

Water Fluoridation

The major source of dietary fluoride in the United States diet is drinking water. When water is fluoridated, it is adjusted to between 0.7 and 1.2 mg of fluoride per liter or 0.7 to 1.2 ppm. This concentration has been found to decrease the incidence of dental caries while minimizing the risk of dental fluorosis and other adverse effects. Approximately 62% of the U.S. population consumes water with sufficient fluoride for the prevention of dental caries. The average fluoride intake for adults living in fluoridated communities ranges from 1.4 to 3.4 mg/d. Because well water can vary greatly in its fluoride content, people who consume water from wells should have the fluoride content of their water tested by the local water district or health department. Water fluoride testing may also be warranted in households that use home water treatment systems. Although water softeners are not thought to change water fluoride levels, reverse osmosis systems, distillation units, and some water filters have been found to remove significant amounts of fluoride from water. However, Brita-type filters do not remove fluoride.[5,18]

Food Sources

The fluoride content of most foods is low (less than 0.05 mg/100 g). Rich sources of fluoride include tea, which concentrates fluoride in its leaves, and marine fish that are consumed with their bones (e.g., sardines). Foods made with mechanically separated (boned) chicken, such as canned meats, hot dogs, and infant foods, also add fluoride to the diet.[21] Foods generally contribute only 0.3 to 0.6 mg of the daily intake of fluoride. An adult male residing in a community with fluoridated water has an intake range from 1 to 3 mg/d. Intake is less than 1 mg/d in nonfluoridated areas.[2] Table 17–2 provides a range of fluoride contents for a few fluoride-rich foods.[5]

Supplements

Fluoride supplements are available only by prescription and are intended for children living in areas with low water fluoride concentrations, for the purpose of bringing their intake to approximately 1 mg/d.[5] The American Dental Association recommends fluoride supplements for those children living in areas with suboptimal water fluoridation.[22] The supplemental fluoride dosage schedule in Table 17–3 was recommended by the American Dental Association, the American Academy of Pediatric Dentistry, and the American Academy of Pediatrics.[23] It requires knowledge of the fluoride concentration of the local drinking water, as well as other possible sources of fluoride intake.

Toothpaste

Fluoridated toothpastes add considerably to fluoride intake of children, especially young children who are more likely to swallow them. Researchers estimate that children under 6 years of age ingest an average of 0.3 mg of fluoride from toothpaste with each brushing. Children under the age of 6 years who ingest more than two or three times the recommended fluoride intake are at increased risk of a white speckling or mottling of the permanent teeth, known as *dental fluorosis*. The major source of excess fluoride intake in this age group comes from swallowing fluoride-containing toothpaste. To prevent dental fluorosis while providing optimum protection from tooth decay, it is recommended that parents supervise children under 6 years of age while brushing with fluoridated toothpaste. In addition to discouraging the swallowing of toothpaste, parents should encourage children to use no more than a pea-size application of toothpaste, and to rinse their mouths with water after brushing.[1,5]

Safety

Adverse Effects

Fluoridation of public drinking water in the United States was initiated over 50 years ago. Since then, a number of adverse effects have been attributed to water fluoridation. However, extensive scientific research has uncovered no evidence of increased risks of cancer, heart disease, kidney disease, liver disease, Alzheimer's disease, birth defects, or Down syndrome.[24,25] The use of high doses of fluoride to treat osteoporosis has been associated with some adverse effects, which are discussed in the Disease Treatment section.

Acute Toxicity. Fluoride is toxic when consumed in excessive amounts, so concentrated fluoride products should be used and stored with caution to prevent the possibility of acute fluoride poisoning, especially in children and other vulnerable individuals. The lowest dose that could trigger life-threatening symptoms is considered to be 5 mg/kg of body weight.

Nausea, abdominal pain, and vomiting almost always accompany acute fluoride toxicity. Other symptoms like diarrhea, excessive salivation and tearing, sweating, and generalized weakness may also occur.[25] To prevent acute fluoride poisoning, the American Dental Association has recommended that no more than 120 mg of fluoride (224 mg of sodium fluoride) be dispensed at one time.[18]

Dental Fluorosis. The mildest form of dental fluorosis is detectable only to the trained observer and is characterized by small opaque white flecks or spots on the enamel of the teeth. Moderate dental fluorosis is characterized by mottling and mild staining of the teeth, and severe dental fluorosis results in marked staining and pitting of the teeth. In its moderate to severe forms, dental fluorosis becomes a cosmetic concern when it affects the incisors and canines (front teeth). Dental fluorosis is a result of excess fluoride intake prior to the eruption of the first permanent teeth (generally before 8 years of age). It is also a dose-dependent condition, with higher fluoride intakes being associated with more pronounced effects on the teeth. The risk of mild to moderate dental fluorosis appears to increase significantly at an intake two to three times that recommended for children of a susceptible age. Severe dental fluorosis has been seen in the United States only at fluoride intakes about five times the recommended level.[24] The incidence of mild and moderate dental fluorosis has increased over the past 50 years, mainly due to increasing fluoride intake from toothpaste, although inappropriate use of fluoride supplements may also contribute. In 1997, the FNB based the tolerable upper intake levels (UL) for fluoride on the prevention of moderate enamel fluorosis.[5] The UL for each age group is presented in Table 17–4.

Skeletal Fluorosis. Intake of fluoride at excessive levels for long periods of time may lead to changes in bone structure known as *skeletal fluorosis*. The early stages of skeletal fluorosis are characterized by increased bone mass, detectable by X-ray. If high fluoride intake persists over many years, joint pain and stiffness may result from the skeletal changes. The most severe form of skeletal fluorosis is known as

Table 17–4 Tolerable Upper Intake Level (UL) for Fluoride

Life Stage	Age	UL, mg/d
Infants	0–6 months	0.7
Infants	6–12 months	0.9
Children	1–3 years	1.3
Children	4–8 years	2.2
Children	9–13 years	10.0
Boys	14–18 years	10.0
Girls	14–18 years	10.0
Men	19 years and over	10.0
Women	19 years and over	10.0

LPI Recommendation

The safety and public health benefits of optimally fluoridated water for prevention of tooth decay in people of all ages and appropriate fluoride supplementation in children and adolescents where optimally fluoridated water is not available have been well established. The Linus Pauling Institute supports the supplementation recommendations of the American Dental Association and the Centers for Disease Control for children and adolescents 16 years of age and younger.[23] At present, available evidence does not indicate a need for fluoride supplementation in generally healthy individuals over the age of 16, even in communities without optimally fluoridated water supplies.

crippling skeletal fluorosis, which may result in calcification of ligaments, immobility, muscle wasting, and neurological problems related to spinal cord compression. Most estimates indicate that crippling skeletal fluorosis occurs only when fluoride intakes exceed 10 to 25 mg/d for at least 10 years. Crippling skeletal fluorosis is extremely rare in the United States. In fact, only five cases have been confirmed in the last 35 years. Interestingly, studies of communities in the United States where water fluoride concentrations were as high as 20 mg/L (ppm), allowing for fluoride intakes as high as 20 mg/d, did not find evidence of crippling skeletal fluorosis. Such water fluoride concentrations are higher than those known to have resulted in crippling skeletal fluorosis in other countries, suggesting that metabolic or dietary factors might render some populations more susceptible.[5,25]

Older Adults

Available evidence does not support a need for fluoride supplementation in generally healthy older adults (65 years and over), even in communities without optimally fluoridated water supplies.

References

1. Cerklewski FL. Fluoride bioavailability—nutritional and clinical aspects. *Nutr Res* 1997;17:907–929.
2. Nielsen FH. Ultratrace minerals. In: Shils M, Olson JA, Shike M, Ross AC, eds. *Nutrition in Health and Disease,* 9th ed. Baltimore: Williams & Wilkins; 1999:283–303.
3. Cerklewski FL. Fluoride—essential or just beneficial? *Nutrition* 1998;14(5):475–476.
4. Cerklewski FL. Fluorine. In: O'Dell BL, Sunde RA, eds. *Handbook of Nutritionally Essential Minerals.* New York: Marcel Dekker, Inc.; 1997:583–602.
5. Food and Nutrition Board, Institute of Medicine. Fluoride. *Dietary Reference Intakes: Calcium, Phosphorus, Magnesium, Vitamin D, and Fluoride.* Washington, D.C.: National Academy Press; 1997:288–313.
6. Centers for Disease Control. Achievements in public health, 1900–1999: fluoridation of drinking water to prevent dental caries. *MMWR* 1999;48:933–940.
7. DePaola DP. Nutrition in relation to dental medicine. In: Shils M, Olson JA, Shike M, Ross AC, eds. *Nutrition in Health and Disease,* 9th ed. Baltimore: Williams & Wilkins; 1999:1099–1124.
8. Krall EA, Dawson-Hughes B. Osteoporosis. In: Shils M, Olson JA, Shike M, Ross AC, eds. *Nutrition in Health and Disease,* 9th ed. Baltimore: Williams & Wilkins; 1999:1353–1364.
9. Fabiani L, Leoni V, Vitali M. Bone-fracture incidence rate in two Italian regions with different fluoride concentration levels in drinking water. *J Trace Elem Med Biol* 1999;13(4):232–237.
10. Lehmann R, Wapniarz M, Hofmann B, Pieper B, Haubitz I, Allolio B. Drinking water fluoridation: bone

Drug Interactions

Calcium supplements, as well as calcium- and aluminum-containing antacids, can decrease the absorption of fluoride. It is best to take these products 2 hours before or after fluoride supplements.[26]

mineral density and hip fracture incidence. *Bone* 1998;22(3):273–278.

11. Cesar Libanati K-H. Fluoride therapy for osteoporosis. In: Marcus R, ed. *Osteoporosis*. San Diego: Academic Press; 1996:1259–1277.

12. Haguenauer D, Welch V, Shea B, Tugwell P, Adachi JD, Wells G. Fluoride for the treatment of post-menopausal osteoporotic fractures: a meta-analysis. *Osteoporos Int* 2000;11(9):727–738.

13. Riggs BL, Hodgson SF, O'Fallon WM, et al. Effect of fluoride treatment on the fracture rate in post-menopausal women with osteoporosis. *N Engl J Med* 1990;322(12):802–809.

14. Pak CY, Sakhaee K, Adams-Huet B, Piziak V, Peterson RD, Poindexter JR. Treatment of postmenopausal osteoporosis with slow-release sodium fluoride: final report of a randomized controlled trial. *Ann Intern Med* 1995;123(6):401–408.

15. Reginster JY, Meurmans L, Zegels B, et al. The effect of sodium monofluorophosphate plus calcium on vertebral fracture rate in postmenopausal women with moderate osteoporosis: a randomized, controlled trial. *Ann Intern Med* 1998;129(1):1–8.

16. Ringe JD, Kipshoven C, Coster A, Umbach R. Therapy of established postmenopausal osteoporosis with monofluorophosphate plus calcium: dose-related effects on bone density and fracture rate. *Osteoporos Int* 1999;9(2):171–178.

17. Balena R, Kleerekoper M, Foldes JA, et al. Effects of different regimens of sodium fluoride treatment for osteoporosis on the structure, remodeling and mineralization of bone. *Osteoporos Int* 1998;8(5):428–435.

18. American Dietetic Association. Position of the American Dietetic Association: the impact of fluoride on health. *J Am Diet Assoc* 2001;101(1):126–132.

19. Alexandersen P, Riis BJ, Christiansen C. Monofluorophosphate combined with hormone replacement therapy induces a synergistic effect on bone mass by dissociating bone formation and resorption in postmenopausal women: a randomized study. *J Clin Endocrinol Metab* 1999;84(9):3013–3020.

20. Murray TM, Ste-Marie LG. Prevention and management of osteoporosis: consensus statements from the Scientific Advisory Board of the Osteoporosis Society of Canada, VII: Fluoride therapy for osteoporosis. *CMAJ* 1996;155(7):949–954.

21. Fein NJ, Cerklewski FL. Fluoride content of foods made with mechanically separated chicken. *J Agric Food Chem* 2001;49(9):4284–4286.

22. Adair SM. Overview of the history and current status of fluoride supplementation schedules. *J Public Health Dent* 1999;59(4):252–258.

23. Centers for Disease Control and Prevention. Recommendations for using fluoride to prevent and control dental caries in the United States. *MMWR Recomm Rep* 2001;50(RR-14):1–42.

24. National Research Council. *Health Effects of Ingested Fluoride*. Washington, D.C.: National Academy Press; 1993.

25. Whitford GM. *The Metabolism and Toxicity of Fluoride*, Vol. 13. Basel: S. Karger AG; 1996.

26. Minerals. *Drug Facts and Comparisons*. St. Louis: Facts and Comparisons; 2000:27–51.

18 Iodine

Iodine, a nonmetallic trace element, is required by humans for the synthesis of thyroid hormones. Iodine deficiency is an important health problem throughout much of the world. Most of the earth's iodine is found in its oceans. In general, the older an exposed soil surface, the more likely the iodine has been leached away by erosion. Mountainous regions, such as the Himalayas, the Andes, and the Alps, and flooded river valleys, such as the Ganges, are among the most severely iodine-deficient areas in the world.[1]

Function

Iodine is an essential component of the thyroid hormones, triiodothyronine (T_3) and thyroxine (T_4), and is therefore essential for normal thyroid function. To meet the body's demand for thyroid hormones, the thyroid gland traps iodine from the blood and converts it into thyroid hormones that are stored and released into the circulation when needed. In target tissues, such as the liver and the brain, T_3, the physiologically active thyroid hormone, can bind to thyroid receptors in the nuclei of cells and regulate gene expression. T_4, the most abundant circulating thyroid hormone, can be converted to T_3 by enzymes known as *deiodinases* in target tissues. In this manner, thyroid hormones regulate a number of physiologic processes, including growth, development, metabolism, and reproductive function.[1,2]

The regulation of thyroid function is a complex process that involves the brain (hypothalamus) and pituitary gland. In response to thyrotropin-releasing hormone (TRH) secretion by the hypothalamus, the pituitary gland secretes thyroid-stimulating hormone (TSH), which stimulates iodine trapping, thyroid hormone synthesis, and release of T_3 and T_4 by the thyroid gland. The presence of adequate circulating T_4 decreases the sensitivity of the pituitary gland to TRH, limiting its secretion of TSH

(Fig. 18–1). When circulating T_4 levels decrease, the pituitary increases its secretion of TSH, resulting in increased iodine trapping, as well as increased production and release of T_3 and T_4. Iodine deficiency results in inadequate production of T_4. In response to decreased blood levels of T_4, the pituitary gland increases its output of TSH. Persistently elevated TSH levels may lead to hypertrophy (enlargement) of the thyroid gland, also known as *goiter*.[3]

Deficiency

Iodine deficiency is now accepted as the most common cause of preventable brain damage in the world. According to the World Health Organization, iodine deficiency disorders (IDD) affect 740 million people throughout the world, and nearly 50 million people suffer from some degree of IDD-related brain damage. The spectrum of IDD includes mental retardation, hypothyroidism, goiter, and varying degrees of other growth and developmental abnormalities.[1,4] Nearly 2.2 million people throughout the world live in areas of iodine deficiency and risk its consequences. Major international efforts have produced dramatic improvements in the correction of iodine deficiency in the 1990s mainly through the use of iodized salt and iodized vegetable oil in iodine-deficient countries.[5]

Thyroid enlargement, or goiter, is one of the earliest and most visible signs of iodine deficiency. The thyroid enlarges in response to persistent stimulation by TSH. In mild iodine deficiency, this adaptive response may be enough to provide the body with sufficient thyroid hormone. However, more severe cases of iodine deficiency result in hypothyroidism. Adequate iodine intake will generally reduce the size of goiters, but the reversibility of the effects of hypothyroidism depends on an individual's stage of development. Iodine defi-

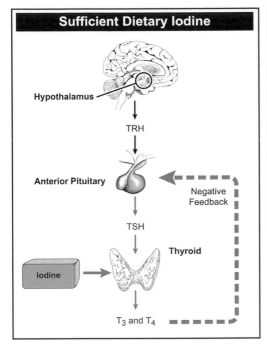

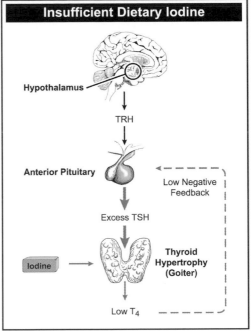

Figure 18–1. Iodine intake and thyroid function. In response to thyrotropin-releasing hormone (TRH) secretion by the hypothalamus, the pituitary gland secretes thyroid-stimulating hormone (TSH), which stimulates iodine trapping, thyroid hormone synthesis, and release of T_3 (triiodothyronine) and T_4 (thyroxine) by the thyroid gland. When dietary iodine intake is sufficient, the presence of adequate circulating T_4 decreases the sensitivity of the pituitary gland to TRH, limiting its secretion of TSH. When circulating T_4 levels decrease, the pituitary increases its secretion of TSH, resulting in increased iodine trapping as well as increased production and release of T_3 and T_4. Dietary iodine deficiency results in inadequate production of T_4. In response to decreased blood levels of T_4, the pituitary gland increases its output of TSH. Persistently elevated TSH levels may lead to hypertrophy of the thyroid gland, also known as *goiter*.

ciency has adverse effects in all stages of development but is most damaging to the developing brain. In addition to regulating many aspects of growth and development, thyroid hormone is important for the myelination of the central nervous system, which is most active before and shortly after birth.[2,5]

The Effects of Iodine Deficiency by Developmental Stage

Prenatal Development. Fetal iodine deficiency is caused by iodine deficiency in the mother. One of the most devastating effects of maternal iodine deficiency is congenital hypothyroidism, a condition that is sometimes referred to as *cretinism* and results in irreversible mental retardation. Congenital hypothyroidism oc-

curs in two forms, although there is considerable overlap between them. The neurologic form is characterized by mental and physical retardation and deafness. It is the result of maternal iodine deficiency that affects the fetus before its own thyroid is functional. The myxedematous or hypothyroid form is characterized by short stature and mental retardation. In addition to iodine deficiency, the hypothyroid form has been associated with selenium deficiency and the presence of goitrogens in the diet that interfere with thyroid hormone production.[6]

Newborns and Infants. Infant mortality is increased in areas of iodine deficiency, and several studies have demonstrated an increase in childhood survival when iodine deficiency is

Table 18–1 Recommended Dietary Allowance (RDA) for Iodine

Life Stage	Age	Males, µg/d	Females, µg/d
Infants	0–6 months	110 (AI)	110 (AI)
Infants	7–12 months	130 (AI)	130 (AI)
Children	1–3 years	90	90
Children	4–8 years	90	90
Children	9–13 years	120	120
Adolescents	14–18 years	150	150
Adults	19 years and older	150	150
Pregnancy	all ages	–	220
Breast-feeding	all ages	–	290

AI, adequate intake level.

corrected.[7] Infancy is a period of rapid brain growth and development. Sufficient thyroid hormone, which depends on adequate iodine intake, is essential for normal brain development. Even in the absence of congenital hypothyroidism, iodine deficiency during infancy may result in abnormal brain development and, consequently, impaired intellectual development.[8]

Children and Adolescents. Iodine deficiency in children and adolescents is often associated with goiter. The incidence of goiter peaks in adolescence and is more common in girls. School children in iodine-deficient areas show poorer school performance, lower IQs, and a higher incidence of learning disabilities than matched groups from iodine-sufficient areas. A recent meta-analysis of 18 studies concluded that iodine deficiency alone lowered mean IQ scores in children by 13.5 points.[9,10]

Adults. Inadequate iodine intake may also result in goiter and hypothyroidism in adults. Although the effects of hypothyroidism are more subtle in the brains of adults than children, recent research suggests that hypothyroidism results in slower response times and impaired mental function.[1]

Pregnancy and Lactation. Iodine requirements are increased in pregnant and breast-feeding women (Table 18–1).[5] Iodine deficiency during pregnancy has been associated with increased incidence of miscarriage, stillbirth, and birth defects. Moreover, severe iodine deficiency during pregnancy may result in congenital hypothyroidism (cretinism) in the offspring.[6] Iodine-deficient women who are breast-feeding may not be able to provide sufficient iodine to their infants who are particularly vulnerable to the effects of iodine deficiency.[1] A daily prenatal supplement providing 150 µg of iodine will help to ensure that pregnant and breast-feeding women consume sufficient iodine during these critical periods.

Because iodine deficiency results in increased iodine trapping by the thyroid, iodine-deficient individuals of all ages are more susceptible to radiation-induced thyroid cancer as well as to iodine-induced hyperthyroidism.[1]

Nutrient Interactions

Selenium deficiency can exacerbate the effects of iodine deficiency. Iodine is essential for the synthesis of thyroid hormone, but selenium-dependent enzymes (iodothyronine deiodinases) are also required for the conversion of T_4 to the biologically active thyroid hormone T_3.[6] Deficiencies of vitamin A or iron may also exacerbate the effects of iodine deficiency.[5]

Goitrogens

Some foods contain substances that interfere with iodine utilization or thyroid hormone production, known as *goitrogens*. The occurrence of goiter in the Democratic Republic of Congo has been related to the consumption of casava, which contains a compound that is metabolized to thiocyanate and blocks thyroidal uptake of iodine. Some species of millet and cruciferous vegetables (for example, cabbage, broccoli, cauliflower, and Brussels sprouts) also contain goitrogens.[1,5] The soybean isoflavones genistein and daidzein have also been found to inhibit thyroid hormone synthesis.[11] Most of these goitrogens are not of clinical importance unless they are consumed in large amounts or there is coexisting iodine deficiency. Recent findings also indicate that tobacco smoking may be associated with an increased risk of goiter in iodine-deficient areas.[12]

Individuals at Risk of Iodine Deficiency

Although the risk of iodine deficiency for populations living in iodine-deficient areas without adequate iodine fortification programs is well recognized, concerns have been raised that certain subpopulations may not consume adequate iodine in countries considered iodine-sufficient. Vegetarian and non-vegetarian diets that exclude iodized salt, fish, and seaweed have been found to contain very little iodine.[1,5,13,14] Urinary iodine excretion studies suggest that iodine intakes are declining in Switzerland, New Zealand, and the United States, possibly due to increased adherence to dietary recommendations to reduce salt intake. Although iodine intake in the United States remains sufficient, further monitoring of iodine intake has been recommended.[15,16]

The Recommended Dietary Allowance

The recommended dietary allowance (RDA) for iodine was reevaluated by the Food and Nutrition Board (FNB) of the Institute of Medicine in 2001 (Table 18–1). The recommended amounts were calculated using several methods, including the measurement of iodine accumulation in the thyroid glands of individuals with normal thyroid function.[5] These recommendations are in agreement with those of the International Council for Control of Iodine Deficiency Disorders, the World Health Organization, and UNICEF.[2]

Disease Prevention

Radiation-Induced Thyroid Cancer

Radioactive iodine, especially ^{131}I, may be released into the environment as a result of nuclear reactor accidents. Thyroid accumulation of radioactive iodine increases the risk of developing thyroid cancer, especially in child-

ren. The increased iodine-trapping activity of the thyroid gland in iodine deficiency results in increased thyroid accumulation of radioactive iodine. Thus, iodine-deficient individuals are at increased risk of developing radiation-induced thyroid cancer because they will accumulate greater amounts of radioactive iodine. Potassium iodide administered in pharmacologic doses (50 to 100 mg for adults) within 48 hours before or 8 hours after radiation exposure from a nuclear reactor accident can significantly reduce thyroid uptake of ^{131}I and decrease the risk of radiation-induced thyroid cancer.[17] The prompt and widespread use of potassium iodide prophylaxis in Poland after the 1986 Chernobyl nuclear reactor accident may explain the lack of a significant increase in childhood thyroid cancer in Poland compared to fallout areas where potassium iodide prophylaxis was not widely used.[18] In the United States the Nuclear Regulatory Commission requires that consideration be given to including potassium iodide as a protective measure for the general public in the case of a major release of radioactivity from a nuclear power plant.[19]

Disease Treatment

Fibrocystic Breast Condition

Fibrocystic breast condition (FCC) is a benign (noncancerous) condition of the breasts, characterized by lumpiness and discomfort in one or both breasts. In estrogen-treated rats, iodine deficiency leads to changes similar to those seen in FCC, and iodine repletion was found to reverse those changes.[20] An uncontrolled study of 233 women with FCC found that treatment with aqueous molecular iodine (I_2) at a dose of 0.08 mg I_2/kg of body weight daily for 6 to 18 months was associated with improvement in pain and other symptoms in over 70 % of those treated.[21] About 10 % of the study participants reported side effects that were described by the investigators as minor. A double-blind, placebo-controlled trial of aqueous molecular iodine (0.07 to 0.09 mg I_2/kg of body weight daily for 6 months) in 56 women with FCC found that 65 % of the women taking molecular iodine reported improvement compared with 33 % of those taking the placebo.[21] Although the investigators recommended larger controlled clinical trials to determine the therapeutic value of molecular iodine in FCC, no further results have been published in the scientific or medical literature. The doses of iodine used in these studies (about 5 mg for a 60 kg person) were several times higher than the tolerable upper level of intake (UL) recommended by the FNB and should only be used under medical supervision.

Sources

Although data from the Total Diet Study indicate that the average iodine intake in the United States is 240 to 300 µg/d for adult men and 190 to 210 µg/d for adult women, iodine intake in the United States has decreased significantly over the past 20 years. Between 1988 and 1994, 11 % of the U.S. population was found to have low urinary iodine concentrations, more than four times the proportion found between 1971 and 1974. Moreover, 6.7 % of pregnant women and 14.5 % of women of childbearing age had urinary iodine concentrations associated with insufficient iodine intake.[16]

Food Sources

The iodine content of most foods depends on the iodine content of the soil in which it was raised. Seafood is rich in iodine because marine animals can concentrate the iodine from seawater. Certain types of seaweed (e.g., wakame) are also very rich in iodine. Processed foods may contain slightly higher levels of iodine due to the addition of iodized salt or food additives, such as calcium iodate and potassium iodate. Dairy products are relatively good sources of iodine because iodine is commonly added to animal feed in the United States. In the United Kingdom and northern Europe, iodine levels in dairy products tend to be lower in summer when cattle are allowed to graze in pastures with low soil iodine content.[5] Table 18–2 lists the iodine content of some iodine-rich foods in micrograms. Because the iodine content of foods can vary considerably, these values should be considered approximate.[22]

Table 18–2   Food Sources of Iodine

Food	Serving	Iodine, µg
Cod	3 ounces*	99
Salt (iodized)	1 g	77
Potato with peel, baked	1 medium	63
Milk	1 cup (8 fluid ounces)	56
Shrimp	3 ounces*	35
Fish sticks	2 fish sticks	35
Navy beans, cooked	1/2 cup	35
Turkey breast, baked	3 ounces*	34
Egg, boiled	1 large	29
Tuna, canned in oil	3 ounces (1/2 can)	17
Seaweed	1 ounce	Variable; may be more than 18,000 µg

*A 3-ounce serving of meat or fish is about the size of a deck of cards.

Supplements

Potassium iodide is available as a nutritional supplement, typically in combination products, such as multivitamin/multimineral supplements. Iodine makes up approximately 77 % of the total weight of potassium iodide.[11] A multivitamin/multimineral supplement that contains 100 % of the daily value for iodine provides 150 µg of iodine. Although most people in the United States consume sufficient iodine in their diets from iodized salt and food additives, an additional 150 µg/d is unlikely to result in excessive iodine intake.

Potassium iodide as well as potassium iodate may be used to iodize salt. In the United States and Canada, iodized salt contains 77 µg of iodine per gram of salt. A more common recommendation for salt iodization is 20 to 40 µg/g depending on variables such as iodine intake from other sources and daily salt consumption. Iodized vegetable oil is also used in some countries as an iodine source.[2,11]

Safety

Acute Toxicity

Acute iodine poisoning is rare and usually occurs only with doses of many grams. Symptoms of acute iodine poisoning include burning of the mouth, throat, and stomach, fever, nausea, vomiting, diarrhea, a weak pulse, and coma.[5]

Iodine Excess

It is rare for diets of natural foods to supply more than 2000 µg of iodine per day, and most diets supply less than 1000 µg/d. People living in the northern coastal regions of Japan, whose diets contain large amounts of seaweed, have been found to have iodine intakes ranging from 50,000 to 80,000 µg (50 to 80 mg) of iodine per day.[1]

In Iodine Deficiency. Iodine supplementation programs in iodine-deficient populations have been associated with an increased incidence of iodine-induced hyperthyroidism (IHH), mainly in older people and those with multinodular goiter. Iodine intakes of 150 to 200 µg/d have been found to increase the incidence of IHH in iodine-deficient populations. Iodine deficiency increases the risk of developing autonomous thyroid nodules that are unresponsive to the normal thyroid regulation system, resulting in hyperthyroidism after iodine supplementation. IHH is considered by some experts to be an iodine deficiency disorder. In general, the large benefit of iodization programs outweighs the small risk of IHH in iodine-deficient populations.[1,23]

In Iodine Sufficiency. In iodine-sufficient populations (e.g., the United States), excess iodine intake is most commonly associated with elevated blood levels of TSH, hypothyroidism, and goiter. Although a slightly elevated TSH level does not necessarily indicate inadequate thyroid hormone production, it is the earliest sign of abnormal thyroid function when iodine intake is excessive. In iodine-sufficient adults, elevated TSH levels have been found at iodine intakes between 1700 and 1800 µg/d. To minimize the risk of developing

Table 18–3 Tolerable Upper Intake Level (UL) for Iodine

Life Stage	Age	UL, µg/d
Infants	0–12 months	Not possible to establish*
Children	1–3 years	200
Children	4–8 years	300
Children	9–13 years	600
Adolescents	14–18 years	900
Adults	19 years and older	1100

*Source of intake should be from food and formula only.

hypothyroidism, the FNB set a UL for iodine at 1100 µg/d for adults. Very high (pharmacologic) doses of iodine may also produce thyroid enlargement (goiter) due to increased TSH stimulation of the thyroid gland. Prolonged intakes of more than 18,000 µg/d (18 mg/d) have been found to increase the incidence of goiter. The UL values for iodine are listed by age group in Table 18–3. The UL is not meant to apply to individuals who are being treated with iodine under medical supervision.[5]

Individuals with Increased Sensitivity to Excess Iodine Intake. Individuals with iodine deficiency, nodular goiter, or autoimmune thyroid disease may be sensitive to intake levels considered safe for the general population and may not be protected by the UL for iodine intake.[5] Children with cystic fibrosis may also be more sensitive to the adverse effects of excess iodine.[11]

Excess Iodine and Thyroid Cancer. Observational studies have found increased iodine intake to be associated with an increased incidence of thyroid papillary cancer. The reasons for this association are not clear. In populations that were previously iodine-deficient, salt iodization programs have resulted in relative increases in thyroid papillary cancers and relative decreases in thyroid follicular cancers. In general, thyroid papillary cancers are less aggressive and have a better prognosis than thyroid follicular cancers.[24]

Drug Interactions

Amiodarone, a medication used to prevent abnormal heart rhythms, contains high levels of iodine and may affect thyroid function. Medications used to treat hyperthyroidism, such as propylthiuracil and methimazole, may increase the risk of hypothyroidism. The use of lithium in combination with pharmacologic doses of potassium iodide may result in hypothyroidism. The use of pharmacologic doses of potassium iodide may decrease the anticoagulant effect of warfarin.[5,11]

LPI Recommendation

The RDA for iodine is sufficient to ensure normal thyroid function. There is presently no evidence that iodine intakes higher than the RDA are beneficial. Most people in the United States consume more than sufficient iodine in their diets, making supplementation unnecessary. Given the importance of sufficient iodine during prenatal development and infancy, pregnant and breast-feeding women should consider taking a supplement providing 150 µg of iodine per day.

Older Adults

Because aging has not been associated with significant changes in the requirement for iodine, our recommendation for iodine is not different for adults over the age of 65.

References

1. Hetzel BS, Clugston GA. Iodine. In: Shils M, Olson JA, Shike M, Ross AC, eds. *Nutrition in Health and Disease,* Vol. 9. Baltimore: Williams & Wilkins; 1999:253–264.
2. Dunn JT. What's happening to our iodine? *J Clin Endocrinol Metab* 1998;83(10):3398–3400.
3. Larsen PR, Davies TF, Hay ID. The thyroid gland. In: Wilson JD, Foster DW, Kronenberg HM, Larsen PR, eds. *Williams Textbook of Endocrinology,* 9th ed. Philadelphia: W.B. Saunders Company; 1998:389–515.
4. World Health Organization. Eliminating iodine deficiency disorders. *World Health Organization* [Web page]. July 23, 2001. Available at: http://www.who.int/nut/idd.htm. Accessed August 23, 2001.
5. Food and Nutrition Board, Institute of Medicine. Iodine. *Dietary Reference Intakes for Vitamin A, Vitamin K, Boron, Chromium, Copper, Iodine, Iron, Manganese, Molybdenum, Nickel, Silicon, Vanadium, and Zinc.* Washington, D.C.: National Academy Press; 2001:258–289.
6. Levander OA, Whanger PD. Deliberations and evaluations of the approaches, endpoints and paradigms for selenium and iodine dietary recommendations. *J Nutr* 1996;126(9 Suppl):2427S–2434S.
7. DeLong GR, Leslie PW, Wang SH, et al. Effect on infant mortality of iodination of irrigation water in a severely iodine-deficient area of China. *Lancet* 1997;350(9080):771–773.
8. Hetzel BS. Iodine and neuropsychological development. *J Nutr* 2000;130(2S Suppl):493S–495S.
9. Bleichrodt N, Shrestha RM, West CE, Hautvast JG, van de Vijver FJ, Born MP. The benefits of adequate iodine intake. *Nutr Rev* 1996;54(4 Pt 2):S72–S78.
10. Tiwari BD, Godbole MM, Chattopadhyay N, Mandal A, Mithal A. Learning disabilities and poor motivation to achieve due to prolonged iodine deficiency. *Am J Clin Nutr* 1996;63(5):782–786.
11. Hendler SS, Rorvik DR, eds. *PDR for Nutritional Supplements.* Montvale, NJ: Medical Economics Company, Inc; 2001.
12. Knudsen N, Bulow I, Laurberg P, Ovesen L, Perrild H, Jorgensen T. Association of tobacco smoking with goiter in a low-iodine-intake area. *Arch Intern Med.* 2002;162(4):439–443.
13. Davidsson L. Are vegetarians an "at risk group" for iodine deficiency? *Br J Nutr* 1999;81(1):3–4.
14. Remer T, Neubert A, Manz F. Increased risk of iodine deficiency with vegetarian nutrition. *Br J Nutr* 1999;81(1):45–49.
15. Thomson CD, Woodruffe S, Colls A, Doyle TD. Urinary iodine and thyroid status of New Zealand residents. In: Roussel AM, Anderson RA, Favier A, eds. *Trace Elements in Man and Animals,* Vol. 10. New York: Kluwer Academic Press; 2000:343–344.
16. Hollowell JG, Staehling NW, Hannon WH, et al. Iodine nutrition in the United States. Trends and public health implications: iodine excretion data from National Health and Nutrition Examination Surveys I and III (1971–1974 and 1988–1994). *J Clin Endocrinol Metab* 1998;83(10):3401–3408.
17. Zanzonico PB, Becker DV. Effects of time of administration and dietary iodine levels on potassium iodide (KI) blockade of thyroid irradiation by 131I from radioactive fallout. *Health Phys* 2000;78(6):660–667.
18. Nauman J, Wolff J. Iodide prophylaxis in Poland after the Chernobyl reactor accident: benefits and risks. *Am J Med* 1993;94(5):524–532.
19. Nuclear Regulatory Commission. Consideration of potassium iodide in emergency plans. Nuclear Regulatory Commission. Final rule. *Fed Regist* 2001;66(13):5427–5440.
20. Eskin BA, Grotkowski CE, Connolly CP, Ghent WR. Different tissue responses for iodine and iodide in rat thyroid and mammary glands. *Biol Trace Elem Res* 1995;49(1):9–19.
21. Ghent WR, Eskin BA, Low DA, Hill LP. Iodine replacement in fibrocystic disease of the breast. *Can J Surg* 1993;36(5):453–460.
22. Pennington JAT, Schoen SA, Salmon GD, Young B, Johnson RD, Marts RW. Composition of core foods of the U.S. food supply, 1982–1991, III: Copper, manganese, selenium, iodine. *J Food Comp Anal* 1995;8:171–217.
23. Delange F. Risks and benefits of iodine supplementation. *Lancet* 1998;351(9107):923–924.
24. Feldt-Rasmussen U. Iodine and cancer. *Thyroid* 2001;11(5):483–486.

19 Iron

Iron has the longest and best described history among all the micronutrients. It is a key element in the metabolism of almost all living organisms. In humans, iron is an essential component of hundreds of proteins and enzymes.[1,2]

Function

Oxygen Transport and Storage

Heme is an iron-containing compound found in a number of biologically important molecules. Hemoglobin and myoglobin are heme-containing proteins that are involved in the transport and storage of oxygen. Hemoglobin is the primary protein found in red blood cells and represents about two thirds of the body's iron. The vital role of hemoglobin in transporting oxygen from the lungs to the rest of the body is derived from its unique ability to acquire oxygen rapidly during the short time it spends in contact with the lungs and to release oxygen as needed during its circulation through the tissues. Myoglobin functions in the transport and short-term storage of oxygen in muscle cells, helping to match the supply of oxygen to the demand of working muscles.[3,4]

Oxygen Sensing

Inadequate oxygen (hypoxia), such as that experienced by those who live at high altitudes or those with chronic lung disease, induces compensatory physiologic responses, including increased red blood cell formation, increased blood vessel growth (angiogenesis), and increased production of enzymes utilized in anaerobic metabolism. Under hypoxic conditions transcription factors, known as hypoxia inducible factors (HIF), bind to response elements in genes that encode various proteins involved in compensatory responses to hypoxia and increase their synthesis. Recent research indicates that an iron-dependent prolyl hydroxylase enzyme plays a critical role in regulating HIF and consequently physiologic responses to hypoxia. When cellular oxygen tension is adequate, newly synthesized HIFα subunits are modified by a prolyl hydroxylase enzyme in an iron-dependent process that targets HIFα for rapid degradation. When cellular oxygen tension drops below a critical threshold, prolyl hydroxylase can no longer target HIFα for degradation, allowing HIFα to bind to HIFβ and form an active transcription factor that is able to enter the nucleus and bind to specific response elements on genes.[5,6]

Electron Transport and Energy Metabolism

Cytochromes are heme-containing compounds that are critical to cellular energy production and therefore life, through their roles in mitochondrial electron transport. They serve as electron carriers during the synthesis of adenosine triphosphate (ATP), the primary energy-storage compound in cells. Nonheme iron-containing enzymes, such as NADH dehydrogenase and succinate dehydrogenase, are also critical to energy metabolism. Cytochrome P450 is a family of enzymes that functions in the metabolism of a number of important biological molecules, as well as the detoxification and metabolism of drugs and pollutants.[3]

Antioxidant and Beneficial Pro-Oxidant Functions

Catalase and peroxidase are heme-containing enzymes that protect against the accumulation of hydrogen peroxide, a potentially damaging reactive oxygen species (ROS), by converting it to water and oxygen. As part of the immune response, some white blood cells engulf bacteria and expose them to ROS to kill them. The synthesis of one such ROS, hypochlorous acid, by neutrophils is catalyzed by the heme-containing enzyme myeloperoxidase.[3,4]

DNA Synthesis

Ribonucleotide reductase is an iron-dependent enzyme that is required for DNA synthesis.[1,2] Thus, iron is required for a number of vital functions, including growth, reproduction, healing, and immune function.

Regulation of Intracellular Iron

Iron response elements are short sequences of nucleotides found in the messenger RNA (mRNA) that code for key proteins in the regulation of iron storage and metabolism. Iron regulatory proteins (IRPs) can bind to iron response elements and affect mRNA translation, thereby regulating the synthesis of specific proteins. It has been proposed that when the iron supply is high, more iron binds to IRPs and prevents them from binding to iron response elements on mRNA. When the iron supply is low, less iron binds to IRPs, allowing increased binding of iron response elements. Thus, when less iron is available, translation of mRNA that codes for the iron storage protein, ferritin, is reduced because iron is not available for storage. Translation of mRNA that codes for the key regulatory enzyme of heme synthesis in immature red blood cells is also reduced to conserve iron. In contrast, IRP binding to iron response elements in mRNA that codes for transferrin receptors inhibits mRNA degradation, resulting in increased synthesis of transferrin receptors and increased iron transport to cells.[4]

Nutrient Interactions

Vitamin A. Vitamin A deficiency may exacerbate iron-deficiency anemia. Vitamin A supplementation has been shown to have beneficial effects on iron-deficiency anemia and improve iron status among children and pregnant women. The combination of vitamin A and iron seems to reduce anemia more effectively than either iron or vitamin A alone.[7,8]

Copper. Adequate copper nutritional status appears to be necessary for normal iron metabolism and red blood cell formation. Anemia is a clinical sign of copper deficiency. Animal studies demonstrate a role for copper in iron absorption,[9] and iron has been found to accumulate in the livers of copper-deficient animals, indicating that copper is required for iron transport to the bone marrow for red blood cell formation.[10]

Zinc. High doses of iron supplements taken together with zinc supplements on an empty stomach can inhibit the absorption of zinc. When taken with food, supplemental iron does not appear to inhibit zinc absorption. Iron-fortified foods have no effect on zinc absorption.[7,11]

Calcium. When consumed together in a single meal, calcium has been found to reduce the absorption of iron. However, little effect has been observed on serum ferritin levels (iron stores) with calcium supplement levels ranging from 1000 to 1500 mg/d.[7,11]

Deficiency

Levels of Iron Deficiency

Iron deficiency is the most common nutrient deficiency in the United States and the world. Three levels of iron deficiency are generally identified and are listed below from least to most severe:[3]

- *Storage iron depletion* Iron stores are depleted, but the functional iron supply is not limited.
- *Early functional iron deficiency* The supply of functional iron is low enough to impair red blood cell formation but not low enough to cause measurable anemia.
- *Iron-deficiency anemia* There is inadequate iron to support normal red blood cell formation, resulting in anemia.

The anemia of iron deficiency is characterized as microcytic and hypochromic, meaning red blood cells are measurably smaller than normal and their hemoglobin content is reduced. At this stage of iron deficiency, symptoms may be a result of inadequate oxygen delivery due to anemia and/or suboptimal function of iron-dependent enzymes. It is important to remember that iron deficiency is not the only cause of anemia and that the diagnosis or treatment of iron deficiency solely on the basis of anemia may lead to misdiagnosis or inappropriate treatment of the underlying cause.[12] See Chapter 2 (on folic acid) and Chapter 9 (on vitamin B_{12}) for information on other nutritional causes of anemia.

Symptoms of Iron Deficiency

Most of the symptoms of iron deficiency are a result of the associated anemia and may include fatigue, rapid heart rate, palpitations, and rapid breathing on exertion. Iron deficiency impairs athletic performance and physical work capacity in several ways. In iron-deficiency anemia, the reduced hemoglobin content of red blood cells results in decreased oxygen delivery to active tissues. Reduced myoglobin levels in muscle cells limit the amount of oxygen that can be delivered to mitochondria for oxidative metabolism. Iron depletion also reduces the oxidative capacity of muscle by reducing the mitochondrial content of cytochromes and other iron-dependent enzymes required for electron transport and ATP synthesis. Lactic acid production is also increased in iron deficiency.[13]

The ability to maintain a normal body temperature on exposure to cold is also impaired in iron-deficient individuals. Severe iron-deficiency anemia may result in brittle and spoon-shaped nails, sores at the corners of the mouth, taste bud atrophy, and sore tongue. In some cases, advanced iron-deficiency anemia may cause difficulty in swallowing due to the formation of webs of tissue in the throat and esophagus. The development of esophageal webs, also known as *Plummer-Vinson syndrome*, may require a genetic predisposition in addition to iron deficiency. Pica, a behavioral disturbance characterized by the consumption of nonfood items, may be a symptom and a cause of iron deficiency.[12]

Individuals at Increased Risk of Iron Deficiency

Infants and Children between the Ages of 6 Months and 4 Years. A full-term infant's iron stores are usually sufficient to last for 6 months. High iron requirements are due to the rapid growth rates sustained during this period.[4]

Adolescents. Early adolescence is another period of rapid growth. In females, the blood loss that occurs with menstruation adds to the increased iron requirement of adolescence.[4]

Pregnant Women. Increased iron utilization by the developing fetus and placenta as well as blood volume expansion significantly increase the iron requirement during pregnancy.[4]

Individuals with Chronic Blood Loss. Chronic bleeding or acute blood loss may result in iron deficiency. One milliliter of blood with a hemoglobin concentration of 150 g/L contains 0.5 mg of iron. Thus, chronic loss of very small amounts of blood may result in iron deficiency. A common cause of chronic blood loss and iron deficiency in developing countries is intestinal parasitic infection. Individuals who donate blood frequently, especially menstruating women, may need to increase their iron intake to prevent deficiency because each 500 mL of blood donated contains between 200 and 250 mg of iron.[1]

Individuals with *Helicobacter pylori* Infection. *H. pylori* infection is associated with iron-deficiency anemia, especially in children, even in the absence of gastrointestinal bleeding.[14]

Vegetarians. Because iron from plant sources is less efficiently absorbed than that from animal sources, the U.S. Food and Nutrition Board (FNB) has estimated that the bioavailability of iron from a vegetarian diet is only 10%, and it is 18% from a mixed diet. Therefore, the recommended dietary allowance (RDA) for iron from a completely vegetarian diet should be adjusted as follows: 14 mg/d for adult men and postmenopausal women, 33 mg/d for premenopausal women, and 26 mg/d for adolescent girls.[11]

Table 19–2   Food Sources of Iron

Food	Serving	Iron, mg
Tofu, firm	$^1/_4$ block (~ $^1/_2$ cup)	6.22
Oysters	6 medium	5.04
Bran cereal with raisins	1 cup, dry	5.00–18.0
Potato, with skin	1 medium potato, baked	2.75
Kidney beans	$^1/_2$ cup, cooked	2.60
Black-strap molasses	1 tablespoon	3.50
Lentils	$^1/_2$ cup, cooked	3.30
Beef	3 ounces,* cooked	2.31
Prune juice	6 fluid ounces	2.27
Cashew nuts	1 ounce	1.70
Shrimp	8 large, cooked	1.36
Tuna, light	3 ounces, canned	1.30
Chicken, dark meat	3 ounces, cooked	1.13
Prunes, dried	~5 prunes (1.5 ounces)	1.06
Raisins, seedless	1 small box (1.5 ounces)	0.89

*A 3-ounce serving of meat or fish is about the size of a deck of cards.

influenced by other dietary factors than that of nonheme iron.[2,7]

Nonheme Iron. Plants, dairy products, meat, and iron salts added to foods are all sources of nonheme iron. The absorption of nonheme iron is strongly influenced by enhancers and inhibitors present in the same meal.[3,7]

Enhancers of Nonheme Iron Absortion

Vitamin C (Ascorbic Acid). Vitamin C strongly enhances the absorption of nonheme iron by reducing dietary ferric iron (Fe^{3+}) to ferrous iron (Fe^{2+}) and forming an absorbable iron-ascorbic acid complex.

Other Organic Acids. Citric, malic, tartaric, and lactic acids have some enhancing effects on nonheme iron absorption.

Meat, Fish, and Poultry. Aside from providing highly absorbable heme iron, meat, fish, and poultry also enhance nonheme iron absorption. The mechanism for this enhancement of nonheme iron absorption is not clear.[7,11]

Inhibitors of Nonheme Iron Absorption

Phytic Acid (Phytate). Phytic acid is present in legumes, grains, and rice and is an inhibitor of nonheme iron absorption. Small amounts of phytic acid (5 to 10 mg) can reduce nonheme iron absorption by 50%. The absorption of iron from legumes, such as soybeans, black beans, lentils, mung beans, and split peas, has been shown to be as low as 2%.[1,11]

Polyphenols. Polyphenols, found in some fruits, vegetables, coffee, tea, wines, and spices, can markedly inhibit the absorption of nonheme iron. This effect is reduced by the presence of vitamin C.[1,11]

Soy Protein. Soy protein, such as that found in tofu, has an inhibitory effect on iron absorption that is independent of its phytic acid content.[11]

Typical Dietary Intake

National surveys in the United States indicate that the average dietary iron intake is 16 to 18 mg/d in men, 12 mg/d in pre- and postmenopausal women, and about 15 mg/d in pregnant women.[11] Thus, the majority of premenopausal and pregnant women in the United States consume less than the RDA for iron and many men consume more than the RDA. In the United States, most grain products are fortified with iron. The iron content of some relatively iron-rich foods is listed in milligrams in Table 19–2.

Supplements

Iron supplements are indicated for the prevention and treatment of iron deficiency. Individuals who are not at risk of iron deficiency (e.g., adult men and postmenopausal women) should not take iron supplements without an appropriate medical evaluation for iron deficiency. A number of iron supplements are available, and different forms provide different proportions of elemental iron. Ferrous sulfate (heptahydrate) is 22% elemental iron; ferrous sulfate (monohydrate) is 33% elemental iron; ferrous gluconate is 12% elemental iron; ferrous fumarate is 33% elemental iron.[23] If not stated otherwise, all of the iron doses discussed in this chapter represent elemental iron.

Iron Overload

Several genetic disorders may lead to pathological accumulation of iron in the body. Hereditary hemochromatosis results in iron overload despite normal iron intake, and sub-Saharan African hemochromatosis appears to require a combination of high iron intake and a genetic predisposition.

Hereditary Hemochromatosis

Up to 1 in 200 individuals of northern European descent are affected by a genetic disorder known as hereditary hemochromatosis (HH). It is characterized by iron deposition in the liver and other tissues as a result of a small increase in intestinal iron absorption over many years. If untreated, tissue iron accumulation may lead to cirrhosis of the liver, diabetes, heart muscle damage (cardiomyopathy), or arthritis. HH was known to be a genetic disorder affecting intestinal iron absorption for many years, but the gene (HFE) and the mutation resulting in HH were only recently identified in 1996.[24] At present, the exact role of the protein encoded by the HFE gene in intestinal iron absorption is not well understood.[25] Iron overload in HH is treated by phlebotomy, the removal of 500 ml of blood at a time, at intervals determined by the severity of the iron overload. Individuals with HH are advised to avoid supplemental iron but are not generally advised to avoid iron-rich foods. Alcohol consumption is strongly discouraged due to the increased risk of cirrhosis of the liver.[1] Genetic testing, which requires a blood sample, is available for those who may be at risk for HH, for example, individuals with a family history of hemochromatosis.

Sub-Saharan African Hemochromatosis

Iron overload in black people of South Africa is associated with chronic exposure to diets containing too much iron derived mainly from cooking pots and steel barrels used to ferment beer. This form of iron overload is usually more severe in adult men, whose beer consumption tends to be higher and whose iron intake may exceed 100 mg/d. Like HH, it may also result in cirrhosis of the liver or diabetes. Unlike HH, Sub-Saharan African hemochromatosis appears to require high iron intake in association with a genetic factor that has not yet been identified.[1,26] African Americans may also incur significant iron overload, and it has been suggested that the mutation associated with Sub-Saharan African hemochromatosis may also occur in Americans of African descent. Unfortunately, the true incidence and the causes of iron overload among African Americans have yet to be determined.[27]

Hereditary Anemias

Iron overload may occur in individuals with severe hereditary anemias that are not caused by iron deficiency. Excessive dietary absorption of iron may occur in response to the body's continued efforts to form red blood cells. Anemic patients at risk of iron overload include those with sideroblastic anemia, pyruvate kinase deficiency, and thalassemia major, especially when they are treated with numerous transfusions. Patients with hereditary spherocytosis and thalassemia minor do not usually develop iron overload, unless they are misdiagnosed as having iron deficiency and treated with large doses of iron over many years.[1] The thalassemias (major and minor) are common in individuals of Mediterranean descent. It has been hypothesized that a Mediterranean form of iron overload, distinct from HH, also exists.[28]

Iron overload due to prolonged iron supplementation is very rare in healthy individuals without a genetic predisposition. This fact emphasizes the degree to which the body's tight control of intestinal iron absorption protects it from the adverse effects of iron overload.[1] However, supplementation of individuals who are not iron deficient should be avoided due to the frequency of hereditary hemochromatosis and recent concerns about the more subtle effects of chronic excess iron intake.

Safety

Toxicity

Overdose. Accidental overdose of iron-containing products is the single largest cause of poisoning fatalities in children under 6 years of age. Although the oral lethal dose of elemental iron is approximately 200 to 250 mg/kg of body weight, considerably less has been fatal. Symptoms of acute toxicity may occur with iron doses of 20 to 60 mg/kg of body weight. Iron overdose is an emergency situation because the severity of iron toxicity is related to the amount of elemental iron absorbed. Acute iron poisoning produces symptoms in four stages: (1) Within 1 to 6 hours of ingestion, symptoms may include nausea, vomiting, abdominal pain, tarry stools, lethargy, weak and rapid pulse, low blood pressure, fever, difficulty breathing, and coma. (2) If not immediately fatal, symptoms may subside for about 24 hours. (3) Symptoms may return 12 to 48 hours after iron ingestion and may include serious signs of failure in the following organ systems: cardiovascular, kidney, liver, hematologic (blood), and central nervous systems. (4) Long-term damage to the central nervous system, liver (cirrhosis), and stomach may develop 2 to 6 weeks after ingestion.[11,23]

Adverse Effects. At therapeutic levels for iron deficiency, iron supplements may cause

Table 19–3 Tolerable Upper Intake Level (UL) for Iron

Life Stage	Age	UL, mg/d
Infants	0–12 months	40
Children	1–13 years	40
Adolescents	14–18 years	45
Adults	19 years and older	45

gastrointestinal irritation, nausea, vomiting, diarrhea, or constipation. Stools will often appear darker in color. Iron-containing liquids can temporarily stain teeth, but diluting the liquid helps to prevent this effect. Taking iron supplements with food instead of on an empty stomach may relieve gastrointestinal effects.[23] The FNB based the tolerable upper levels of intake (UL) for iron on the prevention of gastrointestinal distress (Table 19–3). The UL for adolescents and adults over the age of 14 years, including pregnant and breast-feeding women, is 45 mg/d. It should be noted that the UL is not meant to apply to individuals being treated with iron under close medical supervision. Individuals with hereditary hemochromatosis or other conditions of iron overload, as well as individuals with alcoholic cirrhosis and other liver diseases, may experience adverse effects at iron intake levels below the UL.[11]

Diseases Associated with Iron Excess

Cardiovascular Diseases. Animal studies suggest a role for iron-induced oxidative stress in the pathology of atherosclerosis and myocardial infarction (heart attack).[29] However, epidemiologic studies of iron nutritional status and cardiovascular diseases in humans have yielded conflicting results. A systematic review of 12 prospective epidemiologic studies including 7800 cases of coronary heart disease (CHD) did not find good evidence to support the existence of strong associations between a number of different measures of iron status and CHD.[30] Serum ferritin concentration is the measure of iron status thought to best reflect iron stores. However, the same review found no difference in the risk of CHD between individuals with serum ferritin concentrations of 200 µg/L or higher and those with ferritin concentrations of less than 200 µg/L in the five prospective studies that measured serum ferritin. Two large prospective studies found increased dietary heme iron, but not total dietary iron, to be associated with increased risk of myocardial infarction.[31,32] When iron stores are high, nonheme iron absorption is inhibited more effectively than heme iron absorption, suggesting that iron from animal sources may play a more important role than total iron intake in CHD risk.[29] Although the relationship between iron stores and CHD requires further clarification, it would be prudent for those who are not at risk of iron deficiency (e.g., adult men and postmenopausal women) to avoid excess iron intake.

Cancer. A dramatically increased risk of liver cancer (hepatocellular carcinoma) in individuals with cirrhosis due to iron overload in hereditary hemochromatosis has been well documented. However, the relationship between dietary iron and cancer risk in individuals without hemochromatosis is less clear.[11] Several epidemiologic studies reported associations between measures of increased iron status and the incidence of colorectal cancer or the occurrence of precancerous polyps, but the associations were not consistent. Dietary iron intake appears to be more consistently related to the risk of colorectal cancer than measures of iron status or iron stores.[33,34] Increased red meat consumption has been associated with an increased risk of colorectal cancer, but there are a number of potential mechanisms by which increased meat consumption could affect cancer risk other than increasing iron intake. For example, increased red meat consumption increases the secretion of bile acids, which can be toxic to colonic cells, and increases exposure to carcinogenic compounds generated when meat is cooked.[35] Increased iron in the contents of the colon, rather than increased body iron stores, could increase the risk of colon cancer by exposing colonic cells to potentially damaging ROS derived from iron-catalyzed reactions, especially in the presence of a high fat diet. Although this possibility is presently under investigation, the relationship between dietary iron intake, iron stores, and the risk of colorectal cancer remains unclear.

Neurodegenerative Disease. Iron is required for normal brain and nerve function through its involvement in cellular metabolism, as well as the synthesis of neurotransmitters and myelin. However, accumulation of excess iron can result in increased oxidative stress, and the brain is particularly susceptible to oxidative damage. Iron accumulation and oxidative injury are presently under consideration as potential contributors to a number of neurodegenerative diseases, such as Alzheimer's disease and Parkinson's disease.[36] The abnormal accumulation of iron in the brain does not appear to be a result of increased dietary iron, but rather a disruption in the complex process of cellular iron regulation. Although the mechanisms for this disruption in iron regulation are not yet known, it is presently an active area of biomedical research.[37]

Drug Interactions

Medications that decrease stomach acidity, such as antacids, histamine (H_2) receptor antagonists (e.g., cimetidine, ranitidine), and proton pump inhibitors (e.g., omeprazole, lansoprazole), may impair iron absorption. Taking iron supplements at the same time as the following medications may result in decreased absorption and efficacy of the medication: levodopa, levothyroxine, methyldopa, penicillamine, quinolones, tetracyclines, and bisphosphonates. Therefore, it is best to take these medications 2 hours apart from iron supplements. Cholestyramine resin, used to lower blood cholesterol levels, should also be taken 2 hours apart from iron supplements because it interferes with iron absorption. Allopurinol, a medication used to treat gout, may increase iron storage in the liver and should not be used in combination with iron supplements.[23,38]

LPI Recommendation

Following the most recent RDA for iron should provide sufficient iron to prevent deficiency without causing adverse effects in most individuals. Although sufficient iron can be obtained through a varied diet, a considerable number of people do not consume adequate iron to prevent deficiency. A multivitamin/multimineral supplement containing 100 % of the daily value for iron provides 18 mg of elemental iron. Although this amount of iron may be beneficial for premenopausal women, it is well above the RDA for men and most postmenopausal women.

Adult Men and Postmenopausal Women

Because hereditary hemochromatosis is relatively common and the effects of long-term dietary iron excess on chronic disease risk are not yet clear, men and postmenopausal women who are not at risk of iron deficiency should take a multivitamin/mineral supplement without iron. A number of multivitamins formulated specifically for men or those over 50 years of age do not contain iron.

Older Adults

A recent study in an elderly population (65 years and older) found that high iron stores were much more common than iron deficiency.[39] Thus, older adults should not generally take nutritional supplements containing iron unless they have been diagnosed with iron deficiency. Moreover, it is extremely important to determine the underlying cause of the iron deficiency, rather than simply treating it with iron supplements.

References

1. Fairbanks VF. Iron in medicine and nutrition. In: Shils M, Olson JA, Shike M, Ross AC, eds. *Nutrition in Health and Disease*, 9th ed. Baltimore: Williams & Wilkins; 1999:223–239.
2. Beard JL, Dawson HD. Iron. In: O'Dell BL, Sunde RA, eds. *Handbook of Nutritionally Essential Minerals*. New York: Marcel Dekker, Inc; 1997:275–334.
3. Yip R, Dallman PR. Iron. In: Ziegler EE, Filer LJ, eds. *Present Knowledge in Nutrition*, Vol. 7. Washington, D.C.: ILSI Press; 1996:277–292.
4. Brody T. *Nutritional Biochemistry*, 2nd ed. San Diego: Academic Press; 1999.
5. Ivan M, Kondo K, Yang H, et al. HIFα targeted for VHL-mediated destruction by proline hydroxylation: implications for O_2 sensing. *Science* 2001;292(5516):464–468.
6. Jaakkola P, Mole DR, Tian YM, et al. Targeting of HIF-alpha to the von Hippel-Lindau ubiquitylation complex by O_2-regulated prolyl hydroxylation. *Science* 2001;292(5516):468–472.
7. Lynch SR. Interaction of iron with other nutrients. *Nutr Rev* 1997;55(4):102–110.
8. Suharno D, West CE, Muhilal, Karyadi D, Hautvast JG. Supplementation with vitamin A and iron for nutritional anaemia in pregnant women in West Java, Indonesia. *Lancet* 1993;342(8883):1325–1328.
9. Vulpe CD, Kuo YM, Murphy TL, et al. Hephaestin, a ceruloplasmin homologue implicated in intestinal iron transport, is defective in the sla mouse. *Nat Genet* 1999;21(2):195–199.
10. Turnlund JR. Copper. In: Shils M, Olson JA, Shike M, Ross AC, eds. *Nutrition in Health and Disease*, 9th ed. Baltimore: Williams & Wilkins; 1999:241–252.
11. Food and Nutrition Board, Institute of Medicine. Iron.

Dietary Reference Intakes for Vitamin A, Vitamin K, Boron, Chromium, Copper, Iodine, Iron, Manganese, Molybdenum, Nickel, Silicon, Vanadium, and Zinc. Washington, D.C.: National Academy Press; 2001:290–393.
12. Lee GR. Disorders of iron metabolism and heme synthesis. In: Lee GR, Foerster J, Paraskevas F, Greer JP, Rogers GM, eds. *Wintrobe's Clinical Hematology*, 10th ed. Baltimore: Williams and Wilkins; 1999:979–1070.
13. Beard JL. Iron biology in immune function, muscle metabolism and neuronal functioning. *J Nutr* 2001;131(2S-2):568S–579S.
14. Sherman PM, Macarthur C. Current controversies associated with *Helicobacter pylori* infection in the pediatric population. *Front Biosci* 2001;6:E187–E192.
15. Grantham-McGregor S, Ani C. A review of studies on the effect of iron deficiency on cognitive development in children. *J Nutr* 2001;131(2S-2):649S–666S.
16. Wright RO. The role of iron therapy in childhood plumbism. *Curr Opin Pediatr* 1999;11(3):255–258.
17. Rasmussen K. Is there a causal relationship between iron deficiency or iron-deficiency anemia and weight at birth, length of gestation and perinatal mortality? *J Nutr* 2001;131(2S-2):590S–601S.
18. Yip R. Significance of an abnormally low or high hemoglobin concentration during pregnancy: special consideration of iron nutrition. *Am J Clin Nutr* 2000;72(1 Suppl):272S–279S.
19. Oppenheimer SJ. Iron and its relation to immunity and infectious disease. *J Nutr* 2001;131(2S-2):616S–633S.
20. National Heart, Lung, and Blood Institute Working Group on Restless Legs Syndrome. Restless legs syndrome: detection and management in primary care. *Am Fam Physician* 2000;62(1):108–114.
21. Earley CJ, Connor JR, Beard JL, Malecki EA, Epstein DK, Allen RP. Abnormalities in CSF concentrations of ferritin and transferrin in restless legs syndrome. *Neurology* 2000;54(8):1698–1700.
22. Allen RP, Barker PB, Wehrl F, Song HK, Earley CJ. MRI measurement of brain iron in patients with restless legs syndrome. *Neurology* 2001;56(2):263–265.
23. Minerals. *Drug Facts and Comparisons*. St. Louis: Facts and Comparisons; 2000:27–51.
24. Feder JN, Gnirke A, Thomas W, et al. A novel MHC class I-like gene is mutated in patients with hereditary haemochromatosis. *Nat Genet* 1996;13(4):399–408.
25. Anderson GJ, Powell LW. Of metals, mice, and men: what animal models can teach us about body iron loading. *J Clin Invest* 2000;105(9):1185–1186.
26. Walker AR, Segal I. Iron overload in Sub-Saharan Africa: to what extent is it a public health problem? *Br J Nutr* 1999;81(6):427–434.
27. Wurapa RK, Gordeuk VR, Brittenham GM, Khiyami A, Schechter GP, Edwards CQ. Primary iron overload in African Americans. *Am J Med* 1996;101(1):9–18.
28. Pietrangelo A. Hemochromatosis 1998: is one gene enough? *J Hepatol* 1998;29(3):502–509.
29. de Valk B, Marx JJ. Iron, atherosclerosis, and ischemic heart disease. *Arch Intern Med* 1999;159(14):1542–1548.
30. Danesh J, Appleby P. Coronary heart disease and iron status: meta-analyses of prospective studies. *Circulation* 1999;99(7):852–854.
31. Ascherio A, Willett WC, Rimm EB, Giovannucci EL, Stampfer MJ. Dietary iron intake and risk of coronary

disease among men. *Circulation* 1994;89(3):969–974.

32. Klipstein-Grobusch K, Grobbee DE, den Breeijen JH, Boeing H, Hofman A, Witteman JC. Dietary iron and risk of myocardial infarction in the Rotterdam Study. *Am J Epidemiol* 1999;149(5):421–428.

33. Kato I, Dnistrian AM, Schwartz M, et al. Iron intake, body iron stores and colorectal cancer risk in women: a nested case-control study. *Int J Cancer* 1999;80(5):693–698.

34. Wurzelmann JI, Silver A, Schreinemachers DM, Sandler RS, Everson RB. Iron intake and the risk of colorectal cancer. *Cancer Epidemiol Biomarkers Prev* 1996;5(7):503–507.

35. Bostick R. Diet and nutrition in the prevention of colon cancer. In: Bendich A, Deckelbaum RJ, eds. *Preventive Nutrition: The Comprehensive Guide for Health Professionals*, 2nd ed. Totowa: Humana Press, Inc; 2001:57–95.

36. Pinero DJ, Hu J, Connor JR. Alterations in the interaction between iron regulatory proteins and their iron responsive element in normal and Alzheimer's diseased brains. *Cell Mol Biol (Noisy-le-grand)* 2000; 46(4):761–776.

37. Sayre LM, Perry G, Atwood CS, Smith MA. The role of metals in neurodegenerative diseases. *Cell Mol Biol (Noisy-le-grand)* 2000;46(4):731–741.

38. Hendler SS, Rorvik DR, eds. *PDR for Nutritional Supplements*. Montvale, NJ: Medical Economics Company, Inc; 2001.

39. Fleming DJ, Jacques PF, Tucker KL, et al. Iron status of the free-living, elderly Framingham Heart Study cohort: an iron-replete population with a high prevalence of elevated iron stores. *Am J Clin Nutr* 2001; 73(3):638–646.

20 Magnesium

Magnesium plays important roles in the structure and function of the human body. The adult human body contains about 25 g of magnesium. Over 60% of all the magnesium in the body is found in the skeleton, about 27% is found in muscle, 6 to 7% is found in other cells, and less than 1% is found outside of cells.[1]

Function

Magnesium is involved in more than 300 essential metabolic reactions, some of which are discussed below.[2]

Energy Production

The metabolism of carbohydrates and fats to produce energy requires numerous magnesium-dependent chemical reactions. Magnesium is required by the adenosine triphosphate (ATP) synthesizing protein in mitochondria. ATP, the molecule that provides energy for almost all metabolic processes, exists primarily as a complex with magnesium (MgATP).

Synthesis of Essential Biomolecules

Magnesium is required at a number of steps during the synthesis of nucleic acids and proteins. A number of enzymes participating in the synthesis of carbohydrates and lipids require magnesium for their activity. Glutathione, an important antioxidant, requires magnesium for its synthesis.

Structural Roles

Magnesium plays a structural role in bone, cell membranes, and chromosomes. Magnesium is required for the active transport of ions like potassium and calcium across cell membranes. Through its role in ion transport systems, magnesium affects the conduction of nerve impulses, muscle contraction, and the normal rhythm of the heart.

Cell Signaling

Cell signaling requires MgATP for the phosphorylation of proteins and the formation of the cell signaling molecule, cyclic adenosine monophosphate (cAMP). cAMP is involved in many processes, including the secretion of parathyroid hormone (PTH) from the parathyroid glands. See Chapter 11 (on vitamin D) and Chapter 14 (on calcium) for more detail on the role of PTH.

Cell Migration

Calcium and magnesium levels in the fluid surrounding cells affect the migration of a number of different cell types. Such effects on cell migration may be important in wound healing.

Nutrient Interactions

Zinc. High doses of zinc in supplement form appear to interfere with the absorption of magnesium. A zinc supplement of 142 mg/d in healthy adult males significantly decreased magnesium absorption and magnesium balance (the difference between magnesium intake and magnesium loss).[3]

Fiber. Large increases in the intake of dietary fiber have been found to decrease magnesium utilization in experimental studies. However, the extent to which dietary fiber affects magnesium nutritional status in individuals with a varied diet outside the laboratory is not clear.[2,4]

Protein. Dietary protein may affect magnesium absorption. One study found that magnesium absorption was lower when protein intake was less than 30 g/d, and higher protein intakes

(93 g/d vs. 42 g/d) were associated with improved magnesium absorption in adolescents.[4]

Vitamin D and Calcium. The active form of vitamin D (calcitriol) may increase the intestinal absorption of magnesium to a small extent. However, magnesium absorption does not seem to be calcitriol-dependent as is the absorption of calcium and phosphate. High calcium intake has not been found to affect magnesium balance in most studies. Inadequate blood magnesium levels are known to result in low blood calcium levels, resistance to PTH, and resistance to some of the effects of vitamin D.[2,4]

Deficiency

Overt or symptomatic magnesium deficiency in healthy individuals who are consuming a balanced diet is quite rare because magnesium is abundant in both plant and animal foods and because the kidneys are able to limit urinary excretion of magnesium when intake is low. The following conditions increase the risk of magnesium deficiency[1]:

- *Gastrointestinal disorders* Prolonged diarrhea, Crohn's disease, malabsorption syndromes, surgical removal of a portion of the intestine, and intestinal inflammation due to radiation may all lead to magnesium depletion.
- *Renal disorders (magnesium wasting)* Diabetes mellitus and long-term use of certain diuretics may result in increased urinary loss of magnesium.
- *Chronic alcoholism* Poor dietary intake, gastrointestinal problems, and increased urinary loss of magnesium may all contribute to magnesium depletion, which is frequently encountered in alcoholics.
- *Older age* Several studies have found that elderly people have relatively low dietary intakes of magnesium. Because intestinal magnesium absorption tends to decrease and urinary magnesium excretion tends to increase in older individuals, suboptimal dietary magnesium intake may increase the risk of magnesium depletion in the elderly.[4]

Though severe magnesium deficiency is uncommon, it has been induced experimentally. When magnesium deficiency was induced in humans, the earliest sign was decreased blood magesium levels (hypomagnesemia). Over time blood calcium levels also began to decrease (hypocalcemia) despite adequate dietary calcium. Hypocalcemia persisted despite increased PTH secretion. Usually, increased PTH secretion quickly results in the mobilization of calcium from bone and normalization of blood calcium levels. As the magnesium depletion progressed, PTH secretion diminished to low levels. Along with hypomagnesemia, signs of severe magnesium deficiency included hypocalcemia, low blood potassium levels (hypokalemia), retention of sodium, low circulating levels of PTH, neurological and muscular symptoms (tremor, muscle spasms, tetany), loss of appetite, nausea, vomiting, and personality changes.[2]

A large national survey indicated that the average magnesium intake for men (about 320 mg/d) and the average intake for women (about 230 mg/d) were significantly below the current recommended dietary allowance (RDA). In men and women over 70 years of age magnesium intakes were even lower.[4] Such findings suggest that marginal magnesium deficiency may be relatively common in the United States.

The Recommended Dietary Allowance

In 1997, the Food and Nutrition Board (FNB) of the Institute of Medicine increased the RDA for magnesium, based on the results of recent, tightly controlled balance studies that utilized more accurate methods of measuring magnesium (Table 20–1).[4] Balance studies are useful for determining the amount of a nutrient that will prevent deficiency but give little information regarding the amount required for chronic disease prevention or optimum health.

Table 20–1   Recommended Dietary Allowance (RDA) for Magnesium

Life Stage	Age	Males, mg/d	Females, mg/d
Infants	0–6 months	30 (AI)	30 (AI)
Infants	7–12 months	75 (AI)	75 (AI)
Children	1–3 years	80	80
Children	4–8 years	130	130
Children	9–13 years	240	240
Adolescents	14–18 years	410	360
Adults	19–30 years	400	310
Adults	31 years and older	420	320
Pregnancy	18 years and younger	–	400
Pregnancy	19–30 years	–	350
Pregnancy	31 years and older	–	360
Breast-feeding	18 years and younger	–	360
Breast-feeding	19–30 years	–	310
Breast-feeding	31 years and older	–	320

AI, adequate intake level.

Disease Prevention

Hypertension

Large epidemiologic studies suggest a relationship between magnesium and blood pressure. However, the fact that foods high in magnesium (fruits, vegetables, whole grains) are frequently high in potassium and dietary fiber has made it difficult to evaluate independent effects of magnesium on blood pressure. A study of more than 30,000 male health professionals found an inverse association between dietary fiber, potassium, and magnesium, and the development of hypertension over a 4-year period.[5] In a similar study of more than 40,000 female registered nurses, dietary fiber and dietary magnesium were inversely associated with systolic and diastolic blood pressures in those who did not develop hypertension over the 4-year study period, but neither dietary fiber nor magnesium was related to the risk of developing hypertension.[6] The Atherosclerosis Risk in Communities study examined the dietary intake and blood levels of magnesium in 7731 men and women and the development of hypertension over a 6-year period.[7] The risk of developing hypertension in men and women decreased as blood magnesium levels increased but the trend was only statistically significant in women. Although the investigators found no association between dietary magnesium and the incidence of hypertension, they suggested that low blood magnesium levels may play a modest role in the development of hypertension.

Cardiovascular Diseases

A number of studies have found decreased mortality from cardiovascular diseases in populations who routinely consume "hard" water. Hard (alkaline) water is generally high in magnesium but may also contain more calcium and fluoride than "soft" water, making the cardioprotective effects of hard water difficult to attribute to magnesium alone.[8] One large prospective study (almost 14,000 men and women) found a significant trend for increasing blood magnesium levels to be associated with decreased risk of coronary heart disease in women but not in men. However, the risk of coronary heart disease in the lowest quartile of dietary magnesium intake was not significantly different than the risk in the highest quartile in men or women.[9] Presently, the relationship between dietary magnesium intake and the risk of cardiovascular diseases remains unclear.

Disease Treatment

The use of pharmacologic doses of magnesium to treat specific diseases is discussed below. Although many of the studies cited utilized supplemental magnesium in doses considerably higher than the tolerable upper level of intake (UL) of 350 mg/d recommended by the FNB for healthy individuals, it is important to note that they were all conducted under medical supervision. Because of the potential risk of high doses of supplemental magnesium, especially in the presence of renal insufficiency, any trial of magnesium supplementation for disease treatment above the UL should be conducted under medical supervision.

Hypertension

The results from intervention studies using magnesium supplements to treat hypertension have been conflicting.[4] In uncontrolled trials, hypertensive patients on thiazide diuretics experienced decreases in blood pressure when given magnesium supplements. In general, placebo-controlled trials have not been supportive of a blood pressure–lowering effect for magnesium supplementation.[2] Modest but significant blood pressure–lowering effects have been reported in two placebo-controlled studies using 485 mg/d of supplemental magnesium in individuals with mild to moderate hypertension for at least 2 months,[10,11] but a number of other studies failed to find any blood pressure–lowering effects with magnesium supplementation. One double-blind placebo-controlled study found magnesium supplementation to be beneficial in lowering the blood pressure of individuals with low magnesium status, suggesting that oral magnesium supplementation may be helpful in hypertensive individuals who are depleted of magnesium due to chronic diuretic use, inadequate dietary intake, or both.[12]

Preeclampsia-Eclampsia

Preeclampsia-eclampsia is a disease that is unique to pregnancy and may occur anytime after 20 weeks of pregnancy and up to 6 weeks after birth. Approximately 7% of pregnant women in the United States develop preeclampsia-eclampsia. Preeclampsia is defined as the presence of elevated blood pressure, protein in the urine, and severe swelling (edema) during pregnancy. Eclampsia occurs with the addition of seizures to the above triad of symptoms. Approximately 5% of women with preeclampsia go on to develop eclampsia, which is a significant cause of maternal death.[13] For many years, high-dose intravenous magnesium sulfate has been the treatment of choice for preventing eclamptic convulsions that may occur in association with preeclampsia-eclampsia late in pregnancy or during labor. Magnesium is believed to relieve cerebral blood vessel spasm, increasing blood flow to the brain.[2]

Cardiovascular Diseases

Myocardial Infarction. Results of a meta-analysis of randomized placebo-controlled trials indicated that an intravenous (IV) magnesium infusion given early after suspected myocardial infarction (MI) could decrease the risk of death. The most influential study included in the meta-analysis was a randomized, placebo-controlled trial in 2316 patients that found a significant reduction in mortality (7.8 vs. 10.3% in the placebo group) in those patients who were given IV magnesium sulfate within 24 hours of suspected MI.[14] Follow-up from 1 to 5 years after treatment revealed that the mortality from cardiovascular disease was 21% lower in the magnesium-treated group.[15] However, a larger placebo-controlled trial that included more than 58,000 patients found no significant reduction in 5-week mortality in those patients treated with IV magnesium sulfate within 24 hours of suspected MI, resulting in controversy regarding the efficacy of the treatment.[16] A more recent survey of the treatment of more than 173,000 patients with acute MI in the United States found that only 5% were given IV magnesium in the first 24 hours after the MI and that mortality was higher in those patients treated with IV magnesium.[17] Thus, the use of IV magnesium sulfate in the therapy of acute MI remains controversial.

Endothelial Dysfunction. Vascular endothelial cells line the walls of arteries where they are in contact with the blood that flows through the circulatory system. Normally functioning vascular endothelium promotes vasodilation when needed, for example, during exercise, and inhibits the formation of blood clots. With cardiovascular disease, arteries develop atherosclerotic plaque. Atherosclerosis impairs normal endothelial function, increasing the risk of vasoconstriction and clot formation, which may lead to a heart attack or a stroke. Recent research indicates that pharmacologic doses of oral magnesium may improve endothelial function in individuals with cardiovascular disease. A randomized double-blind placebo-controlled trial in 50 men and women with stable coronary artery disease found that 6 months of oral magnesium supplementation (730 mg/d) resulted in a 12% improvement in flow-mediated vasodilation compared to placebo.[18] In other words, the normal dilation response of the brachial (arm) artery to increased blood flow was improved. Magnesium supplementation also resulted in increased exercise tolerance during an exercise stress test compared with placebo. In another study of 42 patients with coronary artery disease who were already taking low-dose aspirin (an inhibitor of platelet aggregation), 3 months of oral magnesium supplementation (800 to 1200 mg/d) improved some laboratory measures of the propensity of their blood to form clots.[19] Although preliminary, these studies suggest that magnesium may be of benefit in improving endothelial function in individuals with cardiovascular disease.

Diabetes Mellitus

Magnesium depletion is commonly associated with both insulin-dependent and non-insulin–dependent diabetes mellitus. Between 25 and 38% of diabetics have been found to have decreased blood levels of magnesium (hypomagnesemia).[20] One cause of the depletion may be increased urinary loss of magnesium as a result of the increased urinary excretion of glucose that accompanies poorly controlled diabetes. Magnesium depletion has been shown to increase insulin resistance in a few studies and may adversely affect blood glucose control in diabetes. Dietary magnesium supplements (400 mg/d) were also found to improve glucose tolerance in elderly individuals.[21] Presently, there is little scientific evidence supporting routine magnesium supplementation for diabetics. However, a few studies suggest that correcting magnesium depletion in elderly and diabetic individuals may improve glucose tolerance.

Osteoporosis

Although decreased bone mineral density (BMD) is the primary feature of osteoporosis, other osteoporotic changes in the collagenous matrix and mineral components of bone may result in bones that are brittle and more susceptible to fracture. Magnesium comprises about 1% of bone mineral and is known to influence both bone matrix and bone mineral metabolism. As the magnesium content of bone mineral decreases, bone crystals become larger and more brittle. Some studies have found lower magnesium content and larger bone crystals in bones of osteoporotic women compared with nonosteoporotic controls.[22] Inadequate serum magnesium levels are known to result in low serum calcium levels, resistance to PTH, and resistance to some of the effects of vitamin D, all of which can lead to increased bone loss (see Chapter 14 on calcium). A recent study of over 900 elderly men and women found higher dietary magnesium intake to be associated with increased bone mineral density at the hip in both men and women. However, because they are present in many of the same foods the effect of dietary magnesium could not be separated from the effect of dietary potassium.[23] Few studies have addressed the effect of magnesium supplementation on BMD or osteoporosis in humans. In a small group of postmenopausal women with osteoporosis, magnesium supplementation of 750 mg/d for the first 6 months followed by 250 mg/d for 18 more months resulted in increased BMD at the wrist after 1 year, with no further increase after 2 years of supplementation.[24] Another study found that supplementation with 500 mg/d of magnesium and 600 mg/d of calcium in postmenopausal women who were also taking estrogen replacement therapy and a multivitamin resulted in increased bone density at the heel compared with postmenopausal women receiving only estrogen replacement therapy.[25] Presently, the potential for increased magnesium intake to influence calcium and bone metabolism warrants more research with particular attention to its role in the prevention and treatment of osteoporosis.

Migraine Headaches

Individuals who suffer from recurrent migraine headaches have been found to have lower intracellular magnesium levels (demonstrated in both red blood cells and white blood cells) than individuals who do not experience migraines. Oral magnesium supplementation has been shown to increase intracellular magnesium levels in individuals with migraine, leading to the hypothesis that magnesium supplementation might be helpful in decreasing the frequency and severity of migraine headaches. Two placebo-controlled trials have demonstrated modest decreases in the frequency of migraine headaches after supplementation with 600 mg/d of magnesium compared with placebo.[26,27] However, another placebo-controlled study found no benefit compared with placebo of 485 mg/d of magnesium in reducing the frequency of migraine headaches.[28] Although no serious adverse effects were noted during these migraine headache trials, the investigators did note adverse effects such as diarrhea and gastric (stomach) irritation in about 20 to 40 % of the individuals taking the magnesium supplements.

Asthma

Several clinical trials have examined the effect of intravenous magnesium infusions on acute asthma attacks. One double-blind placebo-controlled trial in 38 adults who did not respond to initial treatment in the emergency room found improved lung function and decreased likelihood of hospitalization when IV magnesium sulfate was infused compared with a placebo.[29] However, in another placebo-controlled double-blind study in 48 adults, IV infusion of magnesium sulfate did not improve lung function in patients experiencing an acute asthma attack.[30] Measurements of serum and red blood cell levels of magnesium have not been found to be lower in asthmatic patients than nonasthmatic individuals even during acute asthmatic attacks. At present, available evidence indicates that intravenous magnesium infusion may have a minimal role in the treatment of acute asthma, but oral magnesium supplementation is of no known value in the management of chronic asthma.[31]

Table 20–2 Food Sources of Magnesium

Food	Serving	Magnesium, mg
100 % bran cereal (e.g., All Bran)	¹/₂ cup	128.7
Oat bran	¹/₂ cup dry	96.4
Brown rice	1 cup, cooked	83.8
Almonds	1 ounce (22 almonds)	81.1
Spinach, chopped	¹/₂ cup, cooked	78.3
Swiss chard, chopped	¹/₂ cup, cooked	75.2
Lima beans	¹/₂ cup, cooked	62.9
Shredded wheat	2 biscuits	54.3
Peanuts	1 ounce	49.8
Hazelnuts	1 ounce	49.0
Okra, sliced	¹/₂ cup, cooked	45.6
Molasses, black-strap	1 tablespoon	43.0
Black-eyed peas	¹/₂ cup, cooked	42.8
Banana	1 medium	34.2
Milk 1 % fat	8 fluid ounces	33.7

Sources

Food Sources

Because magnesium is part of chlorophyll, the green pigment in plants, green leafy vegetables are rich in magnesium. Unrefined grains and nuts also have high magnesium content. Meats and milk have an intermediate magnesium content, and refined foods generally have the lowest magnesium content. Water is a variable source of intake; harder water usually has a higher concentration of magnesium salts.[4] Some foods that are relatively rich in magnesium are listed in Table 20–2 along with their magnesium content in milligrams.

Supplements

Magnesium supplements are available as magnesium oxide, magnesium gluconate, magnesium chloride, and magnesium citrate salts, as well as a number of amino acid chelates, including magnesium aspartate. Magnesium hydroxide is used as an ingredient in a number of antacids.[32]

Safety

Toxicity

Adverse effects have not been identified from magnesium occurring naturally in food. However, adverse effects from excess magnesium have been observed with intakes of various magnesium salts (supplemental magnesium). The initial manifestation of excess magnesium supplementation is diarrhea, a well-known side effect of magnesium, which is used therapeutically as a laxative. Individuals with impaired kidney function are at higher risk for adverse effects from magnesium supplementation, and symptoms of magnesium toxicity have occurred in people with impaired kidney function taking moderate doses of magnesium-containing laxatives or antacids. Elevated blood levels of magnesium (hypermagnesemia) may result in a fall in blood pressure (hypotension). Some of the later effects of magnesium toxicity, such as lethargy, confusion, disturbances in normal cardiac rhythm, and deterioration of kidney function, are related to severe hypotension. As hypermagnesemia progresses, muscle weakness and difficulty breathing may occur. Severe hypermagnesemia may result in cardiac arrest.[2,4]

The FNB set the UL for supplemental magnesium intake in generally healthy adolescents and adults at 350 mg/d (Table 20–3). This UL represents the highest level of daily supplemental magnesium intake likely to pose no risk of diarrhea or gastrointestinal disturbance in almost all individuals. The FNB cautions that individuals with renal impairment are at higher risk of adverse effects from excess supplemental magnesium intake. However, the FNB also notes that there are some conditions that may warrant higher doses of magnesium under medical supervision.[4]

Drug Interactions

Magnesium interferes with the absorption of digoxin (a heart medication), nitrofurantoin (an antibiotic), and certain antimalarial drugs, potentially reducing their efficacy. Bisphosphonates (e.g., alendronate and etidronate), drugs used to treat osteoporosis, and magnesium should be taken 2 hours apart so the absorption of the bisphosphonate is not inhibited. Magnesium has also been found to reduce the efficacy of chlorpromazine (a tranquilizer), penicillamine, oral anticoagulants, and the quinolone and tetracycline classes of antibiotics. Because intravenous magnesium has increased the effects of certain muscle relaxing medications used during anesthesia for surgery, it is advisable to let medical staff know if you are taking oral magnesium supplements, laxatives, or antacids prior to anesthesia. High doses of furosemide (lasix) and some thiazide diuretics (e.g., hydrochlorthiazide) over long periods of time may result in magnesium depletion.[32,33]

Table 20–3 Tolerable Upper Intake Level (UL) for Supplemental Magnesium

Life Stage	Age	UL, mg/d
Infants	0–12 months	not possible to establish*
Children	1–3 years	65
Children	4–8 years	110
Children	9–13 years	350
Adolescents	14–18 years	350
Adults	19 years and older	350

*Source of intake should be from food and formula only.

LPI Recommendation

The Linus Pauling Institute supports the latest RDA for magnesium intake (420 mg/d for men over 30 years of age and 320 mg/d for women over 30 years of age). Following the Linus Pauling Institute recommendation to take a daily multivitamin/multimineral supplement will ensure an intake of at least 100 mg of magnesium per day. Few multivitamin/multimineral supplements contain more than 100 mg of magnesium due to its bulk. Because magnesium is plentiful in foods, eating a varied diet that provides green vegetables and whole grains daily should provide the rest of an individual's magnesium requirement.

Older Adults

Older adults (65 years and older) are less likely than younger adults to consume enough magnesium to meet their needs and should therefore take care to eat magnesium-rich foods in addition to taking a multivitamin/mineral supplement daily. Because older adults are more likely to have impaired kidney function, they should avoid taking more than 350 mg/d of supplemental magnesium without medical consultation.

References

1. Shils ME. Magnesium. In: O'Dell BL, Sunde RA, eds. *Handbook of Nutritionally Essential Minerals.* New York: Marcel Dekker, Inc; 1997:117–152.
2. Shils ME. Magnesium. In: Shils M, Olson JA, Shike M, Ross AC, eds. *Nutrition in Health and Disease,* 9th ed. Baltimore: Williams & Wilkins; 1999:169–192.
3. Spencer H, Norris C, Williams D. Inhibitory effects of zinc on magnesium balance and magnesium absorption in man. *J Am Coll Nutr* 1994;13(5):479–484.
4. Food and Nutrition Board, Institute of Medicine. Magnesium. *Dietary Reference Intakes: Calcium, Phosphorus, Magnesium, Vitamin D, and Fluoride.* Washington, D.C.: National Academy Press; 1997:190–249.
5. Ascherio A, Rimm EB, Giovannucci EL, et al. A prospective study of nutritional factors and hypertension among US men. *Circulation* 1992;86(5):1475–1484.
6. Ascherio A, Hennekens C, Willett WC, et al. Prospective study of nutritional factors, blood pressure, and hypertension among US women. *Hypertension* 1996; 27(5):1065–1072.
7. Peacock JM, Folsom AR, Arnett DK, Eckfeldt JH, Szklo M. Relationship of serum and dietary magnesium to incident hypertension: the Atherosclerosis Risk in Communities (ARIC) Study. *Ann Epidemiol* 1999; 9(3):159–165.
8. Marx A, Neutra RR. Magnesium in drinking water and ischemic heart disease. *Epidemiol Rev* 1997;19(2): 258–272.
9. Liao F, Folsom AR, Brancati FL. Is low magnesium concentration a risk factor for coronary heart disease? The Atherosclerosis Risk in Communities (ARIC) Study. *Am Heart J* 1998;136(3):480–490.
10. Witteman JC, Grobbee DE, Derkx FH, Bouillon R, de Bruijn AM, Hofman A. Reduction of blood pressure with oral magnesium supplementation in women with mild to moderate hypertension. *Am J Clin Nutr* 1994;60(1):129–135.
11. Kawano Y, Matsuoka H, Takishita S, Omae T. Effects of magnesium supplementation in hypertensive patients: assessment by office, home, and ambulatory blood pressures. *Hypertension* 1998;32(2):260–265.
12. Shils ME. Magnesium. In: Ziegler EE, Filer LJ, eds. *Present Knowledge in Nutrition,* 7th ed. Washington, D.C.: ILSI Press; 1996:256–264.
13. Crombleholme WR. Obstetrics. In: Tierney LM, McPhee SJ, Papadakis MA, eds. *Current Medical Treatment and Diagnosis,* 37th ed. Stamford: Appleton and Lange; 1998:731–734.
14. Woods KL, Fletcher S, Roffe C, Haider Y. Intravenous magnesium sulphate in suspected acute myocardial infarction: results of the second Leicester Intravenous Magnesium Intervention Trial (LIMIT-2). *Lancet* 1992;339(8809):1553–1558.
15. Woods KL, Fletcher S. Long-term outcome after intravenous magnesium sulphate in suspected acute myocardial infarction: the second Leicester Intravenous Magnesium Intervention Trial (LIMIT-2). *Lancet* 1994;343(8901):816–819.
16. ISIS-4 Collaborative. ISIS-4: a randomised factorial trial assessing early oral captopril, oral mononitrate, and intravenous magnesium sulphate in 58,050 patients with suspected acute myocardial infarction. ISIS-4 (Fourth International Study of Infarct Survival) Collaborative Group. *Lancet* 1995;345(8951):669–685.
17. Ziegelstein RC, Hilbe JM, French WJ, Antman EM, Chandra-Strobos N. Magnesium use in the treatment of acute myocardial infarction in the United States (observations from the Second National Registry of Myocardial Infarction). *Am J Cardiol* 2001;87(1):7–10.
18. Shechter M, Sharir M, Labrador MJ, Forrester J, Silver B, Bairey Merz CN. Oral magnesium therapy improves endothelial function in patients with coronary artery disease. *Circulation* 2000;102(19):2353–2358.
19. Shechter M, Merz CN, Paul-Labrador M, et al. Oral magnesium supplementation inhibits platelet-dependent thrombosis in patients with coronary artery disease. *Am J Cardiol* 1999;84(2):152–156.
20. Tosiello L. Hypomagnesemia and diabetes mellitus: a review of clinical implications. *Arch Intern Med* 1996;156(11):1143–1148.
21. Paolisso G, Sgambatos S, Gambardella A, et al. Daily magnesium supplements impair glucose handling in elderly subjects. *Am J Clin Nutr* 1992;55(6):1161–1167.
22. Sojka JE, Weaver CM. Magnesium supplementation and osteoporosis. *Nutr Rev* 1995;53(3):71–74.
23. Tucker KL, Hannan MT, Chen H, Cupples LA, Wilson PW, Kiel DP. Potassium, magnesium, and fruit and vegetable intakes are associated with greater bone mineral density in elderly men and women. *Am J Clin Nutr* 1999;69(4):727–736.
24. Stendig-Lindberg G, Tepper R, Leichter I. Trabecular bone density in a two year controlled trial of peroral magnesium in osteoporosis. *Magnes Res* 1993;6(2): 155–163.
25. Abraham GE, Grewal H. A total dietary program emphasizing magnesium instead of calcium: effect on the mineral density of calcaneous bone in postmenopausal women on hormonal therapy. *J Reprod Med* 1990;35(5):503–507.
26. Peikert A, Wilimzig C, Kohne-Volland R. Prophylaxis of migraine with oral magnesium: results from a prospective, multi-center, placebo-controlled and double-blind randomized study. *Cephalalgia* 1996; 16(4):257–263.
27. Mauskop A, Altura BM. Role of magnesium in the pathogenesis and treatment of migraines. *Clin Neurosci* 1998;5(1):24–27.
28. Pfaffenrath V, Wessely P, Meyer C, et al. Magnesium in the prophylaxis of migraine—a double-blind placebo-controlled study. *Cephalalgia* 1996;16(6):436–440.
29. Skobeloff EM, Spivey WH, McNamara RM, Greenspon L. Intravenous magnesium sulfate for the treatment of acute asthma in the emergency department. *JAMA* 1989;262(9):1210–1213.

30. Tiffany BR, Berk WA, Todd IK, White SR. Magnesium bolus or infusion fails to improve expiratory flow in acute asthma exacerbations. *Chest* 1993;104(3):831–834.

31. Monteleone CA, Sherman AR. Nutrition and asthma. *Arch Intern Med* 1997;157(1):23–34.

32. Hendler SS, Rorvik DR, eds. *PDR for Nutritional Supplements*. Montvale, NJ: Medical Economics Company, Inc; 2001.

33. Minerals. *Drug Facts and Comparisons*. St. Louis: Facts and Comparisons; 2000:27–51.

21 Manganese

Manganese is a mineral element that is both nutritionally essential and potentially toxic. The derivation of its name from the Greek word for magic remains appropriate because scientists are still working to understand the diverse effects of manganese deficiency and manganese toxicity in living organisms.[1]

Function

Manganese plays an important role in a number of physiologic processes as a constituent of some enzymes and an activator of other enzymes.[2]

Antioxidant Function

Manganese superoxide dismutase (MnSOD) is the principal antioxidant enzyme of mitochondria. Because mitochondria consume over 90% of the oxygen used by cells, they are especially vulnerable to oxidative stress. The superoxide radical is one of the reactive oxygen species produced in mitochondria during adenosine triphosphate synthesis. MnSOD catalyzes the conversion of superoxide radicals to hydrogen peroxide, which can be reduced to water by other antioxidant enzymes.[3]

Metabolism

A number of manganese-activated enzymes play important roles in the metabolism of carbohydrates, amino acids, and cholesterol.[4] Pyruvate carboxylase, a manganese-containing enzyme, and phosphoenolpyruvate carboxykinase, a manganese-activated enzyme, play critical roles in gluconeogenesis, the production of glucose from noncarbohydrate precursors. Arginase, another manganese-containing enzyme, is required by the liver for the urea cycle, a process that detoxifies ammonia generated during amino acid metabolism.[3]

Bone Development

Manganese deficiency results in abnormal skeletal development in a number of animal species. Manganese is the preferred cofactor of enzymes called *glycosyltransferases*, which are required for the synthesis of proteoglycans that are needed for the formation of healthy cartilage and bone.[5]

Wound Healing

Wound healing is a complex process that requires increased production of collagen. Manganese is required for the activation of prolidase, an enzyme that functions to provide the amino acid proline for collagen formation in human skin cells.[6] A genetic disorder known as *prolidase deficiency* results in abnormal wound healing, among other problems, and is characterized by abnormal manganese metabolism.[5] Glycosaminoglycan synthesis, which requires manganese-activated glycosyltransferases, may also play an important role in wound healing.[7]

Nutrient Interactions

Iron. Although the specific mechanisms for manganese absorption and transport have not been determined, some evidence suggests that iron and manganese can share common absorption and transport pathways. Absorption of manganese from a meal is reduced as the meal's iron content is increased.[5] Iron supplementation (60 mg/d for 4 months) was associated with decreased blood manganese levels and decreased MnSOD activity in white blood cells, indicating a reduction in manganese nutritional status.[8] An individual's iron status can affect manganese bioavailability. Intestinal absorption of manganese is increased during iron deficiency, and increased iron stores (ferritin levels) are associated with decreased manganese absorption.[9] The finding that men generally absorb less manganese than women may be related to the fact that men usually have higher iron stores than women.[10]

Magnesium. Supplemental magnesium (200 mg/d) decreased manganese bioavailability slightly, either by decreasing manganese absorption or by increasing its loss in healthy adults.[11]

Calcium. In one set of studies, supplemental calcium (500 mg/d) resulted in slightly lower manganese bioavailability in healthy adults. As a source of calcium, milk had the least effect, and calcium carbonate and calcium phosphate had the greatest effect.[11] Several other studies have found the effect of supplemental calcium on manganese metabolism to be minimal.[12]

Deficiency

Manganese deficiency has been observed in a number of animal species. Signs of manganese deficiency include impaired growth, impaired reproductive function, skeletal abnormalities, impaired glucose tolerance, and altered carbohydrate and lipid metabolism. In humans, demonstration of a manganese deficiency syndrome has been less clear.[2,5] A child on long-term total parenteral nutrition that lacked manganese developed bone demineralization and impaired growth that were corrected by manganese supplementation.[13] Young men who were fed a low-manganese diet developed decreased serum cholesterol levels and a transient skin rash.[14] Blood calcium, phosphorus, and alkaline phosphatase levels were also elevated, which may indicate increased bone remodeling as a consequence of insufficient dietary manganese. Young women fed a manganese-poor diet developed mildly abnormal glucose tolerance in response to an intravenous infusion of glucose.[12]

The Adequate Intake Level

Because there was not enough information on manganese requirements to set a recommended dietary allowance, the Food and Nutrition Board (FNB) of the Institute of Medi-

Table 21–1   The Adequate Intake (AI) for Manganese

Life Stage	Age	Males, mg/d	Females, mg/d
Infants	0–6 months	0.003	0.003
Infants	7–12 months	0.6	0.6
Children	1–3 years	1.2	1.2
Children	4–8 years	1.5	1.5
Children	9–13 years	1.9	1.6
Adolescents	14–18 years	2.2	1.6
Adults	19 years and older	2.3	1.8
Pregnancy	all ages	–	2.0
Breastfeeding	all ages	–	2.6

cine set an adequate intake level (AI). Because symptoms of manganese deficiency have only been documented in humans on total parenteral nutrition or fed experimental diets deficient in manganese, the FNB based the AI on average dietary intakes of manganese determined by the Total Diet Study, an annual survey of the mineral content of representative diets of Americans (Table 21–1).[4]

Disease Prevention

Manganese and Chronic Diseases

Low dietary manganese or low levels of manganese in blood or tissue have been associated with several chronic diseases. Although manganese insufficiency is not currently thought to cause the diseases discussed following, more research may be warranted to determine whether suboptimal manganese nutritional status contributes to certain disease processes.

Osteoporosis

Women with osteoporosis have been found to have decreased plasma levels of manganese and an enhanced plasma response to an oral dose of manganese,[15] suggesting they may have lower manganese status than women without osteoporosis. A study in healthy post-menopausal women found that a supplement containing manganese (5 mg/d), copper (2.5 mg/d), and zinc (15 mg/d) in combination with a calcium supplement (1000 mg/d) was more effective than the calcium supplement alone in preventing spinal bone loss over a period of 2 years.[16] However, the presence of other trace elements in the supplement makes it impossible to determine whether manganese supplementation was the beneficial agent for maintaining bone mineral density.

Diabetes Mellitus

Manganese deficiency results in glucose intolerance similar to diabetes mellitus in some animal species, but studies examining the manganese status of diabetic humans have generated mixed results. Whole blood manganese levels did not differ significantly between 57 diabetics and 28 nondiabetic controls.[17] However, urinary manganese excretion tended to be slightly higher in 185 diabetics compared with 185 nondiabetic controls.[18] Additionally, a study of functional manganese status found the activity of the antioxidant enzyme MnSOD to be lower in the white blood cells of diabetics than in those of nondiabetic controls.[19] Neither 15 nor 30 mg of oral manganese improved glucose tolerance in diabetics or nondiabetic controls when given at the same time as an oral glucose challenge.[20] Although manganese appears to play a role in glucose metabolism, there is little evidence that manganese supplementation improves glucose tolerance in diabetic or nondiabetic individuals.

Seizure Disorders

Manganese-deficient rats are more susceptible to seizures, and rats that are genetically prone to epilepsy have lower than normal brain and blood manganese levels. Certain subgroups of humans with epilepsy have been found to have lower whole blood manganese levels than nonepileptic controls. One study found blood manganese levels of individuals with epilepsy of unknown origin to be lower than those of individuals whose epilepsy was induced by trauma (e.g., head injury) or disease, suggest-ing a possible genetic relationship between epilepsy and abnormal manganese metabolism. Although manganese deficiency does not appear to be a cause of epilepsy in humans, the relationship between manganese metabolism and epilepsy deserves further research.[5,21]

Disease Treatment

Presently, there is insufficient evidence to support the use of manganese to treat diseases or health conditions other than frank manganese deficiency, which is quite rare in humans.

Sources

Food Sources

Estimated average dietary manganese intakes in the United States range from 2.1 to 2.3 mg/d for men and 1.6 to 1.8 mg/d for women. People eating vegetarian diets and Western diets emphasizing whole grains may have manganese intakes as high as 10.9 mg/d.[4] Rich sources of manganese include whole grains, nuts, leafy vegetables, and teas. Foods high in phytic acid, such as beans, seeds, nuts, whole grains, and soy products, or foods high in oxalic acid, such as cabbage, spinach, and sweet potatoes, may slightly inhibit manganese absorption. Although teas are rich sources of manganese, the polyphenols present in tea may moderately reduce the absorption of manganese.[11] The manganese content of some manganese-rich foods is listed in milligrams in Table 21–2.

Supplements

Several forms of manganese are found in supplements, including manganese gluconate, manganese sulfate, manganese ascorbate, and amino acid chelates of manganese. Manganese is available as a stand-alone supplement or in combination products.[22] Relatively high levels of manganese ascorbate may be found in a bone/joint health product containing chondroitin sulfate and glucosamine hydrochloride (see Safety).

Table 21–2   Food Sources of Manganese

Food	Serving	Manganese, mg
Bran cereal with raisins	1 cup	1.44–2.55
Pineapple, raw	1/2 cup, diced	1.28
Pineapple juice	1/2 cup (4 ounces)	1.24
Instant oatmeal (prepared with water)	1 packet	1.20
Pecans	1 ounce	1.12
Brown rice, cooked	1/2 cup	0.88
Spinach, cooked	1/2 cup	0.84
Almonds	1 ounce	0.74
Bread, whole wheat	1 slice	0.65
Peanuts	1 ounce	0.59
Sweet potato, cooked	1/2 cup, mashed	0.55
Navy beans, cooked	1/2 cup	0.51
Pinto beans, cooked	1/2 cup	0.48
Lima beans, cooked	1/2 cup	0.48
Tea, green	1 cup (8 ounces)	0.41–1.58
Tea, black	1 cup (8 ounces)	0.18–0.77

Safety

Toxicity

Inhaled Manganese. Manganese toxicity may result in multiple neurological problems and is a well-recognized health hazard for people who inhale manganese dust.[1,4] Unlike ingested manganese, inhaled manganese is transported directly to the brain before it can be metabolized in the liver.[23] The symptoms of manganese toxicity generally appear slowly over a period of months to years. In its worst form, manganese toxicity can result in a permanent neurological disorder with symptoms similar to those of Parkinson's disease, including tremors, difficulty walking, and facial muscle spasms. This syndrome is sometimes preceded by psychiatric symptoms, such as irritability, aggressiveness, and even hallucinations.[24]

Methylcyclopentadienyl Manganese Tricarbonyl. Methylcyclopentadienyl manganese tricarbonyl (MMT) is a manganese-containing compound used in gasoline as an antiknock additive. Although it has been used for this purpose in Canada for more than 20 years, uncertainty about adverse health effects from inhaled exhaust emissions kept the U.S. Environmental Protection Agency (EPA) from approving its use in unleaded gasoline. In 1995, a U.S. court decision made MMT available for widespread use in unleaded gasoline.[23] A recent study in Montreal, where MMT had been used for more than 10 years, found airborne manganese levels to be similar to those in areas where MMT was not used.[25] However, the impact of long-term exposure to low levels of MMT combustion products has not been thoroughly evaluated and will require additional study.[26]

Ingested Manganese. Limited evidence suggests that high manganese intakes from drinking water may be associated with neurological symptoms similar to those of Parkinson's disease. Severe neurological symptoms were reported in 25 people who drank water contaminated with manganese and probably other contaminants from dry cell batteries for 2 to 3 months.[27] Water manganese levels were found to be 14 mg/L almost 2 months after symptoms began and may already have been declining.[1] A study of older adults in Greece found a high prevalence of neurological symptoms in those exposed to water manganese levels of 1.8 to 2.3 mg/L,[28] although a study of people in Germany drinking water with manganese levels ranging from 0.3 to 2.2 mg/L found no evidence of increased neurological symptoms compared with those drinking water containing less than 0.05 mg/L.[29] Manganese in drinking water may be more bioavailable than manganese in food. However, none of the studies measured dietary manganese, so total manganese intake in these cases is unknown.[1,4] In the United States, the EPA recommends 0.05 mg/L as the maximum allowable manganese concentration in drinking water.[30]

A single case of manganese toxicity was reported in a person who took large amounts of mineral supplements for years,[31] and another case was reported as a result of taking a

Chinese herbal supplement.[24] Manganese toxicity resulting from foods alone has not been reported in humans, even though certain vegetarian diets could provide up 20 mg/d of manganese.[4,31]

Individuals with Increased Susceptibility to Manganese Toxicity

Chronic Liver Disease. Manganese is eliminated from the body mainly in bile. Thus, impaired liver function may lead to decreased manganese excretion. Manganese accumulation in individuals with cirrhosis or liver failure may contribute to neurological problems and Parkinson's disease–like symptoms.[1,22]

Newborns. The newborn brain may be more susceptible to manganese toxicity due to a greater expression of receptors for the manganese transport protein (transferrin) in developing nerve cells and the immaturity of the liver's bile elimination system.[4]

Due to the severe implications of manganese neurotoxicity, the FNB set very conservative upper levels of intake for manganese, which are listed in Table 21–3.[4]

Drug Interactions

Magnesium-containing antacids and laxatives and the antibiotic medication tetracycline may decrease the absorption of manganese if taken together with manganese-containing foods or supplements.[22]

High Levels of Manganese in Supplements Marketed for Bone/Joint Health

Two recent studies have found that supplements containing a combination of glucosamine hydrochloride, chondroitin sulfate, and manganese ascorbate are beneficial in relieving pain due to mild or moderate osteoarthritis of the knee when compared with a placebo.[32,33] The dose of elemental manganese supplied by the supplements was 30 mg/d for 8 weeks in one study[33] and 40 mg/d for 6 months in the other.[32] No adverse effects were reported during either study, and blood man-

Table 21–3 Tolerable Upper Intake Level (UL) for Manganese

Life Stage	Age	UL, mg/d
Infants	0–12 months	not possible to establish*
Children	1–3 years	2
Children	4–8 years	3
Children	9–13 years	6
Adolescents	14–18 years	9
Adults	19 years and older	11

*Source of intake should be from food and formula only.

ganese levels were not measured. Neither study compared the treatment containing manganese ascorbate to a treatment containing glucosamine hydrochloride and chondroitin sulfate without manganese ascorbate, so it is impossible to determine whether the supplement would have resulted in the same benefit without high doses of manganese.

LPI Recommendation

The AI for manganese (2.3 mg/d for adult men and 1.8 mg/d for adult women) appears sufficient to prevent deficiency in most individuals. The daily intake of manganese most likely to promote optimum health is not known. Following the Linus Pauling Institute recommendation to take a multivitamin/multimineral supplement containing 100 % of the daily values (DV) of most nutrients will generally provide 2 mg/d of manganese in addition to that in foods. Because of the potential for toxicity and the lack of information regarding benefit, manganese supplementation beyond 100 % of the DV (2 mg/d) is not recommended. There is presently no evidence that the consumption of a manganese-rich plant-based diet results in manganese toxicity.

Older Adults

The requirement for manganese is not known to be higher for adults 65 years and older. However, liver disease is more common in older adults and may increase the risk of manganese toxicity by decreasing the elimination of manganese from the body. Manganese supplementation beyond 100 % of the DV (2 mg/d) is not recommended.

References

1. Keen CL, Ensunsa JL, Watson MH, et al. Nutritional aspects of manganese from experimental studies. *Neurotoxicology* 1999;20(2–3):213–223.
2. Nielsen FH. Ultratrace minerals. In: Shils M, Olson JA, Shike M, Ross AC, eds. *Nutrition in Health and Disease,* 9th ed. Baltimore: Williams & Wilkins; 1999:283–303.
3. Leach RM, Harris ED. Manganese. In: O'Dell BL, Sunde RA, eds. *Handbook of Nutritionally Essential Minerals.* New York: Marcel Dekker, Inc; 1997:335–355.
4. Food and Nutrition Board, Institute of Medicine. Manganese. *Dietary Reference Intakes for Vitamin A, Vitamin K, Boron, Chromium, Copper, Iodine, Iron, Manganese, Molybdenum, Nickel, Silicon, Vanadium, and Zinc.* Washington, D.C.: National Academy Press; 2001:394–419.
5. Keen CL, Zidenberg-Cherr S. Manganese. In: Ziegler EE, Filer LJ, eds. *Present Knowledge in Nutrition,* 7th ed. Washington, D.C.: ILSI Press; 1996:334–343.
6. Muszynska A, Palka J, Gorodkiewicz E. The mechanism of daunorubicin-induced inhibition of prolidase activity in human skin fibroblasts and its implication to impaired collagen biosynthesis. *Exp Toxicol Pathol* 2000;52(2):149–155.
7. Shetlar MR, Shetlar CL. The role of manganese in wound healing. In: Klimis-Tavantzis DL, ed. *Manganese in Health and Disease.* Boca Raton: CRC Press, Inc.; 1994:145–157.
8. Davis CD, Greger JL. Longitudinal changes of manganese-dependent superoxide dismutase and other indexes of manganese and iron status in women. *Am J Clin Nutr* 1992;55(3):747–752.
9. Finley JW. Manganese absorption and retention by young women is associated with serum ferritin concentration. *Am J Clin Nutr* 1999;70(1):37–43.
10. Finley JW, Johnson PE, Johnson LK. Sex affects manganese absorption and retention by humans from a diet adequate in manganese. *Am J Clin Nutr* 1994;60(6):949–955.
11. Kies C. Bioavailability of manganese. In: Klimis-Tavantzis DL, ed. *Manganese in Health and Disease.* Boca Raton, FL: CRC Press, Inc; 1994:39–58.
12. Johnson PE, Lykken GI. Manganese and calcium absorption and balance in young women fed diets with varying amounts of manganese and calcium. *J Trace Elem Exp Med* 1991;4:19–35.
13. Norose N, Terai M, Norose K. Manganese deficiency in a child with very short bowel syndrome receiving long-term parenteral nutrition. *J Trace Elem Exp Med* 1992;5:100–101.
14. Friedman BJ, Freeland-Graves JH, Bales CW, et al. Manganese balance and clinical observations in young men fed a manganese-deficient diet. *J Nutr* 1987;117(1):133–143.
15. Freeland-Graves J, Llanes C. Models to study manganese deficiency. In: Klimis-Tavantzis DL, ed. *Manganese in Health and Disease.* Boca Raton, FL: CRC Press, Inc; 1994.
16. Strause L, Saltman P, Smith KT, Bracker M, Andon MB. Spinal bone loss in postmenopausal women supplemented with calcium and trace minerals. *J Nutr* 1994;124(7):1060–1064.
17. Walter RM, Jr., Uriu-Hare JY, Olin KL, et al. Copper, zinc, manganese, and magnesium status and complications of diabetes mellitus. *Diabetes Care* 1991;14(11):1050–1056.
18. el-Yazigi A, Hannan N, Raines DA. Urinary excretion of chromium, copper, and manganese in diabetes mellitus and associated disorders. *Diabetes Res* 1991;18(3):129–134.
19. Nath N, Chari SN, Rathi AB. Superoxide dismutase in diabetic polymorphonuclear leukocytes. *Diabetes* 1984;33(6):586–589.
20. Walter RM, Aoki TT, Keen CL. Acute oral manganese does not consistently affect glucose tolerance in nondiabetic and type II diabetic humans. *J Trace Elem Exp Med* 1991;4:73–79.
21. Carl GF, Gallagher BB. Manganese and epilepsy. In: Klimis-Tavantzis DL, ed. *Manganese in Health and Disease.* Boca Raton, FL: CRC Press, Inc; 1994:133–157.
22. Hendler SS, Rorvik DR, eds. *PDR for Nutritional Supplements.* Montvale, NJ: Medical Economics Company, Inc.; 2001.
23. Davis JM. Methylcyclopentadienyl manganese tricarbonyl: health risk uncertainties and research directions. *Environ Health Perspect* 1998;106(Suppl 1):191–201.
24. Pal PK, Samii A, Calne DB. Manganese neurotoxicity: a review of clinical features, imaging and pathology. *Neurotoxicology* 1999;20(2–3):227–238.
25. Zayed J, Thibault C, Gareau L, Kennedy G. Airborne manganese particulates and methylcyclopentadienyl manganese tricarbonyl (MMT) at selected outdoor sites in Montreal. *Neurotoxicology* 1999;20(2–3):151–157.
26. Aschner M. Manganese: brain transport and emerging research needs. *Environ Health Perspect* 2000;108 (Suppl 3):429–432.
27. Kawamura R. Intoxication by manganese in well water. *Kisasato Archives of Experimental Medicine* 1941;18:145–169.
28. Kondakis XG, Makris N, Leotsinidis M, Prinou M, Papapetropoulos T. Possible health effects of high manganese concentration in drinking water. *Arch Environ Health* 1989;44(3):175–178.
29. Vieregge P, Heinzow B, Korf G, Teichert HM, Schleifenbaum P, Mosinger HU. Long-term exposure to manganese in rural well water has no neurological effects. *Can J Neurol Sci* 1995;22(4):286–289.
30. EPA Office of Water. Current Drinking Water Standards. *Environmental Protection Agency* [Web page]. May 31, 2001. Available at: http://www.epa.gov/safewater/mcl.html. Accessed August 8, 2001.
31. Keen CL, Zidenberg-Cherr S. Manganese toxicity in humans and experimental animals. In: Klimis-Tavantzis DL, ed. *Manganese in Health and Disease.* Boca Raton, FL: CRC Press, Inc; 1994:193–205.
32. Das A, Jr., Hammad TA. Efficacy of a combination of FCHG49 glucosamine hydrochloride, TRH122 low molecular weight sodium chondroitin sulfate and manganese ascorbate in the management of knee osteoarthritis. *Osteoarthritis Cartilage* 2000;8(5):343–350.
33. Leffler CT, Philippi AF, Leffler SG, Mosure JC, Kim PD. Glucosamine, chondroitin, and manganese ascorbate for degenerative joint disease of the knee or low back: a randomized, double-blind, placebo-controlled pilot study. *Mil Med* 1999;164(2):85–91.

22 Molybdenum

Molybdenum is an essential trace element for virtually all life forms. It functions as a cofactor for a number of enzymes that catalyze important chemical transformations in the global carbon, nitrogen, and sulfur cycles.[1] Thus, molybdenum-dependent enzymes are not only required for the health of the earth's people, but for the health of its ecosystems as well.

Function

The biological form of molybdenum present in almost all molybdenum-containing enzymes (molybdoenzymes) is an organic molecule known as the *molybdenum cofactor*.[2] In humans, molybdenum is known to function as a cofactor for three enzymes. *Sulfite oxidase* catalyzes the transformation of sulfite to sulfate, a reaction that is necessary for the metabolism of sulfur-containing amino acids, such as cysteine. *Xanthine oxidase* and *aldehyde oxidase* catalyze hydroxylation reactions involving a number of different molecules with similar structures. Xanthine oxidase catalyzes the breakdown of nucleotides (precursors to DNA and RNA) to form uric acid, which contributes to the antioxidant capacity of the blood. Xanthine oxidase and aldehyde oxidase also play a role in the metabolism of drugs and toxins. Of these three enzymes, only sulfite oxidase is known to be crucial for human health.[3,4]

Interaction with Copper

Excess dietary molybdenum has been found to result in copper deficiency in grazing animals (ruminants). In ruminants, the formation of compounds containing sulfur and molybdenum, known as thiomolybdates, appears to prevent the absorption of copper. This interaction between thiomolybdates and copper does not occur to a significant degree in humans. One early study reported that molybdenum intakes of 500 and 1500 μg/d from sorghum increased urinary copper excretion.[2] However, the results of a more recent and well-controlled study of molybdenum intake and copper metabolism in eight healthy young men indicated that very high dietary molybdenum intakes (up to 1500 μg/d) did not adversely affect copper nutritional status.[5]

Deficiency

Dietary molybdenum deficiency has never been observed in healthy people.[2] The only documented case of acquired molybdenum deficiency occurred in a patient with Crohn's disease on long-term total parenteral nutrition (TPN) without molybdenum added to the TPN solution.[6] The patient developed rapid heart and respiratory rates, headache, and night blindness, and ultimately became comatose. He also demonstrated biochemical signs of molybdenum deficiency, including low blood uric acid levels, decreased urinary excretion of uric acid and sulfate, and increased urinary excretion of sulfite. The symptoms disappeared when the administration of amino acid solutions was discontinued. Molybdenum supplementation (160 μg/d) reversed the amino acid intolerance and improved his clinical condition.

Current understanding of the essentiality of molybdenum in humans is based largely on the study of individuals with very rare inborn errors of metabolism that result in a deficiency of the molybdoenzyme sulfite oxidase. Two forms of sulfite oxidase deficiency have been identified: (1) isolated sulfite oxidase deficiency, in which only sulfite oxidase activity is affected, and (2) molybdenum cofactor deficiency, in which the activity of all three molybdoenzymes is affected. Because molybdenum functions only in the form of the molybdenum cofactor in humans, any disturbance of molybdenum cofactor metabolism can disrupt the

Table 22–1   Recommended Dietary Allowance (RDA) for Molybdenum

Life Stage	Age	Males, µg/d	Females, µg/d
Infants	0–6 months	2 (AI)	2 (AI)
Infants	7–12 months	3 (AI)	3 (AI)
Children	1–3 years	17	17
Children	4–8 years	22	22
Children	9–13 years	34	34
Adolescents	14–18 years	43	43
Adults	19 years and older	45	45
Pregnancy	all ages	–	50
Breastfeeding	all ages	–	50

AI, adequate intake level.

function of all molybdoenzymes. Together, molybdenum cofactor deficiency and isolated sulfite oxidase deficiency have been diagnosed in more than 100 individuals worldwide. Both disorders result from recessive traits, meaning that only individuals who inherit two copies of the abnormal gene (one from each parent) develop the disease. Individuals who inherit only one copy of the abnormal gene are known as carriers of the trait but do not exhibit any symptoms. The symptoms of isolated sulfite oxidase deficiency and molybdenum cofactor deficiency are identical and usually include severe brain damage, which appears to be due to the loss of sulfite oxidase activity. At present, it is not clear whether the neurologic effects are a result of the accumulation of a toxic metabolite, such as sulfite, or inadequate sulfate production. Isolated sulfite oxidase deficiency and molybdenum cofactor deficiency can be diagnosed relatively early in pregnancy (10 to 14 weeks of gestation) through chorionic villus sampling, and in some cases, carriers of molybdenum cofactor deficiency can be identified through genetic testing. No cure is presently available for either disorder, although antiseizure medications and dietary restriction of sulfur-containing amino acids may be beneficial in some cases.[7]

The Recommended Dietary Allowance

The recommended dietary allowance (RDA) for molybdenum was most recently revised in January 2001.[2] It was based on the results of nutritional balance studies conducted in eight healthy young men under controlled laboratory conditions. The RDA values for molybdenum are listed in Table 22–1 in micrograms per day by age and gender.[8,9]

Disease Prevention

Gastroesophageal Cancer

Linxian is a small region in northern China where the incidence of cancer of the esophagus and stomach is very high (10 times higher than the average in China and 100 times higher than the average in the United States). The soil in this region is low in molybdenum and other mineral elements, so dietary molybdenum is also low. Increased intake of nitrosamines, which are known carcinogens, may be one of a number of dietary and environmental factors that contributes to the development of gastroesophageal cancer in this population. Plants require molybdenum to synthesize nitrate reductase, a molybdoenzyme necessary for converting nitrates from the soil to amino acids. When soil molybdenum content is low, plant conversion of nitrates to nitrosamines increases, resulting in increased nitrosamine exposure for those who consume the plants. Adding molybdenum to the soil in the form of ammonium molybdenate may help decrease the risk of gastroesophageal cancer by limiting nitrosamine exposure. It is not clear whether dietary molybdenum supplementation is beneficial in decreasing the risk of gastroesophageal cancer. In a large intervention trial, dietary supplementation of molybdenum (30 µg/d) and vitamin C (120 mg/d) did not decrease the incidence of gastroesophageal cancer or other cancers in residents of Linxian over a 5-year period.[10]

Disease Treatment

Presently, there is insufficient evidence to support the use of molybdenum to treat diseases or health conditions other than frank molybdenum deficiency, which is very rare.

Sources

Food Sources

The Total Diet Study, an annual survey of the mineral content of representative diets of Americans, indicates that the dietary intake of molybdenum averages 76 μg/d for women and 109 μg/d for men. Thus, usual molybdenum intakes are well above the RDA for molybdenum. Legumes, such as beans, lentils, and peas, are the richest sources of molybdenum. Grain products and nuts are considered good sources, and animal products, fruits, and many vegetables are generally low in molybdenum.[2] Because the molybdenum content of plants depends on the soil molybdenum content and environmental conditions, the molybdenum content of foods can vary considerably.[11]

Supplements

Molybdenum in nutritional supplements is generally in the form of sodium molybdate or ammonium molybdate.[12]

Safety

Toxicity

The toxicity of molybdenum compounds appears to be relatively low in humans. Increased blood uric acid levels and goutlike symptoms have been reported in occupationally exposed workers in a copper-molybdenum plant and an Armenian population consuming 10 to 15 mg of molybdenum from food daily.[13] In other studies, blood and urinary uric acid levels were not elevated by molybdenum intakes of up to 1.5 mg/d.[2] There is one report of an acute toxic reaction associated with molybdenum from a dietary supplement. An adult male, reported to have consumed a total of 13.5 mg of molyb-

Table 22–2 Tolerable Upper Intake Level (UL) for Molybdenum

Life Stage	Age	UL, μg/d
Infants	0–12 months	not possible to establish*
Children	1–3 years	300
Children	4–8 years	600
Children	9–13 years	1100 (1.1 mg/d)
Adolescents	14–18 years	1700 (1.7 mg/d)
Adults	19 years and older	2000 (2.0 mg/d)

*Source of intake should be from food and formula only.

denum over a period of 18 days (300 to 800 μg/d), developed acute psychosis with hallucinations, seizures, and other neurologic symptoms.[12] However, a controlled study found no serious adverse effects of molybdenum intakes of up to 1.5 mg/d (1500 μg/d) for 24 days in four healthy young men.[9]

The Food and Nutrition Board (FNB) of the Institute of Medicine found little evidence that molybdenum excess was associated with adverse health outcomes in generally healthy people. To determine the tolerable upper level of intake, the FNB selected adverse reproductive effects in rats as the most sensitive index of toxicity and applied a large uncertainty factor because animal data were used.[2] Tolerable upper intake levels (UL) for molybdenum are listed by age group in Table 22–2.

Drug Interactions

High doses of molybdenum have been found to inhibit the metabolism of acetaminophen in rats.[14] However, it is not known whether this occurs at clinically relevant doses in humans.

LPI Recommendation

The RDA for molybdenum (45 µg/d for adults) is sufficient to prevent deficiency. Although the intake of molybdenum most likely to promote optimum health is not known, there is presently no evidence that intakes higher than the RDA are beneficial. Most people in the United States consume more than sufficient molybdenum in their diets, making supplementation unnecessary. Following the Linus Pauling Institute's general recommendation to take a multivitamin/multimineral supplement that contains 100% of the daily values (DV) for most nutrients is likely to provide 75 µg/d of molybdenum because the DV for molybdenum has not been revised to reflect the most recent RDA. Although the amount of molybdenum presently found in most multivitamin/multimineral supplements is higher than the RDA, it is well below the tolerable upper intake level (UL) of 2000 µg/d and should be safe for adults.

Older Adults

Because aging has not been associated with significant changes in the requirement for molybdenum, our recommendation for molybdenum is the same for adults over 65 years.

References

1. Wuebbens MM, Liu MT, Rajagopalan K, Schindelin H. Insights into molybdenum cofactor deficiency provided by the crystal structure of the molybdenum cofactor biosynthesis protein MoaC. *Structure Fold Des* 2000;8(7):709–718.
2. Food and Nutrition Board, Institute of Medicine. Molybdenum. *Dietary Reference Intakes for Vitamin A, Vitamin K, Boron, Chromium, Copper, Iodine, Iron, Manganese, Molybdenum, Nickel, Silicon, Vanadium, and Zinc*. Washington, D.C.: National Academy Press; 2001:420–441.
3. Nielsen FH. Ultratrace minerals. In: Shils M, Olson JA, Shike M, Ross AC, eds. *Nutrition in Health and Disease*, 9th ed. Baltimore: Williams & Wilkins; 1999:283–303.
4. Beedham C. Molybdenum hydroxylases as drug-metabolizing enzymes. *Drug Metab Rev* 1985;16(1–2):119–156.
5. Turnlund JR, Keyes WR. Dietary molybdenum: Effect on copper absorption, excretion, and status in young men. In: Roussel AM, ed. *Trace Elements in Man and Animals*, Vol. 10. New York: Kluwer Academic Press; 2000:951–953.
6. Abumrad NN, Schneider AJ, Steel D, Rogers LS. Amino acid intolerance during prolonged total parenteral nutrition reversed by molybdate therapy. *Am J Clin Nutr* 1981;34(11):2551–2559.
7. Johnson JL, Duran M. Molybdenum cofactor deficiency and isolated sulfite deficiency. In: Scriver RC, ed. *Metabolic and Molecular Bases of Inherited Disease*. New York: McGraw-Hill; 2001:3163–3177.
8. Turnlund JR, Keyes WR, Peiffer GL, Chiang G. Molybdenum absorption, excretion, and retention studied with stable isotopes in young men during depletion and repletion. *Am J Clin Nutr* 1995;61(5):1102–1109.
9. Turnlund JR, Keyes WR, Peiffer GL. Molybdenum absorption, excretion, and retention studied with stable isotopes in young men at five intakes of dietary molybdenum. *Am J Clin Nutr* 1995;62(4):790–796.
10. Blot WJ, Li JY, Taylor PR, et al. Nutrition intervention trials in Linxian, China: supplementation with specific vitamin/mineral combinations, cancer incidence, and disease-specific mortality in the general population. *J Natl Cancer Inst* 1993;85(18):1483–1492.
11. Mills CF, Davis GK. Molybdenum. In: Mertz W, ed. *Trace Elements in Human and Animal Nutrition*, 5th ed. San Diego: Academic Press; 1987:429–463.
12. Hendler SS, Rorvik DR, eds. *PDR for Nutritional Supplements*. Montvale, NJ: Medical Economics Company, Inc; 2001.
13. Vyskocil A, Viau C. Assessment of molybdenum toxicity in humans. *J Appl Toxicol* 1999;19(3):185–192.
14. Boles JW, Klaassen CD. Effects of molybdate and pentachlorophenol on the sulfation of acetaminophen. *Toxicology* 2000;146(1):23–35.

23 Phosphorus

Phosphorus is an essential mineral that is required by every cell in the body for normal function.[1] The majority of the phosphorus in the body is found as phosphate (PO_4). Approximately 85% of the body's phosphorus is found in bone.[2]

Function

Phosphorus is a major structural component of bone in the form of a calcium phosphate salt called *hydroxyapatite*. Phospholipids (e.g., phosphatidylcholine) are major structural components of cell membranes. All energy production and storage are dependent on phosphorylated compounds, such as adenosine triphosphate and creatine phosphate. Nucleic acids, responsible for the storage and transmission of genetic information, are long chains of phosphate-containing molecules. A number of enzymes, hormones, and cell-signaling molecules depend on phosphorylation for their activation. Phosphorus also helps to maintain normal acid–base balance (pH) in its role as one of the body's most important buffers. The phosphorus-containing molecule 2,3-diphosphoglycerate binds to hemoglobin in red blood cells and affects oxygen delivery to the tissues of the body.[1]

Nutrient Interactions

Fructose. A recent study of 11 adult men found that a diet high in fructose (20% of total calories) resulted in increased urinary loss of phosphorus and a negative phosphorus balance (i.e., daily loss of phosphorus was higher than daily intake). This effect was more pronounced if the diet was also low in magnesium.[3] A potential mechanism for this effect is the lack of feedback inhibition of the conversion of fructose to fructose-1-phosphate in the liver. In other words, increased accumulation of fructose-1-phosphate in the cell does not inhibit the enzyme that phosphorylates fructose, using up large amounts of phosphate. This phenomenon is known as *phosphate trapping*.[1] This finding is relevant because fructose consumption in the United States has been increasing rapidly since the introduction of high-fructose corn syrup in 1970, while magnesium intake has decreased over the past century.[3]

Calcium and Vitamin D. Dietary phosphorus is readily absorbed in the small intestine, and any excess phosphorus absorbed is excreted by the kidneys. The regulation of blood calcium and phosphorus levels is interrelated through the actions of parathyroid hormone (PTH) and vitamin D (Fig. 23–1). A slight drop in blood calcium levels (e.g., in the case of inadequate calcium intake) is sensed by the parathyroid glands, resulting in their increased secretion of PTH. PTH stimulates increased conversion of vitamin D to its active form (calcitriol) in the kidneys. Increased calcitriol levels result in increased intestinal absorption of both calcium and phosphorus. Both PTH and vitamin D stimulate bone resorption, resulting in the release of bone mineral (calcium and phosphate) into the blood. Although PTH stimulation results in decreased urinary excretion of calcium, it also results in increased urinary excretion of phosphorus. The increased urinary excretion of phosphorus is advantageous in bringing blood calcium levels up to normal because high blood levels of phosphate suppress the conversion of vitamin D to its active form in the kidneys.[4]

Is High Phosphorus Intake Detrimental to Bone Health? Some investigators are concerned about the increasing amounts of phosphates in the diet, which can be attributed to phosphoric acid in soft drinks and phosphate additives in a number of commercially prepared foods.[5,6] Because phosphorus is not as tightly regulated by the body as calcium, blood phosphate levels

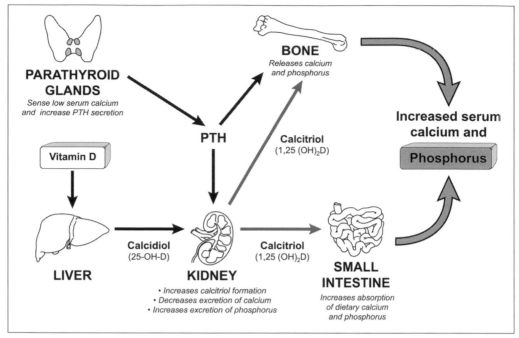

Figure 23–1. Calcium and phosphorus homeostasis. Calcium-sensing proteins in the parathyroid glands sense serum calcium levels. In response to slight declines in serum calcium, the parathyroid glands secrete parathyroid hormone (PTH). PTH stimulates the activity of the 1-hydroxylase enzyme in the kidney, resulting in increased production of calcitriol, the biologically active form of vitamin D. Calcitriol activates the vitamin D–dependent transport system in the small intestine, increasing the absorption of dietary calcium and phosphorus. Calcitriol and PTH act on the skeleton to increase the mobilization of calcium and phosphorus into the circulation. In the kidneys, calcitriol and PTH increase calcium reabsorption and increase phosphorus excretion.

can rise slightly with a high phosphorous diet, especially after meals. High blood phosphate levels reduce the formation of the active form of vitamin D (calcitriol) in the kidneys, reduce blood calcium, and lead to increased PTH release by the parathyroid glands. However, high blood phosphorus levels also lead to decreased urinary calcium excretion.[2] If sustained, elevated PTH levels could have an adverse effect on bone mineral content, but this effect has only been observed in humans on diets that were high in phosphorus and low in calcium. Moreover, similarly elevated PTH levels have been reported in diets that were low in calcium without being high in phosphorus.[7] Recently, a controlled trial in young women found no adverse effects of a phosphorus-rich diet (3000 mg/d) on bone-related hormones and biochemical markers of bone resorption when dietary calcium intakes were maintained at almost 2000 mg/d.[8] At present there is no convincing evidence that the dietary phosphorus levels experienced in the United States adversely affect bone mineral density in humans. However, the substitution of phosphate-containing soft drinks and snack foods for milk and other calcium-rich foods does represent a serious risk to bone health.

Deficiency

Inadequate phosphorus intake results in abnormally low blood phosphate levels (hypophosphatemia). The effects of hypophosphatemia may include loss of appetite, anemia, muscle weakness, bone pain, rickets (in children), osteomalacia (in adults), increased susceptibility to infection, numbness and tingling of the extremities, and difficulty

Table 23–1   Recommended Dietary Allowance (RDA) for Phosphorus

Life Stage	Age	Males, mg/d	Females, mg/d
Infants	0–6 months	100 (AI)	100 (AI)
Infants	7–12 months	275 (AI)	275 (AI)
Children	1–3 years	460	460
Children	4–8 years	500	500
Children	9–13 years	1250	1250
Adolescents	14–18 years	1250	1250
Adults	19 years and older	700	700
Pregnancy	18 years and younger	–	1250
Pregnancy	19 years and older	–	700
Breastfeeding	18 years and younger	–	1250
Breastfeeding	19 years and older	–	700

AI, adequate intake level.

walking. Severe hypophosphatemia may result in death. Because phosphorus is so widespread in food, dietary phosphorus deficiency is usually seen only in cases of near total starvation. Other individuals at risk of hypophosphatemia include alcoholics, diabetics recovering from an episode of diabetic ketoacidosis, and starving or anorexic patients on refeeding regimens that are high in calories but too low in phosphorus.[1,2]

The Recommended Dietary Allowance

The recommended dietary allowance (RDA) for phosphorus was based on the maintenance of normal blood phosphate levels in adults, which was felt to represent adequate phosphorus intake to meet cellular and bone formation needs (Table 23–1).[2]

Disease Prevention

Presently, there is insufficient evidence to support the use of phosphorus to prevent diseases or health conditions other than hypophosphatemia.

Disease Treatment

Presently, there is insufficient evidence to support the use of phosphorus to treat diseases or health conditions other than hypophosphatemia.

Sources

Food Sources

Phosphorus is found in most foods because it is a critical component of all living organisms. Dairy products, meat, and fish are particularly rich sources of phosphorus. Phosphorus is also a component of many polyphosphate food additives and is present in most soft drinks as phosphoric acid. Dietary phosphorus derived from food additives is not calculated in most food databases, so the total amount of phosphorus consumed by the average person in the United States is not entirely clear. A large survey of nutrient consumption in the United States found the average phosphorus intake in men to be 1495 mg/d and the average phosphorus intake in women to be 1024 mg/d. The Food and Nutrition Board estimates phosphorus consumption in the United States has increased 10 to 15% over the past 20 years.[2]

The phosphorus in all plant seeds (beans, peas, cereals, and nuts) is present in a storage form of phosphate called *phytic acid* or *phytate*. Only about 50% of the phosphorus from phytate is available to humans because we lack enzymes (phytases) that liberate it from phytate.[9] Yeasts possess phytases, so whole grains incorporated into leavened breads have more bioavailable phosphorus than whole grains incorporated into breakfast cereals or flat breads.[2] Table 23–2 lists a number of phosphorus-rich foods along with their phosphorus content in milligrams.

Table 23–2   Food Sources of Phosphorus

Food	Serving	Phosphorus, mg
Yogurt, plain non-fat	8 ounces	383
Lentils*	1/2 cup, cooked	356
Fish, salmon	3 ounces, cooked[†]	252
Milk, skim	8 ounces	247
Fish, halibut	3 ounces, cooked[†]	242
Beef	3 ounces, cooked[†]	173
Turkey	3 ounces, cooked[†]	173
Chicken	3 ounces, cooked[†]	155
Almonds*	1 ounce	139
Cheese, mozarella; part skim	1 ounce	131
Egg	1 large, cooked	104
Peanuts*	1 ounce	101
Bread, whole wheat	1 slice	64
Carbonated cola drink	12 ounces	44
Bread, enriched white	1 slice	24

*Phosphorus from nuts, seeds, and grains is about 50% less bioavailable than phosphorus from other sources.
[†]A 3-ounce serving of meat or fish is about the size of a deck of cards.

Supplements

Sodium phosphate and potassium phosphate salts are used for the treatment of hypophosphatemia, and their use requires medical supervision. Calcium phosphate salts are sometimes used as calcium supplements.[10]

Safety

Toxicity

The most serious adverse effect of abnormally elevated blood levels of phosphate (hyperphosphatemia) is the calcification of nonskeletal tissues, most commonly the kidneys. Such calcium phosphate deposition can lead to organ damage, especially kidney damage. Because the kidneys are very efficient at eliminating excess phosphate from the circulation, hyperphosphatemia from dietary causes is a problem mainly in people with severe kidney failure (end-stage renal disease) or hypoparathyroidism. When kidney function is only 20% of normal, even typical levels of dietary phosphorus may lead to hyperphosphatemia. Pronounced hyperphosphatemia has also occurred due to increased intestinal absorption of phosphate salts taken by mouth, as well as due to colonic absorption of the phosphate salts in enemas.[1] To avoid the adverse effects of hyperphosphatemia, the Food and Nutrition Board of the Institute of Medicine set a tolerable upper intake level (UL) of oral phosphorus intake for generally healthy individuals (Table 23–3).[2] The lower UL for individuals over 70 years of age reflects the increased likelihood of impaired kidney function above age 70. The UL does not apply to individuals with significantly impaired kidney function or other health conditions known to increase the risk of hyperphosphatemia.

Drug Interactions

Aluminum-containing antacids reduce the absorption of dietary phosphorus by forming aluminum phosphate, which is unabsorbable. When consumed in high doses, aluminum-containing antacids can produce abnormally low blood phosphate levels (hypophosphatemia), as well as aggravate phosphate deficiency due to other causes.[11] As little as 1 ounce of aluminum hydroxide gel three times a day for several weeks can diminish blood phosphate levels and lead to increased urinary calcium loss.[1] Excessively high doses of calcitriol, the active form of vitamin D, or its analogs may result in hyperphosphatemia.[2]

Table 23–3 Tolerable Upper Intake Level (UL) for Phosphorus

Life Stage	Age	UL, g/d
Infants	0–12 months	not possible to establish*
Children	1–8 years	3
Children	9–13 years	4
Adolescents	14–18 years	4
Adults	19–70 years	4
Adults	70 years and older	3
Pregnancy	–	3.5
Breast-feeding	–	4

*Source of intake should be from food and formula only.

Potassium supplements or potassium-sparing diuretics taken together with a phosphate may result in high serum levels of potassium (hyperkalemia). Hyperkalemia can be a serious problem, resulting in life-threatening heart rhythm abnormalities (arrhythmias). People on such a combination need to be sure their health care provider is aware of it, and they should have their serum potassium levels checked regularly.[11]

LPI Recommendation

The Linus Pauling Institute supports the RDA for phosphorus (700 mg/d for adults). Though few multivitamin/multimineral supplements contain more than 15% of the current RDA for phosphorus, a varied diet should easily provide adequate phosphorus for most people.

Older Adults

At present there is no evidence that the phosphorus requirement of adults 65 and older differs from that of younger adults (700 mg/d). Though few multivitamin/multimineral supplements contain more than 15% of the current RDA for phosphorus, a varied diet should easily provide adequate phosphorus for most people.

References

1. Knochel JP. Phosphorus. In: Shils M, Olson JA, Shike M, Ross AC, eds. *Nutrition in Health and Disease*, 9th ed. Baltimore: Williams & Wilkins; 1999:157–167.
2. Food and Nutrition Board, Institute of Medicine. Phosphorus. *Dietary Reference Intakes: Calcium, Phosphorus, Magnesium, Vitamin D, and Fluoride.* Washington, D.C.: National Academy Press; 1997:146–189.
3. Milne DB, Nielsen FH. The interaction between dietary fructose and magnesium adversely affects macro-mineral homeostasis in men. *J Am Coll Nutr* 2000;19(1):31–37.
4. Bringhurst FR, Demay MB, Kronenberg HM. Hormones and disorders of mineral metabolism. In: Wilson JD, Foster DW, Kronenberg HM, Larsen PR, eds. *Williams Textbook of Endocrinology*, 9th ed. Philadelphia: W.B. Saunders Company; 1998:1155–1210.
5. Calvo MS, Park YK. Changing phosphorus content of the U.S. diet: potential for adverse effects on bone. *J Nutr* 1996;126(4 Suppl):1168S–1180S.
6. Calvo MS. Dietary considerations to prevent loss of bone and renal function. *Nutrition* 2000;16(7–8):564–566.
7. Weaver CM, Heaney RP. Calcium. In: Shils M, Olson JA, Shike M, Ross AC, eds. *Nutrition in Health and Disease*, 9th ed. Baltimore: Williams & Wilkins; 1999:141–155.
8. Grimm M, Muller A, Hein G, Funfstuck R, Jahreis G. High phosphorus intake only slightly affects serum minerals, urinary pyridinium crosslinks and renal function in young women. *Eur J Clin Nutr* 2001;55(3):153–161.
9. National Research Council, Food and Nutrition Board. *Recommended Dietary Allowances*, 10th ed. Washington, D.C.: National Academy Press; 1989.
10. Hendler SS, Rorvik DR, eds. *PDR for Nutritional Supplements.* Montvale, NJ: Medical Economics Company, Inc; 2001.
11. Minerals. *Drug Facts and Comparisons.* St. Louis: Facts and Comparisons; 2000:27–51.

24 Potassium

Potassium is an essential dietary mineral that is also known as an electrolyte. The term *electrolyte* refers to a substance that dissociates into ions (charged particles) in solution, making it capable of conducting electricity. The normal functioning of our bodies depends on the tight regulation of potassium concentrations both inside and outside of cells.[1]

Function

Maintenance of Membrane Potential

Potassium (K+) is the principal positively charged ion (cation) in the fluid inside of cells, and sodium (Na+) is the principal cation in the fluid outside of cells. Potassium concentrations are about 30 times higher inside than outside cells, and sodium concentrations are more than 10 times lower inside than outside cells. The concentration differences between potassium and sodium across cell membranes create an electrochemical gradient known as the *membrane potential*. A cell's membrane potential is maintained by ion pumps in the cell membrane, especially the Na+, K+ ATPase pumps. These pumps use adenosine triphosphate (ATP) to pump Na+ out of the cell in exchange for K+ (Fig. 24–1). Their activity has been estimated to account for 20 to 40% of the resting energy expenditure in a typical adult. The large proportion of energy dedicated to maintaining Na+/K+ concentration gradients emphasizes the importance of this function in sustaining life. Tight control of cell membrane potential is critical for nerve impulse transmission, muscle contraction, and heart function.[2,3]

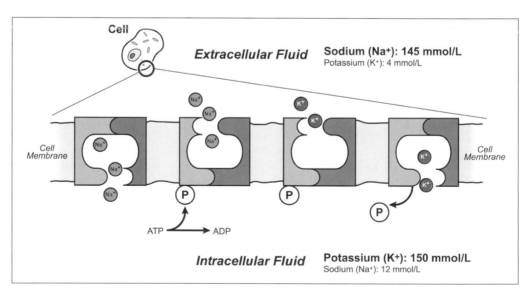

Figure 24–1. A simplified model of the Na+, K+ ATPase pump. The concentration differences between potassium (K+) and sodium (Na+) across cell membranes create an electrochemical gradient known as the membrane potential. Adenosine triphosphate (ATP) provides the energy to pump three Na+ ions out of the cell in exchange for two K+ ions, thus maintaining the membrane potential.

Cofactor for Enzymes

A limited number of enzymes require the presence of potassium for their activity. The activation of Na⁺, K⁺ ATPase requires the presence of sodium and potassium. The presence of potassium is also required for the activity of pyruvate kinase, an important enzyme in carbohydrate metabolism.[2]

Deficiency

An abnormally low serum potassium concentration is referred to as *hypokalemia*. Hypokalemia is most commonly a result of excessive loss of potassium (e.g., from prolonged vomiting, the use of some diuretics, some forms of kidney disease, or disturbances of metabolism). The symptoms of hypokalemia are related to alterations in membrane potential and cellular metabolism. They include fatigue, muscle weakness and cramps, and intestinal paralysis, which may lead to bloating, constipation, and abdominal pain. Severe hypokalemia may result in muscular paralysis or abnormal heart rhythms (cardiac arrhythmias) that can be fatal.[2,4]

Conditions That Increase the Risk of Hypokalemia

Conditions that increase the risk of hypokalemia include the following: the use of potassium-wasting diuretics (e.g., thiazide diuretics or furosemide), alcoholism, severe vomiting or diarrhea, overuse or abuse of laxatives, anorexia nervosa or bulimia, magnesium depletion, and congestive heart failure. In rare cases, habitual consumption of large amounts of black licorice has resulted in hypokalemia. Licorice contains a compound (glycyrrhizic acid) with similar physiologic effects to those of aldosterone, a hormone that increases urinary excretion of potassium.[5]

Low dietary intakes of potassium do not generally result in hypokalemia. However, recent research indicates that insufficient dietary potassium increases the risk of a number of chronic diseases.

Table 24–1   Minimum Requirement for Potassium

Life Stage	Age	Minimum Requirement, mg/d
Infants	0–5 months	500
Infants	6–11 months	700
Children	1 year	1000
Children	2–5 years	1400
Children	6–9 years	1600
Children	10–18 years	2000
Adults	over 18 years	2000

The Minimum Requirements

In 1989, the Food and Nutrition Board (FNB) of the Institute of Medicine estimated the minimum requirement for potassium in adults to be 2000 mg/d (Table 24–1). However, they also noted that an increase in fruit and vegetable consumption that would raise potassium intake to about 3500 mg/d would exert a beneficial effect on hypertension (high blood pressure).[4] Updated recommendations for potassium intake by the FNB are expected in 2003.

Disease Prevention

The diets of Western industrialized cultures are quite different from those of prehistoric cultures and the few remaining isolated primitive cultures. Among other differences, the daily intake of sodium chloride (salt) in Western industrialized cultures is about three times higher than the daily intake of potassium on a molar basis, and salt intakes in primitive cultures are about seven times lower than potassium intakes.[6] The relative deficiency of dietary potassium in the modern diet may play a role in the pathology of some chronic diseases.

Stroke

Several large epidemiologic studies have suggested that increased potassium intake is associated with decreased risk of stroke. A prospective study of more than 43,000 men followed for 8 years found that men in the top fifth of dietary potassium intake (averaging 4300 mg/d) were only 62% as likely to have a stroke as those in the lowest fifth of potassium intake (averaging 2400 mg/d).[7] The inverse association was especially high in men with hypertension. However, a similar prospective study of more than 85,000 women followed for 14 years found a much more modest association between potassium intake and the risk of stroke.[8] Another large study that followed more than 9000 people for an average of 16 years found that potassium intake was inversely related to stroke only in black men and men with hypertension.[9] However, black men and women reported significantly lower potassium intakes than white men and women (1606 mg/d vs. 2178 mg/d). More recent data from the same population indicate that those with potassium intakes higher than 1352 mg/d were only 72% as likely to have a stroke as those with potassium intakes lower than 1352 mg/d.[10] Taken together, the epidemiologic data suggest that a modest increase in fruit and vegetable intake (rich sources of dietary potassium), especially in those with hypertension and/or relatively low potassium intakes, could significantly reduce the risk of stroke.

Osteoporosis

Four cross-sectional studies have reported significant positive associations between dietary potassium intake and bone mineral density (BMD) in populations of premenopausal, peri-menopausal, and postmenopausal women and elderly men.[11-13] The average dietary potassium intakes of the study participants ranged from about 3000 to 3400 mg/d; the highest potassium intakes exceeded 6000 mg/d, and the lowest intakes ranged from 1400 to 1600 mg/d. In all of these studies, BMD was also positively and significantly associated with fruit and vegetable intake. The only study to examine changes in BMD over time found that higher dietary potassium intakes (and fruit and vegetable intakes) were associated with significantly less decline in BMD at the hip in men but not in women over a period of 4 years.[13] Potassium-rich foods, such as fruits and vegetables, are also rich in precursors to bicarbonate ions, which serve to buffer acids in the body. The modern Western diet tends to be relatively low in sources of alkali (fruits and vegetables) and high in sources of acid (fish and meat). When the quantity of bicarbonate ions is insufficient to maintain normal pH, the body is capable of mobilizing alkaline calcium salts from bone to neutralize acids consumed in the diet and generated by metabolism.[14] Increased consumption of fruits and vegetables reduces the net acid content of the diet and may preserve calcium in bones, which might otherwise be mobilized to maintain normal pH. Support for this theory was provided by a study of 18 postmenopausal women, which found that potassium bicarbonate supplementation decreased urinary acid and calcium excretion while increasing biomarkers of bone formation and decreasing biomarkers of bone resorption.[15]

Kidney Stones

Abnormally high urinary calcium (hypercalciuria) increases the risk of developing kidney stones. In individuals with a history of developing calcium-containing kidney stones, increased dietary acid load was significantly associated with increased urinary calcium excretion.[16] Increasing dietary potassium (and alkali) intake by increasing fruit and vegetable intake or by taking potassium bicarbonate supplements has been found to decrease urinary calcium excretion. Additionally, potassium deprivation has been found to increase urinary calcium excretion.[17,18] A large prospective study of more than 45,000 men followed for 4 years found that men whose potassium intake averaged more than 4042 mg/d were only half as likely to develop symptomatic kidney stones as men whose intake averaged less than 2895 mg per day.[19] A similar study that followed more than 90,000 women over a period of 12 years found that women in the highest fifth of potassium intake (averaging 3458 mg/d) were only 65% as likely to develop symptomatic kidney stones as women in the lowest fifth of potassium intake (averaging 2703 mg/d).[20] In both these prospective studies, dietary potassium intake was derived almost entirely from potassium-rich foods, such as fruits and vegetables.

Disease Treatment

Hypertension

A number of studies indicate that groups with relatively high dietary potassium intakes have lower blood pressures than comparable groups with relatively low potassium intakes.[21] Data on over 17,000 adults who participated in the Third National Health and Nutritional Examination Survey indicated that higher dietary potassium intakes were associated with significantly lower blood pressures.[22] The results of the Dietary Approaches to Stop Hypertension (DASH) trial provided further support for the beneficial effects of a potassium-rich diet on blood pressure.[23] Compared to a control diet providing only 3.5 servings per day of fruits and vegetables and 1700 mg/d of potassium, consumption of a diet that included 8.5 servings per day of fruits and vegetables and 4100 mg/d of potassium lowered blood pressure by an average of 2.8/1.1 mm Hg (systolic BP/diastolic BP) in people with normal blood pressure and by an average of 7.2/2.8 mm Hg in people with hypertension. Increasing dietary calcium intake by 800 mg/d in the DASH trial lowered systolic and diastolic BP still further (see Chapter 14 on calcium).

In 1997, a meta-analysis of 33 randomized controlled trials including 2609 individuals assessed the effects of increased potassium intake, mostly in the form of potassium chloride (KCl) supplements, on blood pressure.[24] Increased potassium intake (2300 to 3900 mg/d) resulted in slight but significant blood pressure reductions that averaged 1.8/1 mm Hg in people with normal blood pressure and 4.4/2.5 mm Hg in people with hypertension. Subgroup analysis indicated that the blood pressure–lowering effect of potassium was more pronounced in individuals with higher salt intakes and in trials where black individuals were a majority of the participants. A recent clinical trial in 150 Chinese men and women with borderline to mild hypertension found that moderate supplementation with 500 mg/d of potassium chloride for 12 weeks resulted in a significant 5 mm Hg reduction in systolic BP but not diastolic BP compared with placebo.[25] Like many Western diets, the customary diet of this population was high in sodium and low in potassium.

Sources

Food Sources

The richest sources of potassium are fruits and vegetables. People who eat large amounts of fruits and vegetables have a high potassium intake (8 to 11 g/d).[4] A recent dietary survey in the United States indicated that the average dietary potassium intake in women is about 2300 mg/d for adult women and 3100 mg/d for adult men.[22] The potassium content of some relatively potassium-rich foods is listed in milligrams in Table 24–2.

Supplements

Multivitamin/multimineral supplements in the United States do not contain more than 99 mg of potassium per serving. Higher doses of supplemental potassium are generally prescribed to prevent and treat potassium depletion and hypokalemia. The use of more potent potassium supplements in potassium deficiency requires close monitoring of plasma potassium concentrations. Potassium supplements are available as a number of different salts, including potassium chloride, citrate, gluconate, bicarbonate, aspartate, and orotate.[26] Because of the potential for serious side effects the decision to use a potent potassium supplement should be made in collaboration with one's health care provider.

Safety

Toxicity (Excess)

Abnormally elevated serum potassium concentrations are referred to as *hyperkalemia*. Hyperkalemia occurs when potassium intake exceeds the capacity of the kidneys to eliminate it. Acute or chronic renal (kidney) failure, the use of potassium-sparing diuretics, and insufficient aldosterone secretion (hypoaldosteronism) may result in the accumulation of excess potassium in the plasma due to decreased urinary potassium excretion. Oral doses greater than 18 g taken at one time in individuals not accustomed to high intakes may lead to severe hyperkalemia, even in those

Table 24–2   Food Sources of Potassium

Food	Serving	Potassium, mg
Potato, baked with skin	1 medium	721
Prunes, dried	$1/2$ cup	633
Raisins	$1/2$ cup	598
Prune juice	6 fluid ounces	530
Lima beans, cooked	$1/2$ cup	478
Banana	1 medium	467
Acorn squash, cooked	$1/2$ cup (cubed)	448
Artichoke, cooked	1 medium	425
Spinach, cooked	$1/2$ cup	419
Tomato juice	6 fluid ounces	400
Orange juice	6 fluid ounces	354
Molasses	1 tablespoon	293
Tomato	1 medium	273
Sunflower seeds	1 ounce	241
Orange	1 medium	237
Bran cereal with raisins	1 ounce	227–360
Almonds	1 ounce	211

Table 24–3   Medications Associated with Hyperkalemia[27]

Medication Family	Specific Medications
Potassium-sparing agents	spironolactone, triamterene, amiloride
Angiotensin-converting enzyme inhibitors	captopril, enalapril, fosinopril
Nonsteroidal anti-inflammatory agents	indomethacin, ibuprofen, ketorolac
Anti-infective agents	trimethoprim-sulfamethoxazole, pentamidine
Anticoagulant	heparin
Cardiac glycoside	digitalis
Antihypertensive agents	beta-blockers, alpha- and beta-blockers
Angiotensin receptor blockers	losartan, valsartan, irbesartan, candesartan

with normal kidney function.[4] Hyperkalemia may also result from a shift of intracellular potassium into the circulation, which may occur with the rupture of red blood cells (hemolysis) or tissue damage (e.g., trauma or severe burns). Symptoms of hyperkalemia may include tingling of the hands and feet, muscular weakness, and temporary paralysis. The most serious complication of hyperkalemia is the development of an abnormal heart rhythm (cardiac arrhythmia), which can lead to cardiac arrest.[27]

Adverse Reactions to Potassium Supplements

Gastrointestinal symptoms are the most common side effects of potassium supplements, including nausea, vomiting, abdominal discomfort, and diarrhea. Intestinal ulceration has been reported after the use of enteric-coated potassium chloride tablets. Taking potassium with meals or taking a microencapsulated form of potassium may reduce gastrointestinal side effects. The most serious adverse reaction to potassium supplementation is hyperkalemia. Individuals with abnormal kidney function and those on potassium-sparing medications should be monitored closely to prevent hyperkalemia.[5,26]

Drug Interactions

The classes of medication listed in Table 24–3 are known to increase the risk of hyperkalemia (elevated serum potassium),[27] and the medications listed in Table 24–4 are known to increase the risk of hypokalemia (low serum potassium).[5]

Table 24–4 Medications Associated with Hypokalemia[5]

Medication Family	Specific Medications
Beta-adrenergic agonists	epinephrine
Decongestants	pseudoephedrine, phenylpropanolamine
Bronchodilators	albuterol, terbutaline, pirbuterol, isoetharine, fenoterol, ephedrine, isoproterenol, meta-proterenol, theophylline
Tocolytic (labor-suppressing) agents	ritodrine, nylidrin
Diuretics	acetazolamide, thiazides, chlorthalidone, indapamide, metolazone, quinethazone, bumetanide, ethycrinic acid, furosemide, torsemide
Mineralocorticoids	fludrocortisone
Substances with mineralocorticoid effects	licorice, carbenoxolone, gossypol
High-dose glucocorticoids	
High-dose antibiotics	penicillin, nafcillin, carbenicillin
Other	caffeine, sodium polystyrene sulfonate

LPI Recommendation

Although the potassium intake most likely to promote optimum health is not known, there is considerable evidence that a diet supplying more than 4000 mg/d of potassium is associated with decreased risk of stroke, hypertension, osteoporosis, and kidney stones. Fruits and vegetables are among the richest sources of dietary potassium, and a large body of evidence supports the association of increased fruit and vegetable intakes with reduced risk of chronic disease.[28,29] Consequently, the Linus Pauling Institute recommends increasing potassium intake by increasing consumption of potassium-rich foods, especially fruits, vegetables, and nuts.

Older Adults

The above recommendations are especially important for older adults (65 years and older) as they frequently consume less than five servings of fruits and vegetables daily and are more likely to take medications that affect potassium status.

References

1. Peterson LN. Potassium in nutrition. In: O'Dell BL, Sunde RA, eds. *Handbook of Nutritionally Essential Minerals.* New York: Marcel Dekker, Inc.; 1997:153–183.
2. Sheng H-W. Sodium, chloride and potassium. In: Stipanuk M, ed. *Biochemical and Physiological Aspects of Human Nutrition.* Philadelphia: W.B. Saunders Company; 2000:686–710.
3. Brody T. *Nutritional Biochemistry*, 2nd ed. San Diego: Academic Press; 1999.
4. National Research Council, Food and Nutrition Board. *Recommended Dietary Allowances*, 10th ed. Washington, D.C.: National Academy Press; 1989.
5. Gennari FJ. Hypokalemia. *N Engl J Med* 1998;339(7):451–458.
6. Young DB, Lin H, McCabe RD. Potassium's cardiovascular protective mechanisms. *Am J Physiol* 1995;268(4 Pt 2):R825–R837.
7. Ascherio A, Rimm EB, Hernan MA, et al. Intake of potassium, magnesium, calcium, and fiber and risk of stroke among US men. *Circulation* 1998;98(12):1198–1204.
8. Iso H, Stampfer MJ, Manson JE, et al. Prospective study of calcium, potassium, and magnesium intake and risk of stroke in women. *Stroke* 1999;30(9):1772–1779.
9. Fang J, Madhavan S, Alderman MH. Dietary potassium intake and stroke mortality. *Stroke* 2000;31(7):1532–1537.
10. Bazzano LA, He J, Ogden LG, et al. Dietary potassium intake and risk of stroke in US men and women: National Health and Nutrition Examination Survey I epidemiologic follow-up study. *Stroke* 2001;32(7):1473–1480.
11. New SA, Bolton-Smith C, Grubb DA, Reid DM. Nutritional influences on bone mineral density: a cross-sectional study in premenopausal women. *Am J Clin Nutr* 1997;65(6):1831–1839.
12. New SA, Robins SP, Campbell MK, et al. Dietary influences on bone mass and bone metabolism: further evidence of a positive link between fruit and vegetable consumption and bone health? *Am J Clin Nutr* 2000;71(1):142–151.
13. Tucker KL, Hannan MT, Chen H, Cupples LA, Wilson PW, Kiel DP. Potassium, magnesium, and fruit and vegetable intakes are associated with greater bone mineral density in elderly men and women. *Am J Clin Nutr* 1999;69(4):727–736.
14. Morris RC, Frassetto LA, Schmidlin O, Forman A, Sebastian A. Expression of osteoporosis as determined by diet-disordered electrolyte and acid–base metabo-

lism. In: Burkhardt P, Dawson-Hughes B, Heaney R, eds. *Nutritional Aspects of Osteoporosis*. San Diego: Academic Press; 2001:357–378.

15. Sebastian A, Harris ST, Ottaway JH, Todd KM, Morris RC, Jr. Improved mineral balance and skeletal metabolism in postmenopausal women treated with potassium bicarbonate. *N Engl J Med* 1994;330(25): 1776–1781.

16. Trinchieri A, Zanetti G, Curro A, Lizzano R. Effect of potential renal acid load of foods on calcium metabolism of renal calcium stone formers. *Eur Urol* 2001;39(Suppl 2):33–36.

17. Lemann J, Jr., Pleuss JA, Gray RW. Potassium causes calcium retention in healthy adults. *J Nutr* 1993; 123(9):1623–1626.

18. Morris RC, Jr., Schmidlin O, Tanaka M, Forman A, Frassetto L, Sebastian A. Differing effects of supplemental KCl and KHCO3: pathophysiological and clinical implications. *Semin Nephrol* 1999;19(5):487–493.

19. Curhan GC, Willett WC, Rimm EB, Stampfer MJ. A prospective study of dietary calcium and other nutrients and the risk of symptomatic kidney stones. *N Engl J Med* 1993;328(12):833–838.

20. Curhan GC, Willett WC, Speizer FE, Spiegelman D, Stampfer MJ. Comparison of dietary calcium with supplemental calcium and other nutrients as factors affecting the risk for kidney stones in women. *Ann Intern Med* 1997;126(7):497–504.

21. Barri YM, Wingo CS. The effects of potassium depletion and supplementation on blood pressure: a clinical review. *Am J Med Sci* 1997;314(1):37–40.

22. Hajjar IM, Grim CE, George V, Kotchen TA. Impact of diet on blood pressure and age-related changes in blood pressure in the US population: analysis of NHANES III. *Arch Intern Med* 2001;161(4):589–593.

23. Appel LJ, Moore TJ, Obarzanek E, et al. A clinical trial of the effects of dietary patterns on blood pressure. DASH Collaborative Research Group. *N Engl J Med* 1997;336(16):1117–1124.

24. Whelton PK, He J, Cutler JA, et al. Effects of oral potassium on blood pressure. Meta-analysis of randomized controlled clinical trials. *JAMA* 1997; 277(20):1624–1632.

25. Gu D, He J, Wu X, Duan X, Whelton PK. Effect of potassium supplementation on blood pressure in Chinese: a randomized, placebo-controlled trial. *J Hypertens* 2001;19(7):1325–1331.

26. Hendler SS, Rorvik DR, eds. *PDR for Nutritional Supplements*. Montvale, NJ: Medical Economics Company, Inc; 2001.

27. Mandal AK. Hypokalemia and hyperkalemia. *Med Clin North Am* 1997;81(3):611–639.

28. Liu S, Manson JE, Lee IM, et al. Fruit and vegetable intake and risk of cardiovascular disease: the Women's Health Study. *Am J Clin Nutr* 2000;72(4):922–928.

29. Joshipura KJ, Ascherio A, Manson JE, et al. Fruit and vegetable intake in relation to risk of ischemic stroke. *JAMA* 1999;282(13):1233–1239.

25 Selenium

Selenium is a trace element that is essential in small amounts but can be toxic in larger amounts. Humans and animals require selenium for the function of a number of selenium-dependent enzymes, also known as *selenoproteins.* During selenoprotein synthesis, selenocysteine is incorporated into a very specific location in the amino acid sequence to form a functional protein. Unlike animals, plants do not appear to require selenium for survival. However, when selenium is present in the soil, plants incorporate it nonspecifically into compounds that usually contain sulfur.[1,2]

Function

Selenoproteins

At least 11 selenoproteins have been characterized, and there is evidence that additional selenoproteins exist.

Glutathione Peroxidases. Four selenium-containing glutathione peroxidases (GPx) have been identified: cellular or classical GPx, plasma or extracellular GPx, phospholipid hydroperoxide GPx, and gastrointestinal GPx.[3] Although each GPx is a distinct selenoprotein, they are all antioxidant enzymes that reduce potentially damaging reactive oxygen species, such as hydrogen peroxide and lipid hydroperoxides, to harmless products like water and alcohols by coupling their reduction with the oxidation of glutathione (Fig. 25–1). Sperm mitochondrial capsule selenoprotein, an antioxidant enzyme that protects developing sperm from oxidative damage and later forms a structural protein required by mature sperm, was once thought to be a distinct selenoprotein, but now appears to be phospholipid hydroperoxide GPx.[4]

Thioredoxin Reductase. In conjunction with the compound thioredoxin, thioredoxin reductase participates in the regeneration of several antioxidant systems, including vitamin C.

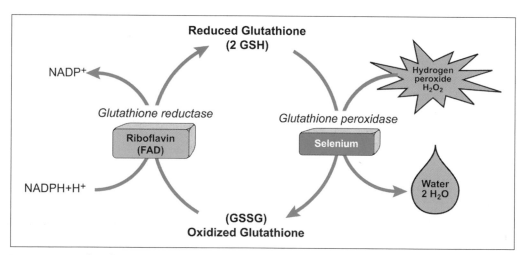

Figure 25–1. The glutathione oxidation reduction (redox) cycle. One molecule of hydrogen peroxide is reduced to two molecules of water while two molecules of glutathione (GSH) are oxidized in a reaction catalyzed by the selenoenzyme glutathione peroxidase. Oxidized glutathione may be reduced by the flavin adenine dinucleotide (FAD)-dependent enzyme, glutathione reductase.

Maintenance of thioredoxin in a reduced form by thioredoxin reductase is important for regulating cell growth and viability.[3,5]

Iodothyronine Deiodinases (Thyroid Hormone Deiodinases). The thyroid gland releases very small amounts of biologically active thyroid hormone (triiodothyronine or T_3) and larger amounts of an inactive form of thyroid hormone (thyroxine or T_4) into the circulation. Most of the biologically active T_3 in the circulation and inside cells is created by the removal of one iodine atom from T_4 in a reaction catalyzed by selenium-dependent iodothyronine deiodinase enzymes. Through their actions on T_3, T_4, and other thyroid hormone metabolites, three different selenium-dependent iodothyronine deiodinases (types I, II, and III) can both activate and inactivate thyroid hormone, making selenium an essential element for normal development, growth, and metabolism through the regulation of thyroid hormones.[3,6]

Selenoprotein P. Selenoprotein P is found in plasma and is also associated with vascular endothelial cells (cells that line the inner walls of blood vessels). Although the function of selenoprotein P has not been clearly delineated, it has been suggested to function as a transport protein, as well as an antioxidant capable of protecting endothelial cells from damage by a reactive nitrogen species called *peroxynitrite*.[3,7]

Selenoprotein W. Selenoprotein W is found in muscle. Although its function is presently unknown, it is thought to play a role in muscle metabolism.[3]

Selenophosphate Synthetase. Incorporation of selenocysteine into selenoproteins is directed by the genetic code and requires the enzyme selenophosphate synthetase. A selenoprotein itself, selenophosphate synthetase catalyzes the synthesis of monoselenium phosphate, a precursor of selenocysteine that is required for the synthesis of selenoproteins.[2,3]

Nutrient Interactions

Antioxidant Nutrients. As an integral part of the glutathione peroxidases and thioredoxin reductase, selenium probably interacts with every nutrient that affects the prooxidant/antioxidant balance of the cell. Other minerals that are critical components of antioxidant enzymes include copper, zinc (as superoxide dismutase), and iron (as catalase). Selenium as glutathione peroxidase also appears to support the activity of vitamin E (α-tocopherol) in limiting the oxidation of lipids. Animal studies indicate that selenium and vitamin E tend to spare one another and that selenium can prevent some of the damage resulting from vitamin E deficiency in models of oxidative stress.[1] Thioredoxin reductase also maintains the antioxidant function of vitamin C by catalyzing its regeneration.[5]

Iodine. Selenium deficiency may exacerbate the effects of iodine deficiency. Iodine is essential for the synthesis of thyroid hormone, but the selenoenzymes, iodothyronine deiodinases, are also required for the conversion of thyroxine (T_4) to the biologically active thyroid hormone triiodothyronine (T_3). Selenium supplementation in a small group of elderly individuals decreased plasma T_4, indicating increased deiodinase activity with increased conversion to T_3.[2]

Deficiency

Insufficient selenium intake results in decreased activity of the glutathione peroxidases. Even when severe, isolated selenium deficiency does not usually result in obvious clinical illness. However, selenium-deficient individuals appear to be more susceptible to additional physiological stresses.[1]

Individuals at Increased Risk of Selenium Deficiency

Clinical selenium deficiency has been observed in chronically ill patients who were receiving total parenteral nutrition without added selenium for prolonged periods of time. Muscular weakness, muscle wasting, and cardiomyopathy (inflammation and damage to the heart muscle) have been observed in these patients. Total parenteral nutritional solutions are now supplemented with selenium to prevent such problems. People who have had a large portion of the small intestine surgically removed or those with severe gastrointestinal problems, such as Crohn's disease, are also at risk for selenium deficiency due to impaired absorption. Specialized medical diets used to treat metabolic disorders, such as phenylketonuria, are often low in selenium. Specialized diets that will be used exclusively over long periods of time should have their selenium content assessed to determine the need for selenium supplementation.[1]

Keshan Disease

Keshan disease is a cardiomyopathy (disease of the heart muscle) that affects young women and children in a selenium-deficient region of China. The acute form of the disease is characterized by the sudden onset of cardiac insufficiency, and the chronic form results in moderate to severe heart enlargement with varying degrees of cardiac insufficiency. The incidence of Keshan disease is closely associated with very low dietary intakes of selenium and poor selenium nutritional status. Selenium supplementation has been found to protect people from developing Keshan disease but cannot reverse heart muscle damage once it occurs.[1,8] Despite the strong evidence that selenium deficiency is a fundamental factor in the etiology of Keshan's disease, the seasonal and annual variation in its occurrence suggests that an infectious agent is involved in addition to selenium. Coxsackievirus is one of the viruses that has been isolated from Keshan patients, and this virus has been found to be capable of causing an inflammation of the heart called *myocarditis* in selenium-deficient mice. Studies in mice indicate that oxidative stress induced by selenium deficiency results in changes in the viral genome capable of converting a relatively harmless viral strain to a myocarditis-causing strain.[9,10] Though not proven in Keshan disease, selenium deficiency may result in a more virulent strain of virus with the potential to invade and damage the heart muscle. (See "Disease Prevention" for more information on selenium and viral infection.)

Table 25–1   Recommended Dietary Allowance (RDA) for Selenium

Life Stage	Age	Males, µg/d	Females, µg/d
Infants	0–6 months	15 (AI)	15 (AI)
Infants	7–12 months	20 (AI)	20 (AI)
Children	1–3 years	20	20
Children	4–8 years	30	30
Children	9–13 years	40	40
Adolescents	14–18 years	55	55
Adults	19 years and older	55	55
Pregnancy	all ages	–	60
Breastfeeding	all ages	–	70

AI, adequate intake level.

Kashin-Beck Disease

Kashin-Beck disease is characterized by the degeneration of the articular cartilage between joints (osteoarthritis) and is associated with poor selenium status in areas of northern China, North Korea, and eastern Siberia. The disease affects children between the ages of 5 and 13. Severe forms of the disease may result in joint deformities and dwarfism due to degeneration of cartilage-forming cells. Unlike Keshan disease, there is little evidence that improving selenium nutritional status prevents Kashin-Beck disease. Thus, the role of selenium deficiency in the etiology of Kashin-Beck disease is less certain. A number of other causative factors have been suggested for Kashin-Beck disease, including fungal toxins in grain, iodine deficiency, and contaminated drinking water.[1,8]

The Recommended Dietary Allowance

The recommended dietary allowance (RDA) was revised in 2000 by the Food and Nutrition Board (FNB) of the Institute of Medicine. The most recent RDA is based on the amount of dietary selenium required to maximize the activity of the antioxidant enzyme glutathione peroxidase in blood plasma (Table 25–1).[11]

Disease Prevention

Immune Function

Selenium deficiency has been associated with impaired function of the immune system. Moreover, selenium supplementation in individuals who are not overtly selenium-deficient appears to stimulate the immune response. In two small studies, healthy[12,13] and immunosuppressed individuals[14] supplemented with 200 µg/d of selenium as sodium selenite for 8 weeks showed an enhanced immune cell response to foreign antigens compared with those taking a placebo. A considerable amount of basic research also indicates that selenium plays a role in regulating the expression of cell-signaling molecules called *cytokines*, which orchestrate the immune response.[15]

Viral Infection

Selenium deficiency appears to enhance the virulence or progression of some viral infections. The increased oxidative stress resulting from selenium deficiency may induce mutations or changes in the expression of some viral genes. When selenium-deficient mice are inoculated with a relatively harmless strain of cocksackievirus, mutations occur in the viral genome that result in a more virulent form of the virus, which causes an inflammation of the heart muscle known as *myocarditis*. Once mutated, this form of the virus also causes myocarditis in mice that are not selenium-deficient, demonstrating that the increased virulence is due to a change in the virus rather than to the effects of selenium deficiency on the host immune system. Recently, a study in mice that lack the cellular glutathione peroxidase enzyme (GPx-1 knockout mice) demonstrated that cellular glutathione peroxidase provides protection against myocarditis resulting from mutations in the genome of a previously benign virus. Selenium deficiency results in decreased activity of glutathione peroxidase, increasing the likelihood of mutations in the viral genome induced by oxidative damage. Cocksackie virus has been isolated from the blood of some sufferers of Keshan disease, suggesting that it may be a cofactor in the development of this cardiomyopathy associated with selenium deficiency in humans.[9,10]

Cancer

Animal Studies. There is a great deal of evidence indicating that selenium supplementation at high levels reduces the incidence of cancer in animals. More than two thirds of over 100 published studies in 20 different animal models of spontaneous, viral, and chemically induced cancers found that selenium supplementation significantly reduced tumor incidence.[16] The evidence indicates that the methylated forms of selenium are the active species against tumors, and these methylated selenium compounds are produced at the greatest amounts with excess selenium intakes. Selenium deficiency does not appear to make animals more susceptible to developing cancerous tumors.[17]

Epidemiologic Studies. Geographic studies have consistently shown a trend for populations that live in areas with low soil selenium and have relatively low selenium intakes to have higher cancer mortality rates. Results of epidemiologic studies of cancer incidence in groups with less variable selenium intakes have been less consistent, but also show a trend for individuals with lower selenium levels (blood and nails) to have a higher incidence of several different types of cancer. However, this trend is less pronounced in women. Chronic infection with viral hepatitis B or C significantly increases the risk of liver cancer. In a study of Taiwanese men with chronic viral hepatitis B or C infection, decreased plasma selenium concentrations were associated with an even greater risk of liver cancer.[18] A case-control study within a prospective study of over 9000 Finnish men and women examined serum selenium levels in 95 individuals subsequently diagnosed with lung cancer and 190 matched controls.[19] Lower serum selenium levels were associated with an increased risk of lung cancer, and the association was more pronounced in smokers. In this Finnish population, selenium levels were only about 60% of selenium levels generally observed in other Western countries. Another case-control study within a prospective study of over 50,000 male health professionals in the United States found a significant inverse relationship between toenail selenium content and the risk of prostate cancer in 181 men diagnosed with advanced prostate cancer and 181 matched controls.[20] In individuals whose toenail selenium content was consistent with an average intake of 159 μg/d, the risk of advanced prostate cancer was only 35% of that of individuals with toenail selenium content consistent with an intake of 86 μg/d. Within a prospective study of more than 9000 Japanese-American men, a case-control study that examined 249 confirmed cases of prostate cancer and 249 matched controls found the risk of developing prostate cancer to be 50% less in men with serum selenium levels in the highest quartile compared with those in the lowest quartile,[21] although another case-control study found that men with prediagnostic plasma selenium levels in the lowest quartile were four to five times more likely to develop prostate cancer than those in the highest quartile.[22] In contrast, one of the largest case-control studies to date found a significant inverse association between toenail selenium and the risk of colon cancer but no associations between toenail selenium and the risk of breast cancer or prostate cancer.[23]

Human Intervention Trials. An intervention trial undertaken among a general population of 130,471 individuals in five townships of Quidong, China, a high-risk area for viral hepatitis B infection and liver cancer, provided table salt enriched with sodium selenite to the population of one township (20,847 people), using the other four townships as controls. During an 8-year follow up period the average incidence of liver cancer was reduced by 35% in the selenium-enriched population while no reduction was found in the control populations. In a clinical trial in the same region, 226 individuals with evidence of chronic hepatitis B infection were supplemented with either 200 μg of selenium in the form of a selenium-enriched yeast tablet or a placebo yeast tablet daily. During the 4-year follow-up period 7 of 113 individuals on the placebo developed primary liver cancer, while none of the 113 subjects supplemented with selenium developed liver cancer.[24]

In the United States, a double-blind, placebo-controlled study of 1250 older adults with a history of skin cancer found that 200 μg/d of selenium-enriched yeast for an average of 7.4 years did not affect the recurrence of skin cancers.[25] However, selenium supplementation was associated with a 52% decrease in prostate cancer incidence and a 33% decrease in total cancer in men. The protective effect of selenium supplementation was greatest in those with lower pretreatment plasma selenium levels. Selenium supplementation did not decrease the risk of cancer in women who made up 25% of the study participants. In response to the generally recognized need to confirm these findings, several large placebo-controlled trials designed to further investigate the role of selenium supplementation in cancer prevention are presently under way.[16]

Possible Mechanisms. Several mechanisms have been proposed for the cancer-prevention effects of selenium: (1) maximizing the activity of antioxidant selenoenzymes and improving antioxidant status, (2) improving immune system function, (3) affecting the metabolism of carcinogens, and (4) increasing the levels of selenium metabolites that inhibit tumor cell growth. A two-stage model has been proposed to explain the different anticarcinogenic activities of selenium at different doses. At nutritional or physiologic doses (~40 to 100 μg/d in adults) selenium maximizes antioxidant selenoenzyme activity and probably enhances immune system function and carcinogen metabolism. At supranutritional or pharmacologic levels (~200 to 300 μg/d in adults) the formation of selenium metabolites, especially methylated forms of selenium, may also exert anticarcinogenic effects.[17]

Cardiovascular Diseases

Theoretically, optimizing selenoenzyme activity could decrease the risk of cardiovascular diseases by decreasing lipid peroxidation and influencing the metabolism of cell-signaling molecules known as *prostaglandins*. However, prospective studies in humans have not demonstrated strong support for the cardioprotective effects of selenium. Although one study found a significant increase in illness and death from cardiovascular diseases in individuals with serum selenium levels below 45 µg/L compared with matched pairs above 45 µg/L,[27] another study, using the same cutoff points for serum selenium, found a significant difference only in deaths from stroke.[28] A study of middle-aged and elderly Danish men found an increased risk of cardiovascular diseases in men with serum selenium levels below 79 µg/L,[29] but several other studies found no clear inverse association between selenium nutritional status and cardiovascular disease risk.[30] In a multicenter study in Europe, toenail selenium levels and risk of myocardial infarction (heart attack) were only associated in the center where selenium levels were the lowest.[31] Although some epidemiologic evidence suggests that low levels of selenium (lower than those commonly found in the United States) may increase the risk of cardiovascular diseases, definitive evidence regarding the role of selenium in preventing cardiovascular diseases will require controlled clinical trials.

Disease Treatment

Human Immunodeficiency Virus

There appears to be a unique interaction between selenium and the human immunodeficiency viruses (HIV) that cause acquired immune deficiency syndrome (AIDS). Declining selenium levels in HIV-infected individuals are sensitive markers of disease progression and severity, even before malnutrition becomes a factor. Low levels of plasma selenium have also been associated with a significantly increased risk of death from HIV. Adequate selenium nutritional status may increase resistance to HIV infection by enhancing the function of important immune system cells known as *T cells* and modifying their production of intracellular messengers known as *cytokines*.[15] In HIV infection, increased oxidative stress appears to favor viral replication, possibly by activating specific transcription pathways. As an integral component of glutathione peroxidase and thioredoxin reductase, selenium plays an important role in decreasing oxidative stress in HIV-infected cells and possibly suppressing the rate of HIV replication.[32] Recent research indicates that HIV may be capable of incorporating host selenium into viral selenoproteins that have glutathione-peroxidase activity. Though the significance of these findings requires further clarification, they suggest that both the human immune system and the activity of the virus are affected by selenium nutritional status.[33,34]

Only a few trials of selenium supplementation in HIV-infected individuals have been published. Two uncontrolled trials of selenium supplementation (one using 400 µg/d of selenium-enriched yeast and the other 80 µg/d of sodium selenite plus 25 mg/d of vitamin C) reported subjective improvement but did not demonstrate any improvement in biological parameters related to AIDS progression.[35] Another trial followed 15 HIV-infected patients supplemented with 100 µg/d of sodium selenite and 22 unsupplemented patients for 1 year and found evidence of decreased oxidative stress and a significant decrease in a biological marker of immunologic activation and HIV progression in the selenium-supplemented patients. However, there were no differences in CD4 T-cell count (an important biological marker of the progress of HIV infection) or mortality between the supplemented and unsupplemented patients.[36,37] At least two double-blind placebo-controlled trials of selenium supplementation in HIV-positive individuals are presently under way.[2]

Sources

Food Sources

The richest food sources of selenium are organ meats and seafood, followed by muscle meats. In general, there is wide variation in the selenium content of plants and grains because plants do not appear to require selenium, so the incorporation of selenium into plant proteins is dependent only on soil selenium content. Brazil nuts grown in areas of Brazil with selenium-rich soil may provide more than 100 µg of selenium in one nut, although those grown in selenium-poor soil may provide 10 times less.[38] In the United States, grains are a good source of selenium, but fruits and vegetables tend to be relatively poor sources of selenium. In general, drinking water is not a significant source of selenium in North America. The average dietary intake of adults in the United States has been found to range from about 80 to 110 µg/d. Because of food distribution patterns in the United States, people living in areas with low soil selenium avoid deficiency because they eat foods produced in areas with higher soil selenium.[1,11] Table 25–2 lists some good food sources of selenium and their selenium content in micrograms.

Supplements

Selenium supplements are available in several forms. Sodium selenite and sodium selenate are inorganic forms of selenium. Selenate is almost completely absorbed, but a significant amount is excreted in the urine before it can be incorporated into proteins. Selenite is only about 50% absorbed but is better retained than selenate once absorbed. Selenomethionine, an organic form of selenium that occurs naturally in foods, is about 90% absorbed.[11] Selenomethionine and selenium-enriched yeast, which mainly supplies selenomethionine, are also available as supplements. The consumer should be aware that some forms of selenium yeast on the market contain yeast plus mainly inorganic forms of selenium. Both inorganic and organic forms of selenium can be metabolized to selenocysteine by the body and incorporated into selenoenzymes.[39] At present, it is not clear whether one form of selenium is preferable to another. Most of the animal studies showing reduced tumor incidence used sodium selenite, as did two human trials showing enhancement of immune cell function. However, the recent placebo-controlled trial in humans that demonstrated a reduction in the incidence of several types of cancer used selenium yeast, which supplied mainly selenomethionine.

Table 25–2   Food Sources of Selenium

Food	Serving	Selenium, µg
Brazil nuts (from selenium-rich soil)	1 ounce (6–8 kernels)	839*
Crab meat	3 ounces[†]	40
Salmon	3 ounces[†]	40
Halibut	3 ounces[†]	40
Noodles, enriched	1 cup, cooked	35
Shrimp	3 ounces[†] (10–12)	34
Pork	3 ounces[†]	33
Chicken, light meat	3 ounces[†]	20
Rice, brown	1 cup, cooked	19
Beef	3 ounces[†]	17
Bread, whole wheat	2 slices	15
Milk	8 ounces (1 cup)	5
Walnuts, black	1 ounce, shelled	5

*Above the tolerable upper intake level (UL) of 400 µg/d.
[†]A 3-ounce serving of meat or fish is about the size of a deck of cards.

Selenium-Enriched Vegetables

Selenium-enriched garlic and ramps (wild leeks) have been shown to reduce chemically induced tumors in rats.[40] Selenium-enriched vegetables are of interest to scientists because some of the forms of selenium they produce (e.g., methylated forms of selenium) may be more potent inhibitors of tumor formation than the forms currently available in supplements.

Safety

Toxicity

Although selenium is required for health, high doses can be toxic. Acute and fatal toxicities have occurred with accidental or suicidal ingestion of gram quantities of selenium. Clinically significant selenium toxicity was reported in 13 individuals after taking supplements that contained 27.3 mg (27,300 µg) per

Table 25–3 Tolerable Upper Intake Level (UL) for Selenium

Life Stage	Age	UL, µg/d
Infants	0–6 months	45
Infants	6–12 months	60
Children	1–3 years	90
Children	4–8 years	150
Children	9–13 years	280
Adolescents	14–18 years	400
Adults	19 years and older	400

tablet due to a manufacturing error. Chronic selenium toxicity (selenosis) may occur with smaller doses of selenium over long periods of time. The most frequently reported symptoms of selenosis are hair and nail brittleness and loss. Other symptoms may include gastrointestinal disturbances, skin rashes, a garlic breath odor, fatigue, irritability, and nervous system abnormalities. In an area of China with a high prevalence of selenosis, toxic effects occurred with increasing frequency when blood selenium concentrations reached a level corresponding to an intake of 850 µg/d. The FNB recently set the tolerable upper intake level (UL) for selenium at 400 µg/d in adults based on the prevention of hair and nail brittleness and loss, early signs of chronic selenium toxicity (Table 25–3).[11] The UL of 400 µg/d includes selenium obtained from food, which averages about 100 µg/d for adults in the United States, as well as selenium from supplements

Drug Interactions

At present, few interactions between selenium and medications are known.[41] The anticonvulsant medication valproic acid has been found to decrease plasma selenium levels. Supplemental sodium selenite has been found to decrease toxicity from the antibiotic nitrofurantoin and the herbicide paraquat in animals.[42]

LPI Recommendation

The RDA for selenium (55 µg/d for adults) is sufficient to prevent deficiency. The average American diet is estimated to provide about 100 µg/d of selenium, an amount that appears sufficient to maximize plasma and cellular glutathione peroxidase activity.

Men

As discussed above, only one controlled clinical trial of the effect of selenium on cancer risk has been completed at this time. That study found that 200 µg/d of supplemental selenium significantly decreased the risk of prostate cancer. Because 200 µg was the only dose tested, it is not certain whether lower doses of supplemental selenium are also effective. For this reason, some experts feel that 200 µg/d of supplemental selenium is the only dose known to be of benefit in preventing cancer in men. Although 100 % of the daily value (DV) for selenium is presently 70 µg/d, the amount of selenium found in multivitamin/multimineral supplements may vary from 20 µg to more than 100 µg. In addition to a daily multivitamin/multimineral supplement, the Linus Pauling Institute recommends an extra selenium supplement for men such that the selenium intake from all supplements is approximately, but not more than, 200 µg/d. If a multivitamin/multimineral contains 100 % of the DV of selenium (70 µg/d), the Linus Pauling Institute recommends an extra selenium supplement of 100 µg/d.

Women

Because there is no evidence that selenium supplementation decreases the risk of cancer in women who are not selenium deficient, the Linus Pauling Institute recommends that women take a multivitamin/multimineral supplement that provides between the RDA (55 µg/d) and the DV (70 µg/d).

Older Adults

Because aging has not been associated with significant changes in the requirement for selenium, the Linus Pauling Institute Recommendation for selenium is the same for men and women 65 years and older.

References

1. Burk RF, Levander OA. Selenium. In: Shils M, Olson JA, Shike M, Ross AC, eds. *Nutrition in Health and Disease*, 9th ed. Baltimore: Williams & Wilkins; 1999:265–276.
2. Rayman MP. The importance of selenium to human health. *Lancet* 2000;356(9225):233–241.
3. Holben DH, Smith AM. The diverse role of selenium within selenoproteins: a review. *J Am Diet Assoc* 1999;99(7):836–843.
4. Ursini F, Heim S, Kiess M, et al. Dual function of the selenoprotein PHGPx during sperm maturation. *Science* 1999;285(5432):1393–1396.
5. Mustacich D, Powis G. Thioredoxin reductase. *Biochem J* 2000;346(Pt 1):1–8.
6. Larsen PR, Davies TF, Hay ID. The thyroid gland. In: Wilson JD, Foster DW, Kronenberg HM, Larsen PR, eds. *Williams Textbook of Endocrinology*, 9th ed. Philadelphia: W.B. Saunders Company; 1998:389–515.
7. Arteel GE, Briviba K, Sies H. Protection against peroxynitrite. *FEBS Lett* 1999;445(2–3):226–230.
8. Foster LH, Sumar S. Selenium in health and disease: a review. *Crit Rev Food Sci Nutr* 1997;37(3):211–228.
9. Beck MA, Esworthy RS, Ho YS, Chu FF. Glutathione peroxidase protects mice from viral-induced myocarditis. *FASEB J* 1998;12(12):1143–1149.
10. Levander OA. Coxsackievirus as a model of viral evolution driven by dietary oxidative stress. *Nutr Rev* 2000;58(2 Pt 2):S17–24.
11. Food and Nutrition Board, Institute of Medicine. Selenium. *Dietary Reference Intakes for Vitamin C, Vitamin E, Selenium, and Carotenoids*. Washington, D.C.: National Academy Press; 2000:284–324.
12. Roy M, Kiremidjian-Schumacher L, Wishe HI, Cohen MW, Stotzky G. Supplementation with selenium and human immune cell functions, I: Effect on lymphocyte proliferation and interleukin 2 receptor expression. *Biol Trace Elem Res* 1994;41(1–2):103–114.
13. Kiremidjian-Schumacher L, Roy M, Wishe HI, Cohen MW, Stotzky G. Supplementation with selenium and human immune cell functions, II: Effect on cytotoxic lymphocytes and natural killer cells. *Biol Trace Elem Res* 1994;41(1–2):115–127.
14. Kiremidjian-Schumacher L, Roy M, Glickman R, et al. Selenium and immunocompetence in patients with head and neck cancer. *Biol Trace Elem Res* 2000; 73(2):97–111.
15. Baum MK, Miguez-Burbano MJ, Campa A, Shor-Posner G. Selenium and interleukins in persons infected with human immunodeficiency virus type 1. *J Infect Dis* 2000;182(Suppl 1):S69–S73.
16. Rayman MP, Clark LC. Selenium in cancer prevention. In: Roussel AM, ed. *Trace Elements in Man and Animals*, 10th ed. New York: Plenum Press; 2000:575–580.
17. Combs GF, Jr., Gray WP. Chemopreventive agents: selenium. *Pharmacol Ther* 1998;79(3):179–192.
18. Yu MW, Horng IS, Hsu KH, Chiang YC, Liaw YF, Chen CJ. Plasma selenium levels and risk of hepatocellular carcinoma among men with chronic hepatitis virus infection. *Am J Epidemiol* 1999;150(4):367–374.
19. Knekt P, Marniemi J, Teppo L, Heliovaara M, Aromaa A. Is low selenium status a risk factor for lung cancer? *Am J Epidemiol* 1998;148(10):975–982.
20. Yoshizawa K, Willett WC, Morris SJ, et al. Study of prediagnostic selenium level in toenails and the risk of advanced prostate cancer. *J Natl Cancer Inst* 1998;90(16):1219–1224.
21. Nomura AM, Lee J, Stemmermann GN, Combs GF, Jr. Serum selenium and subsequent risk of prostate cancer. *Cancer Epidemiol Biomarkers Prev* 2000;9(9):883–887.
22. Brooks JD, Metter EJ, Chan DW, et al. Plasma selenium level before diagnosis and the risk of prostate cancer development. *J Urol* 2001;166(6):2034–2038.
23. Ghadirian P, Maisonneuve P, Perret C, et al. A case-control study of toenail selenium and cancer of the breast, colon, and prostate. *Cancer Detect Prev* 2000; 24(4):305–313.
24. Yu SY, Zhu YJ, Li WG. Protective role of selenium against hepatitis B virus and primary liver cancer in Qidong. *Biol Trace Elem Res* 1997;56(1):117–124.
25. Clark LC, Combs GF, Jr., Turnbull BW, et al. Effects of selenium supplementation for cancer prevention in patients with carcinoma of the skin: a randomized controlled trial. Nutritional Prevention of Cancer Study Group. *JAMA* 1996;276(24):1957–1963.
26. Duffield-Lillico AJ, Reid ME, Turnbull BW, et al. Baseline characteristics and the effect of selenium supplementation on cancer incidence in a randomized clinical trial: a summary report of the Nutrional Prevention of Cancer Trial. *Cancer Epidemiol Biomarkers Prev* 2002;11(7):630–639.
27. Salonen JT, Alfthan G, Huttunen JK, Pikkarainen J, Puska P. Association between cardiovascular death and myocardial infarction and serum selenium in a matched-pair longitudinal study. *Lancet* 1982; 2(8291):175–179.
28. Virtamo J, Valkeila E, Alfthan G, Punsar S, Huttunen JK, Karvonen MJ. Serum selenium and the risk of coronary heart disease and stroke. *Am J Epidemiol* 1985;122(2):276–282.
29. Suadicani P, Hein HO, Gyntelberg F. Serum selenium concentration and risk of ischaemic heart disease in a prospective cohort study of 3000 males. *Atherosclerosis* 1992;96(1):33–42.
30. Salvini S, Hennekens CH, Morris JS, Willett WC, Stampfer MJ. Plasma levels of the antioxidant selenium and risk of myocardial infarction among U.S. physicians. *Am J Cardiol* 1995;76(17):1218–1221.
31. Kardinaal AF, Kok FJ, Kohlmeier L, et al. Association between toenail selenium and risk of acute myocardial infarction in European men. The EURAMIC Study. European Antioxidant Myocardial Infarction and Breast Cancer. *Am J Epidemiol* 1997;145(4):373–379.
32. Look MP, Rockstroh JK, Rao GS, Kreuzer KA, Spengler U, Sauerbruch T. Serum selenium versus lymphocyte subsets and markers of disease progression and inflammatory response in human immunodeficiency virus-1 infection. *Biol Trace Elem Res* 1997;56(1):31–41.
33. Zhang W, Ramanathan CS, Nadimpalli RG, Bhat AA, Cox AG, Taylor EW. Selenium-dependent glutathione peroxidase modules encoded by RNA viruses. *Biol Trace Elem Res* 1999;70(2):97–116.
34. Zhao L, Cox AG, Ruzicka JA, Bhat AA, Zhang W, Taylor EW. Molecular modeling and in vitro activity of an HIV-1-encoded glutathione peroxidase. *Proc Natl Acad Sci USA* 2000;97(12):6356–6361.

35. Constans J, Conri C, Sergeant C. Selenium and HIV infection. *Nutrition* 1999;15(9):719–720.

36. Constans J, Delmas-Beauvieux MC, Sergeant C, et al. One-year antioxidant supplementation with beta-carotene or selenium for patients infected with human immunodeficiency virus: a pilot study. *Clin Infect Dis* 1996;23(3):654–656.

37. Delmas-Beauvieux MC, Peuchant E, Couchouron A, et al. The enzymatic antioxidant system in blood and glutathione status in human immunodeficiency virus (HIV)-infected patients: effects of supplementation with selenium or beta-carotene. *Am J Clin Nutr* 1996;64(1):101–107.

38. Chang JC. Selenium content of brazil nuts from two geographic locations in Brazil. *Chemosphere* 1995; 30:801–802.

39. Schrauzer GN. Selenomethionine: a review of its nutritional significance, metabolism and toxicity. *J Nutr* 2000;130(7):1653–1656.

40. Whanger PD, Ip C, Polan CE, Uden PC, Welbaum G. Tumorigenesis, metabolism, speciation, bioavailability, and tissue deposition of selenium in selenium-enriched ramps (*Allium tricoccum*). *J Agric Food Chem* 2000;48(11):5723–5730.

41. Hendler SS, Rorvik DR, eds. *PDR for Nutritional Supplements*. Montvale, NJ: Medical Economics Company, Inc.; 2001.

42. Flodin NW. Micronutrient supplements: toxicity and drug interactions. *Prog Food Nutr Sci* 1990;14(4):277–331.

26 Sodium Chloride

Salt (sodium chloride) is essential for life. The tight regulation of the body's sodium and chloride concentrations is so important that multiple mechanisms work in concert to control them. Although scientists agree that a minimal amount of salt is required for survival, the health implications of excess salt intake represent an area of considerable controversy among scientists, clinicians, and public health experts.[1]

Function

Sodium (Na^+) and chloride (Cl^-) are the principal ions in the fluid outside of cells (extracellular fluid), which includes blood plasma. As such, they play critical roles in a number of life-sustaining processes.[2]

Maintenance of Membrane Potential

Sodium and chloride are electrolytes that contribute to the maintenance of concentration and charge differences across cell membranes. Potassium (K^+) is the principal positively charged ion (cation) inside of cells, and sodium (Na^+) is the principal cation in extracellular fluid. Potassium concentrations are about 30 times higher inside than outside cells, and sodium concentrations are more than 10 times lower inside than outside cells. The concentration differences between potassium and sodium across cell membranes create an electrochemical gradient known as the *membrane potential*. A cell's membrane potential is maintained by ion pumps in the cell membrane, especially the Na^+, K^+ ATPase pumps (Fig. 26–1). These pumps use adenosine triphosphate (ATP)

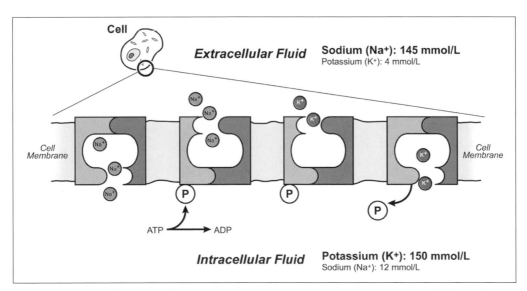

Figure 26–1. A model of the Na^+, K^+ ATPase pump. The concentration differences between potassium (K^+) and sodium (Na^+) across cell membranes create an electrochemical gradient known as the membrane potential. Adenosine triphosphate (ATP) provides the energy to pump three Na^+ ions out of the cell in exchange for two K^+ ions, thus maintaining the membrane potential.

to pump Na^+ out of the cell in exchange for K^+. Their activity has been estimated to account for 20 to 40% of the resting energy expenditure in a typical adult. The large proportion of energy dedicated to maintaining Na^+/K^+ concentration gradients emphasizes the importance of this function in sustaining life. Tight control of cell membrane potential is critical for nerve impulse transmission, muscle contraction, and cardiac function.[3,4]

Nutrient Absorption and Transport

Absorption of sodium in the small intestine plays an important role in the absorption of chloride, amino acids, glucose, and water. Similar mechanisms are involved in the reabsorption of these nutrients after they have been filtered from the blood by the kidneys. Chloride, in the form of hydrochloric acid, is also an important component of gastric juice, which aids the digestion and absorption of many nutrients.[2,5]

Maintenance of Blood Volume and Blood Pressure

Because sodium is the primary determinant of extracellular fluid volume including blood volume, a number of physiological mechanisms that regulate blood volume and blood pressure work by adjusting the body's sodium content. In the circulatory system, pressure receptors (baroreceptors) sense changes in blood pressure and send excitatory or inhibitory signals to the nervous system and/or endocrine glands to affect sodium regulation by the kidneys. In general, sodium retention results in water retention and sodium loss results in water loss.[4,5] Following are descriptions of two of the many systems that affect blood volume and blood pressure through sodium regulation.

Renin–Angiotensin–Aldosterone System. In response to a significant decrease in blood volume or pressure (e.g., serious blood loss or dehydration), the kidneys release renin into the circulation. Renin is an enzyme that splits a small peptide (angiotensin I) from a larger protein (angiotensinogen) produced by the liver. Angiotensin I is split into a smaller peptide (angiotensin II) by angiotensin-converting

enzyme, an enzyme present on the inner surface of blood vessels and in the lungs, liver, and kidneys. Angiotensin II stimulates the constriction of small arteries, resulting in increased blood pressure. Angiotensin II is also a potent stimulator of aldosterone synthesis by the adrenal glands. Aldosterone is a steroid hormone that acts on the kidneys to increase the reabsorption of sodium and the excretion of potassium. Retention of sodium by the kidneys increases the retention of water, resulting in increased blood volume and blood pressure.[4]

Antidiuretic Hormone. Secretion of antidiuretic hormone (ADH) by the posterior pituitary gland is stimulated by a significant decrease in blood volume or pressure. ADH acts on the kidney to increase the reabsorption of water.[4]

Deficiency

Sodium (and chloride) deficiency does not generally result from inadequate dietary intake, even in those on very low-salt diets.[5]

Hyponatremia

Hyponatremia is defined as a serum sodium concentration of less than 136 mmol/L, and may result from increased fluid retention (dilutional hyponatremia) or increased sodium loss. Dilutional hyponatremia may be due to inappropriate ADH secretion, which is associated with disorders affecting the central nervous system and a number of drugs. In some cases, excessive water intake may also lead to dilutional hyponatremia. Conditions that increase the loss of sodium and chloride include severe or prolonged vomiting or diarrhea, excessive and persistent sweating, the use of some diuretics, and some forms of kidney disease. Symptoms of hyponatremia include headache, nausea, vomiting, muscle cramps, fatigue, disorientation, and fainting. Complications of severe and rapidly developing hyponatremia may include cerebral edema (swelling of the brain), seizures, coma, and brain damage. Acute or severe hyponatremia may be fatal without prompt and appropriate medical treatment.[6]

Table 26–1 Minimum Requirement for Sodium and Chloride

Life Stage	Age	Sodium, mg/d	Chloride, mg/d
Infants	0–5 months	120	180
Infants	6–11 months	200	300
Children	1 year	225	350
Children	2–5 years	300	500
Children	6–9 years	400	600
Children	10–18 years	500	750
Adults	over 18 years	500	750

Prolonged Endurance Exercise and Hyponatremia. Hyponatremia has recently been recognized as a potential problem in individuals competing in very long endurance exercise events, such as marathons, ultramarathons, and ironman triathlons. In 1997, 25 of 650 participants in an ironman triathlon (almost 4%) received medical attention for hyponatremia.[7] Participants who developed hyponatremia during an ironman triathlon had evidence of fluid overload despite relatively modest fluid intakes, suggesting that fluid excretion was inadequate and/or the fluid needs of these ultradistance athletes may be less than currently recommended.[8] It has been speculated that the use of nonsteroidal anti-inflammatory drugs may increase the risk of exercise-related hyponatremia by impairing water excretion,[9] but firm evidence is presently lacking.

The Minimum Requirements

In 1989, the Food and Nutrition Board (FNB) of the Institute of Medicine determined minimum requirements for sodium and chloride, which are listed in Table 26–1.[5] These requirements are well below the average dietary intakes of most of the world's people. Updated recommendations for sodium chloride intake by the FNB are expected in 2003.

Disease Prevention (Dietary Salt Reduction)

Gastric Cancer

Epidemiologic studies, conducted mainly in Asian countries, indicate that high intakes of salted, smoked, and pickled foods increase the risk of gastric cancer.[10] Although these foods are high in salt, they may also contain carcinogens, such as nitrosamines. Additionally, populations with high intakes of salted foods tend to have low intakes of fruits and vegetables, which are also associated with increased risk of gastric cancer. The risk of developing stomach cancer is increased by chronic inflammation of the stomach and infection by the bacterium *Helicobacter pylori*. High concentrations of salt may damage the cells lining the stomach, potentially increasing the risk of *H. pylori* infection and of cancer-promoting genetic damage to cells by carcinogens in the stomach. Although there is little evidence that salt is a carcinogen alone, high intakes of certain salted foods, such as salted fish, may increase the risk of gastric cancer in susceptible individuals.[11,12]

Osteoporosis

Osteoporosis is a multifactorial skeletal disorder in which bone strength is compromised, resulting in an increased risk of fracture. Nutrition is one of many factors contributing to the development and progression of osteoporosis. Increased salt intake has been found to increase urinary excretion of calcium. Each 2.3 g increment of sodium (5.8 g of salt) excreted by the kidney has been found to draw about 24 to 40 mg of calcium into the urine.[13] Salt intake has been associated with biochemical markers of bone resorption in some studies but not in others. In general, cross-sectional studies have not found an association between sodium intake and bone mineral density (BMD).[14] However, a 2-year study of postmenopausal women found that increased urinary sodium excretion (an indicator of increased sodium intake) was associated with decreased BMD at the hip.[15] Long-term prospective studies are needed to determine whether decreasing salt intake has clinically significant effects on BMD and fracture risk in individuals at risk for osteoporosis. For more information on osteoporosis, see Chapter 14 on calcium.

Kidney Stones

Most kidney stones contain calcium as a main constituent. Although their cause is often unknown, abnormally elevated urinary calcium (hypercalciuria) increases the risk of developing calcium stones.[16] Increased dietary salt has been found to increase urinary calcium excretion, and this effect may be more pronounced in patients with a history of calcium-containing kidney stones.[17] A large prospective study that followed more than 90,000 women over a 12-year period found that women with a sodium intake averaging 4.9 g/d (12.6 g/d of salt) had a 30% higher risk of developing symptomatic kidney stones than women whose sodium intake averaged 1.5 g/d (4.0 g/d of salt).[18] However, a similar study in men did not find an association between sodium intake and symptomatic kidney stones.[19] Clinical studies have shown that salt restriction reduces urinary calcium in individuals with a tendency to form calcium stones,[20] and a 5-year randomized trial of two different diets in men with recurrent calcium oxalate stones found that a diet low in salt and animal protein significantly decreased stone recurrence compared with a low calcium diet.[21]

Disease Treatment (Dietary Salt Reduction)

Hypertension

Although the reduction of dietary salt has been advocated as a means to prevent and treat hypertension for almost 30 years, the actual benefits of dietary salt reduction are still controversial among scientists and clinicians. Animal studies, as well as cross-cultural studies comparing cultures with very low salt intakes with those with high intakes, suggest that increased salt consumption is associated with increased blood pressure. However, populations in cross-cultural studies may differ in a number of other ways that could affect blood pressure.[22,23]

Clinical Trials and Meta-Analyses. Within populations the evidence relating salt intake to blood pressure is less clear. A number of randomized clinical trials have examined the effect of dietary salt reduction on blood pressure in hypertensive and nonhypertensive (normotensive) individuals. Several investigators have used meta-analysis to analyze the pooled data from many different trials and estimate the magnitude of the effect of dietary salt reduction on blood pressure.[24–26] The most recently published meta-analysis examined data pooled from more than 100 separate studies and more than 5000 hypertensive and normotensive participants.[26] Overall, reducing salt intake by about 6 g/d lowered blood pressure (BP) by 3.9/1.9 mm Hg (systolic BP/diastolic BP) in hypertensive individuals, although even greater reductions in salt intake lowered blood pressure by only 1.2/0.3 mm Hg in normotensive individuals. Although clinicians have questioned the value of such modest blood pressure reductions in hypertensive patients, overviews of observational studies and randomized trials suggest that reducing diastolic BP by an average of 2 mm Hg in the U.S. population would reduce the prevalence of hypertension by 17%, the risk of heart attack by 6%, and the risk of stroke by 15%.[27] Thus, modest reductions in individual risk may translate into significant public health benefits.

Salt Sensitivity. Dietary salt restriction has been reported to lower blood pressure significantly in 30 to 60% of hypertensive individuals and 25 to 50% of normotensive individuals, suggesting that there is a subset of people who are more sensitive to the effects of dietary salt on blood pressure. Salt sensitivity has been reported to be more common in obese and insulin-resistant individuals as well as African-American, elderly, and female hypertensive patients.[28] A multicenter study of 624 hypertensive individuals who were diagnosed as salt-sensitive found that lowering salt intake by 5 to 6 g/day resulted in an average blood pressure decrease of 10/7 mm Hg.[29] Such a reduction is clinically significant and similar to that induced by some blood pressure medications. Although the physiologic mechanisms contributing to salt sensitivity are not yet clear, considerable research is being directed toward the genetic basis for hypertension and salt sensitivity. Common variations in specific genes, known as *polymorphisms*, may contribute to salt sensitivity in hypertension. Genetic polymorphisms currently under investigation include those of genes whose products function prominently in the renin–angiotensin–aldosterone system.[30]

Salt and Target Organ Damage. Chronic hypertension results in damage to the heart, blood vessels, and kidneys, which significantly increases the risk of heart disease and stroke, as well as hypertensive kidney disease. In a number of clinical studies, salt intake has been significantly correlated with left ventricular hypertrophy, an abnormal thickening of the heart muscle, which is implicated in increased mortality from cardiovascular diseases.[22] Recent research indicates that high salt intake may contribute to organ damage in ways that are independent of its effects on blood pressure.[31] For example, studies in animals and humans have found increased salt intake to be associated with pathological changes in the structure and function of large elastic arteries that are independent of changes in blood pressure.[32]

Nutrient Interactions and Hypertension. A multicenter, randomized feeding study, called the DASH (Dietary Approaches to Stop Hypertension) trial, demonstrated that a diet emphasizing fruits, vegetables, whole grains, poultry, fish, nuts, and low-fat dairy products substantially lowered blood pressure in hypertensive (11.4/5.5 mm Hg) and normotensive people (3.5/2.1 mm Hg) compared with a typical U.S. diet.[33] Among other nutrients, the DASH diet was markedly higher in potassium and calcium than the typical U.S. diet. However, sodium levels were kept constant throughout the study to better evaluate the effects of other dietary components. More recently the DASH-sodium trial compared the DASH diet with a typical U.S. (control) diet at three levels of salt intake: low, 2.9 g/d; medium, 5.8 g/d (recommended by U.S. dietary guidelines); and high, 8.7 g/d (typical U.S. intake).[34] The DASH diet significantly lowered systolic and diastolic blood pressures in hypertensive and normotensive people at each level

of salt intake compared with the control diet. Reduction of salt intake resulted in an additional lowering of systolic and diastolic blood pressures in both diets. The combination of the DASH diet and reduced salt intake lowered blood pressure more than either intervention alone. Compared with the high-salt control diet, average blood pressure on the low-sodium DASH diet was decreased 8.9/4.5 mm Hg. The effect of salt reduction was greater in the control diet than in the DASH diet, suggesting that salt reduction may be more beneficial in those who consume typical U.S. diets. The DASH trials support the idea that healthful dietary patterns offer an effective approach to the prevention and treatment of hypertension.[35]

The National High Blood Pressure Education Program and the National Heart, Lung, and Blood Institute of the National Institutes of Health (NIH) recommend consuming no more than 6 g/d of salt, which is 4 g/d less than the national average.[36]

Sources

Food Sources

Most of the sodium and chloride in the diet comes from salt. It has been estimated that 75% of the salt intake in the United States is derived from salt added during food processing or manufacturing, rather than from salt added at the table or during cooking. The lowest salt intakes are associated with diets that emphasize unprocessed foods, especially fruits, vegetables, and legumes. The average American diet provides about 10 g of salt daily (4 g of sodium and 6 g of chloride).[5] The National High Blood Pressure Education Program and the National Heart, Lung, and Blood Institute of the NIH recommend consuming no more than 6 g/d of salt ($\sim$2.4 g/d of sodium) to reduce the risk of hypertension and its complications.[36]

Table 26–2 lists the sodium content in milligrams of some foods that are high in salt, and Table 26–3 lists the sodium content in milligrams of some foods that are relatively low in salt. As the majority of sodium and chloride intake comes from salt, dietary salt content can

Table 26–2   Foods That Are High in Salt

Food	Serving	Sodium, mg
Potato chips, salted	8 ounces (1 bag)	1348
Macaroni and cheese, canned	1 cup	1343
Chicken soup, canned	1 cup	1106
Pretzels, salted	2 ounces (10 pretzels)	1029
Ham	3 ounces*	1023
Corned beef hash	1 cup	1003
Corn dog	1	973
Fish sandwich w/tartar sauce and cheese	1 sandwich	939
Tomato juice, canned (salt added)	1 cup (8 fluid ounces)	877
Dill pickle	1 medium	833
Hot dog, beef	1	458

* A 3-ounce serving of meat or fish is about the size of a deck of cards.

Table 26–3   Foods That Are Low in Salt

Food	Serving	Sodium, mg
Olive oil	1 tablespoon	0.0
Pear, raw	1 medium	0.0
Popcorn, air-popped	1 cup	0.3
Almonds, unsalted	1 cup	1.4
Brown rice	1 cup, cooked	1.9
Orange juice, frozen	1 cup (8 fluid ounces)	2.5
Mango	1 fruit	4.1
Tomato	1 medium	11.1
Fruit cocktail, canned	1 cup	14.9
Potato chips, unsalted	8 ounces (1 bag)	18.2
Carrot	1 medium	21.4
Tomato juice, canned, no salt added	1 cup (8 fluid ounces)	24.3

be estimated from sodium content by multiplying sodium content by 2.5.
[*Example*: 2000 mg of sodium × 2.5 = 5000 mg (5 g) of salt].

Safety

Toxicity

Excessive intakes of sodium chloride lead to an increase in extracellular fluid volume as water is pulled from cells to maintain normal sodium concentrations. However, as long as water needs can be met, normally functioning kidneys can excrete the excess sodium and restore the system to normal.[36] Ingestion of large amounts of salt may lead to nausea, vomiting, diarrhea, and abdominal cramps.[37] Abnormally high serum sodium concentrations (hypernatremia) generally develop from excess water loss, frequently accompanied by an impaired thirst mechanism or lack of access to water. Symptoms of hypernatremia in the presence of excess fluid loss may include dizziness or fainting, low blood pressure, and diminished urine production. Severe hypernatremia may result in edema, hypertension, rapid heart rate, difficulty breathing, convulsions, coma, and death. Hypernatremia is rarely caused by excessive sodium intake (e.g., the ingestion of large amounts of seawater or intravenous infusion of concentrated saline solution). In end-stage renal failure, impaired urinary sodium excretion may lead to fluid retention, resulting in edema, high blood pressure, or congestive heart failure if salt and water intake are not restricted.[2,38]

Drug Interactions

The medications listed in Table 26–4 increase the risk of hyponatremia (abnormally low serum sodium concentration).[6]

Table 26–4 Medications Associated with Hyponatremia[6]

Classes of Medications Associated with Hyponatremia

Medication Class	Examples
Diuretics	hydrochlorthiazide, furosemide
Nonsteroidal anti-inflammatory drugs	ibuprofen, naproxen sodium
Opiate derivatives	codeine, morphine
Phenothiazines	prochlorperazine, promethazine
Serotonin-reuptake inhibitors	fluoxetine, paroxetine
Tricyclic antidepressants	amitriptyline, imipramine

Individual Medications Associated with Hyponatremia

Medication Class	Medication
Anticonvulsant	carbamazepine
Antilipidemic	clofibrate
Antineoplastics	cyclophosphamide vincristine
Hormones	desmopressin oxytocin
Oral hypoglycemic	chlorpropamide

LPI Recommendation

Although the salt intake most likely to promote optimum health is controversial, there is evidence that a diet relatively low in salt and high in potassium is associated with decreased risk of hypertension and its associated cardiovascular and renal complications. Moreover, the DASH trial demonstrated that a diet emphasizing fruits, vegetables, whole grains, nuts, and low-fat dairy products substantially lowered blood pressure, an effect that was enhanced by reducing salt intake to less than 6 g/d. The Linus Pauling Institute recommends a diet that is rich in fruits and vegetables (at least five servings per day) and limits processed foods that are high in salt.

Older Adults

Adults over the age of 65 are at increased risk of hypertension, stroke, and other chronic diseases and may benefit from a diet that is relatively rich in potassium and low in salt. A recent study found that one half of the older adults surveyed consumed less than five servings of fruits and vegetables daily.[39]

References

1. Taubes G. The (political) science of salt. *Science* 1998;281(5379):898–901, 903–897.
2. Harper ME, Willis JS, Patrick J. Sodium and chloride in nutrition. In: O'Dell BL, Sunde RA, eds. *Handbook of Nutritionally Essential Minerals.* New York: Marcel Dekker; 1997:93–116.
3. Brody T. *Nutritional Biochemistry*, 2nd ed. San Diego: Academic Press; 1999.
4. Sheng H-W. Sodium, chloride and potassium. In: Stipanuk M, ed. *Biochemical and Physiological Aspects of Human Nutrition.* Philadelphia: W.B. Saunders Company; 2000:686–710.
5. National Research Council, Food and Nutrition Board. *Recommended Dietary Allowances*, 10th ed. Washington, D.C.: National Academy Press; 1989.
6. Adrogue HJ, Madias NE. Hyponatremia. *N Engl J Med* 2000;342(21):1581–1589.
7. Speedy DB, Rogers IR, Noakes TD, et al. Diagnosis and prevention of hyponatremia at an ultradistance triathlon. *Clin J Sport Med* 2000;10(1):52–58.
8. Speedy DB, Noakes TD, Kimber NE, et al. Fluid balance during and after an ironman triathlon. *Clin J Sport Med* 2001;11(1):44–50.
9. Ayus JC, Varon J, Arieff AI. Hyponatremia, cerebral edema, and noncardiogenic pulmonary edema in marathon runners. *Ann Intern Med* 2000;132(9):711–714.
10. Palli D. Epidemiology of gastric cancer: an evaluation of available evidence. *J Gastroenterol* 2000;35(Suppl 12):84–89.
11. Cohen AJ, Roe FJ. Evaluation of the aetiological role of dietary salt exposure in gastric and other cancers in humans. *Food Chem Toxicol* 1997;35(2):271–293.
12. Hirohata T, Kono S. Diet/nutrition and stomach cancer in Japan. *Int J Cancer* 1997;(Suppl 10):34–36.
13. Weaver CM, Heaney RP. Calcium. In: Shils M, Olson JA, Shike M, Ross AC, eds. *Nutrition in Health and Disease*, 9th ed. Baltimore: Williams & Wilkins; 1999:141–155.
14. Cohen AJ, Roe FJ. Review of risk factors for osteoporosis with particular reference to a possible aetiological role of dietary salt. *Food Chem Toxicol* 2000;38(2–3):237–253.
15. Devine A, Criddle RA, Dick IM, Kerr DA, Prince RL. A longitudinal study of the effect of sodium and calcium intakes on regional bone density in postmenopausal women. *Am J Clin Nutr* 1995;62(4):740–745.
16. Heller HJ. The role of calcium in the prevention of kidney stones. *J Am Coll Nutr* 1999;18(5 Suppl):373S–378S.

17. Audran M, Legrand E. Hypercalciuria. *Joint Bone Spine* 2000;67(6):509–515.

18. Curhan GC, Willett WC, Speizer FE, Spiegelman D, Stampfer MJ. Comparison of dietary calcium with supplemental calcium and other nutrients as factors affecting the risk for kidney stones in women. *Ann Intern Med* 1997;126(7):497–504.

19. Curhan GC, Willett WC, Rimm EB, Stampfer MJ. A prospective study of dietary calcium and other nutrients and the risk of symptomatic kidney stones. *N Engl J Med* 1993;328(12):833–838.

20. Assimos DG, Holmes RP. Role of diet in the therapy of urolithiasis. *Urol Clin North Am* 2000;27(2):255–268.

21. Borghi L, Schianchi T, Meschi T, et al. Comparison of two diets for the prevention of recurrent stones in idiopathic hypercalciuria. *N Engl J Med* 2002;346(2):77–84.

22. Chrysant GS. High salt intake and cardiovascular disease: is there a connection? *Nutrition* 2000;16(7–8):662–664.

23. Tobian L. Dietary sodium chloride and potassium have effects on the pathophysiology of hypertension in humans and animals. *Am J Clin Nutr* 1997;65(2 Suppl):606S–611S.

24. Midgley JP, Matthew AG, Greenwood CM, Logan AG. Effect of reduced dietary sodium on blood pressure: a meta-analysis of randomized controlled trials. *JAMA* 1996;275(20):1590–1597.

25. Cutler JA, Follmann D, Allender PS. Randomized trials of sodium reduction: an overview. *Am J Clin Nutr* 1997;65(2 Suppl):643S–651S.

26. Graudal NA, Galloe AM, Garred P. Effects of sodium restriction on blood pressure, renin, aldosterone, catecholamines, cholesterols, and triglyceride: a meta-analysis. *JAMA* 1998;279(17):1383–1391.

27. Cook NR, Cohen J, Hebert PR, Taylor JO, Hennekens CH. Implications of small reductions in diastolic blood pressure for primary prevention. *Arch Intern Med* 1995;155(7):701–709.

28. Whelton PK, He J, Cutler JA, et al. Effects of oral potassium on blood pressure: meta-analysis of randomized controlled clinical trials. *JAMA* 1997;277(20):1624–1632.

29. Chrysant SG, Weir MR, Weder AB, et al. There are no racial, age, sex, or weight differences in the effect of salt on blood pressure in salt-sensitive hypertensive patients. *Arch Intern Med* 1997;157(21):2489–2494.

30. Giner V, Poch E, Bragulat E, et al. Renin-angiotensin system genetic polymorphisms and salt sensitivity in essential hypertension. *Hypertension* 2000;35(1 Pt 2):512–517.

31. Aviv A. Salt and hypertension: the debate that begs the bigger question. *Arch Intern Med* 2001;161(4):507–510.

32. Safar ME, Thuilliez C, Richard V, Benetos A. Pressure-independent contribution of sodium to large artery structure and function in hypertension. *Cardiovasc Res* 2000;46(2):269–276.

33. Appel LJ, Moore TJ, Obarzanek E, et al. A clinical trial of the effects of dietary patterns on blood pressure. DASH Collaborative Research Group. *N Engl J Med* 1997;336(16):1117–1124.

34. Sacks FM, Svetkey LP, Vollmer WM, et al. Effects on blood pressure of reduced dietary sodium and the Dietary Approaches to Stop Hypertension (DASH) diet. DASH-Sodium Collaborative Research Group. *N Engl J Med* 2001;344(1):3–10.

35. Greenland P. Beating high blood pressure with low-sodium DASH. *N Engl J Med* 2001;344(1):53–55.

36. Chobanian AV, Hill M. National Heart, Lung, and Blood Institute Workshop on Sodium and Blood Pressure: a critical review of current scientific evidence. *Hypertension* 2000;35(4):858–863.

37. Minerals. *Drug Facts and Comparisons*. St. Louis: Facts and Comparisons; 2000:27–51.

38. Okuda T. Fluid and electrolyte disorders. In: Tierney LM, McPhee SJ, Papadakis MA, eds. *Current Medical Diagnosis and Treatment,* 37th ed. Stamford: Appleton & Lange; 1998:824–849.

39. Foote JA, Giuliano AR, Harris RB. Older adults need guidance to meet nutritional recommendations. *J Am Coll Nutr* 2000;19(5):628–640.

27 Zinc

Zinc is an essential trace element for all forms of life. The significance of zinc in human nutrition and public health was recognized relatively recently. Clinical zinc deficiency in humans was first described in 1961, when the consumption of diets with low zinc bioavailability due to high phytic acid content was associated with "adolescent nutritional dwarfism" in the Middle East.[1] Since then, zinc insufficiency has been recognized by a number of experts as an important public health issue, especially in developing countries.[2]

Function

Numerous aspects of cellular metabolism are zinc-dependent. Zinc plays important roles in growth and development, the immune response, neurological function, and reproduction. On the cellular level, the function of zinc can be divided into three categories: (1) catalytic, (2) structural, and (3) regulatory.[3]

Catalytic Role

Nearly 100 different enzymes depend on zinc for their ability to catalyze vital chemical reactions. Zinc-dependent enzymes can be found in all known classes of enzymes.[4]

Structural Role

Zinc plays an important role in the structure of proteins and cell membranes. A fingerlike structure, known as a *zinc finger motif*, stabilizes the structure of a number of proteins. For example, copper provides the catalytic activity for the antioxidant enzyme copper-zinc superoxide dismutase and zinc plays a critical structural role.[4,5] The structure and function of cell membranes are also affected by zinc. Loss of zinc from biological membranes increases their susceptibility to oxidative damage and impairs their function.[6]

Regulatory Role

Zinc finger proteins have been found to regulate gene expression by acting as transcription factors (binding to DNA and influencing the transcription of specific genes). Zinc also plays a role in cell signaling and has been found to influence hormone release and nerve impulse transmission. Recently zinc has been found to play a role in apoptosis (gene-directed cell death), a critical cellular regulatory process with implications for growth and development, as well as a number of chronic diseases.[7]

Nutrient Interactions

Copper. Taking large quantities of zinc (50 mg/d or more) over a period of weeks can interfere with copper bioavailability. High intake of zinc induces the intestinal synthesis of a copper-binding protein called *metallothionein*. Metallothionein traps copper within intestinal cells and prevents its systemic absorption. More typical intakes of zinc do not affect copper absorption and high copper intakes do not affect zinc absorption.[4]

Iron. Supplemental (38 to 65 mg/d of elemental iron) but not dietary levels of iron may decrease zinc absorption. This interaction is of concern in the management of iron supplementation during pregnancy and lactation and has led some experts to recommend zinc supplementation for pregnant and lactating women taking more than 60 mg/d of elemental iron.[8,9]

Calcium. High levels of dietary calcium impair zinc absorption in animals, but it is uncertain whether this occurs in humans. Increasing the calcium intake of postmenopausal women by 890 mg/d in the form of milk or calcium phosphate (total calcium intake 1360 mg/d) reduced zinc absorption and zinc balance in postmenopausal women,[10] but increasing the calcium intake of adolescent girls by 1000 mg/d in the form of calcium citrate malate (total calcium intake 1667 mg/d) did not affect zinc absorption or balance.[11] Calcium in combination with phytic acid reduces zinc absorption. This effect is particularly relevant to individuals consuming a diet that is highly dependent on tortillas made with lime (calcium oxide). For more information on phytic acid, see the section on food sources.

Folic Acid. The bioavailability of dietary folate is increased by the action of a zinc-dependent enzyme, suggesting a possible interaction between zinc and folic acid. In the past, some studies found low zinc intake to decrease folate absorption, although other studies found folic acid supplementation to impair zinc utilization in individuals with marginal zinc status.[4,5] However, a more recent study found that supplementation with a relatively high dose of folic acid (800 μg/d) for 25 days did not alter zinc status in a group of students being fed low-zinc diets (3.5 mg/d), nor did zinc intake impair folate utilization.[12]

Deficiency

Severe Zinc Deficiency

Much of what is known about severe zinc deficiency was derived from the study of individuals born with acrodermatitis enteropathica, a genetic disorder resulting from the impaired uptake and transport of zinc. The symptoms of severe zinc deficiency include the slowing or cessation of growth and development, delayed sexual maturation, characteristic skin rashes, chronic and severe diarrhea, immune system deficiencies, impaired wound healing, diminished appetite, impaired taste sensation, night blindness, swelling and clouding of the corneas, and behavioral disturbances. Before the cause of acrodermatitis enteropathica was known, patients typically died in infancy. Oral zinc therapy results in the complete remission of symptoms, though it must be maintained indefinitely in individuals with the genetic disorder.[5,13] Although dietary zinc deficiency is unlikely to cause severe zinc deficiency in individuals without a genetic disorder, zinc mal-

absorption or conditions of increased zinc loss, such as severe burns or prolonged diarrhea, may also result in severe zinc deficiency.

Mild Zinc Deficiency

More recently, it has become apparent that milder zinc deficiency contributes to a number of health problems, especially common in children who live in developing countries. The lack of a sensitive indicator of mild zinc deficiency hinders the scientific study of its health implications. However, controlled trials of moderate zinc supplementation have demonstrated that mild zinc deficiency contributes to impaired physical and neuropsychological development and increased susceptibility to life-threatening infections in young children.[13]

Individuals at Risk of Zinc Deficiency. Populations at increased risk of zinc deficiency include infants and children; pregnant and lactating women, especially teenagers; patients receiving total parenteral nutrition (intravenous feedings); malnourished individuals, including those with protein-energy malnutrition and anorexia nervosa; individuals with severe or persistent diarrhea; individuals with malabsorption syndromes, including sprue and short bowel syndrome; individuals with inflammatory bowel disease, including Crohn's disease and ulcerative colitis; individuals with alcoholic liver disease; individuals with sickle cell anemia; and older adults (65 years and older).[5]

Strict Vegetarians. The requirement for dietary zinc may be as much as 50 % greater for strict vegetarians whose major food staples are grains and legumes because high levels of phytic acid in these foods reduce the absorption of zinc.[4]

The Recommended Dietary Allowance

Because a sensitive indicator of zinc nutritional status is not readily available, the recommended dietary allowance (RDA) for zinc was based on a number of different indicators of zinc nutritional status and represents the daily intake likely to prevent deficiency in nearly all

Table 27–1   Recommended Dietary Allowance (RDA) for Zinc

Life Stage	Age	Males, mg/d	Females, mg/d
Infants	0–6 months	2 (AI)	2 (AI)
Infants	7–12 months	3	3
Children	1–3 years	3	3
Children	4–8 years	5	5
Children	9–13 years	8	8
Adolescents	14–18 years	11	9
Adults	19 years and older	11	8
Pregnancy	18 years and younger	–	12
Pregnancy	19 years and older	–	11
Breast-feeding	18 years and younger	–	13
Breast-feeding	19 years and older	–	12

AI, adequate intake level.

individuals in a specific age and gender group (Table 27–1).[4]

Disease Prevention

The following health problems and diseases may be avoided by addressing zinc deficiency.

Impaired Growth and Development

Growth Retardation. Significant delays in linear growth and weight gain, known as *growth retardation* or *failure to thrive*, are common features of mild zinc deficiency in children. In the 1970s and 1980s, several randomized placebo-controlled studies of zinc supplementation in young children with significant growth delays were conducted in Denver, Colorado. Modest zinc supplementation (5.7 mg/d) resulted in increased growth rates compared with placebo.[14] More recently, a number of larger studies in developing countries observed similar results with modest zinc supplementation. A meta-analysis of growth data from zinc intervention trials recently confirmed the widespread occurrence of growth limiting zinc deficiency in young children, especially in developing countries.[15] Although the exact mechanism for the growth-limiting effects of zinc deficiency are not known, recent research indicates that zinc availability affects cell-signaling systems that coordinate the response to the growth-regulating hormone, insulin-like growth factor-1.[16]

Delayed Neurological and Behavioral Development in Young Children. Low maternal zinc nutritional status has been associated with diminished attention in the newborn infant and poorer motor function at 6 months of age. Zinc supplementation has been associated with improved motor development in very low birth weight infants, more vigorous activity in Indian infants and toddlers, and more functional activity in Guatemalan infants and toddlers.[17] Additionally, zinc supplementation was associated with better neuropsychologic functioning (e.g., attention) in Chinese first-grade students, but only when zinc was provided with other micronutrients.[18] Two other studies failed to find an association between zinc supplementation and measures of attention in children diagnosed with growth retardation. Although initial studies suggest that zinc deficiency may depress cognitive development in young children, more controlled research is required to determine the nature of the effect and whether zinc supplementation is beneficial.[19]

Increased Susceptibility to Infectious Disease in Children

Adequate zinc intake is essential in maintaining the integrity of the immune system,[20] and zinc-deficient individuals are known to experience increased susceptibility to a variety of infectious agents.[21]

Diarrhea. It is estimated that diarrheal diseases result in the deaths of over 3 million children in developing countries each year. The adverse effects of zinc deficiency on immune system function are likely to increase the susceptibility of children to infectious diarrhea, and persistent diarrhea contributes to zinc deficiency and malnutrition. Recent research indicates that zinc deficiency may also potentiate the effects of toxins produced by diarrhea-causing bacteria like *Escherichia coli*.[22] Zinc supplementation in combination with oral rehydration therapy has been shown to significantly reduce the duration and severity of acute and persistent childhood diarrhea and to increase survival in a number of randomized controlled trials.[23]

Pneumonia. Zinc supplementation may also reduce the incidence of lower respiratory infections, such as pneumonia. A pooled analysis of a number of studies in developing countries demonstrated a substantial reduction in the prevalence of pneumonia in children supplemented with zinc.[24]

Malaria. Several studies have indicated that zinc supplementation may reduce the incidence of clinical attacks of malaria in children.[25] A placebo-controlled trial in preschool children in Papua, New Guinea, found that zinc supplementation reduced the frequency of health center attendance due to *Plasmodium falciparum* malaria by 38%.[26] Additionally, the number of malaria episodes accompanied by high blood levels of the malaria-causing parasite were reduced by 68%, suggesting that zinc supplementation may be of benefit in preventing more severe episodes of malaria. However, a 6-month trial in more than 700 west African children did not find zinc supplementation to reduce morbidity from *P. falciparum* malaria compared with placebo.[27]

Impaired Immune Response in the Elderly

Age-related declines in immune function are similar to those associated with zinc deficiency, and the elderly represent a group that is vulnerable to mild zinc deficiency. However, the results of zinc supplementation trials on immune function in the elderly have been mixed. Certain aspects of immune function in the elderly have been found to improve with zinc supplementation.[28] For example, a randomized placebo-controlled study in men and women over 65 years of age found that a zinc supplement of 25 mg/d for 3 months increased levels of some circulating immune cells (CD4 T cells and cytotoxic T lymphocytes) compared with placebo.[29] However, other studies have not found zinc supplementation to improve parameters of immune function, indicating that more research is required before any recommendations regarding zinc and immune system response in the elderly can be made.

Pregnancy Complications

It has been estimated that 82% of pregnant women worldwide are likely to have inadequate zinc intakes. Poor maternal zinc nutritional status has been associated with a number of adverse outcomes of pregnancy, including low birth weight, premature delivery, and labor and delivery complications. However, the results of maternal zinc supplementation trials in the United States and developing countries have been mixed.[17] Although some studies have found maternal zinc supplementation to increase birth weight and decrease the likelihood of premature delivery, two recent studies in Peruvian and Bangladeshi women found no difference between zinc supplementation and placebo in the incidence of low birth weight or premature delivery.[30,31] Supplementation studies designed to examine the effect of zinc supplementation on labor and delivery complications have also generated mixed results, though few have been conducted in zinc-deficient populations.[17]

Disease Treatment

Common Cold

The use of zinc lozenges within 24 hours of the onset of cold symptoms and continued every 2 to 3 hours while awake until symptoms resolve has been advocated for reducing the duration of the common cold. At least 10 controlled trials of zinc gluconate lozenges for the treatment of common colds in adults have been published. Five studies found that zinc lozenges reduced the duration of cold symptoms, and five studies found no difference between zinc lozenges and placebo lozenges on the duration or severity of cold symptoms. A recent meta-analysis of published randomized controlled trials on the use of zinc gluconate lozenges in colds found that evidence for their effectiveness in reducing the duration of common colds was still lacking.[32] The only study to examine the use of zinc gluconate lozenges in children (ages 6 to 16 years) found that zinc gluconate lozenges were not effective in treating cold symptoms, although the dose used (50 to 60 mg/d) was considerably less than that used in adults.[33] Two recent studies examined the effect of zinc acetate lozenges on cold symptoms. Although one study found that zinc acetate lozenges (12.8 mg of zinc per lozenge) taken every 2 to 3 hours while awake reduced the duration of overall cold symptoms (4.5 vs. 8.1 days) compared with placebo,[34] another study found zinc acetate lozenges no different than placebo in reducing the duration or severity of cold symptoms.[35] Two controlled trials of zinc nasal spray did not find it to affect the duration or severity of cold symptoms.[36,37]

Despite numerous well-controlled clinical trials, the efficacy of zinc lozenges in treating common cold symptoms remains unclear. The physiologic basis for a beneficial effect of high-dose zinc supplementation on cold symptoms is not known. Taking zinc lozenges every 2 to 3 hours while awake often results in daily zinc intakes well above the tolerable upper intake level (UL) of 40 mg/d. Short-term use of zinc lozenges (e.g., 5 days) has not resulted in serious side effects, though some individuals experienced gastrointestinal disturbances and mouth irritation. Use of zinc lozenges for prolonged periods (e.g., 6 to 8 weeks) is likely to result in copper deficiency. For this reason, some experts have recommended that a person who does not show clear evidence of improvement of cold symptoms after 3 to 5 days of zinc lozenge treatment seek medical evaluation.[34]

Age-Related Macular Degeneration

A leading cause of blindness in people over the age of 65 in the United States is a degenerative disease of the macula, known as age-related macular degeneration (AMD). In the back of the eye, the macula is the portion of the retina involved with central vision. Zinc is hypothe-sized to play a role in the development of AMD for several reasons: (1) zinc is found in high concentrations in the part of the retina affected by AMD, (2) retinal zinc content has been shown to decline with age, and (3) the activity of some zinc-dependent retinal enzymes has been shown to decline with age. However, scientific evidence that zinc intake is associated with the development or progression of AMD is limited. Observational studies have not demonstrated clear associations between dietary zinc intake and the incidence of AMD.[38–40] A randomized controlled trial provoked interest when it found that 200 mg/d of zinc sulfate (81 mg/d of elemental zinc) over 2 years reduced the loss of vision in patients with AMD.[41] However, a later trial using the same dose and duration found no beneficial effect in patients with a more advanced form of AMD in one eye.[42] A large randomized controlled trial of daily antioxidant (500 mg of vitamin C, 400 IU of vitamin E, and 15 mg of beta carotene) and high-dose zinc (80 mg of zinc and 2 mg of copper) supplementation found that the antioxidant combination plus high-dose zinc and high-dose zinc alone significantly reduced the risk of advanced macular degeneration compared with placebo in individuals with moderate to severe signs of the disease in at least one eye.[43] At present, there is little evidence that zinc supplementation would be beneficial to people with early signs of macular degeneration, but further randomized controlled trials are warranted.[44]

Diabetes Mellitus

Moderate zinc deficiency may be relatively common in individuals with diabetes mellitus. Increased urinary zinc excretion appears to contribute to the marginal zinc nutritional status that has been observed in diabetics.[45] Although zinc supplementation has been reported to improve immune function in diabetics, zinc supplementation of 50 mg/d adversely affected control of blood glucose in insulin-dependent diabetics.[46] More recently, supplementation of type 2 diabetics with 30 mg/d of zinc for 6 months reduced a nonspecific measure of oxidative stress (plasma TBARS), without significantly affecting blood glucose control.[47] Presently, the influence of zinc on glucose metabolism requires further study before high-dose zinc supplementation can be advocated for diabetics.[5]

Human Immunodeficiency Virus/Acquired Immune Deficiency Syndrome

Sufficient zinc is essential in maintaining immune system function, and human immunodeficiency virus (HIV)-infected individuals are particularly susceptible to zinc deficiency. Decreased serum zinc levels have been associated with more advanced disease and increased mortality in HIV patients.[48,49] In one of the few zinc supplementation studies conducted in acquired immune deficiency syndrome patients, 45 mg/d of zinc for 1 month resulted in a decreased incidence in opportunistic infections compared with placebo.[50] However, the HIV virus also requires zinc, and excessive zinc intake may stimulate the progression of HIV infection. In an observational study of HIV-infected men, increased zinc intake was associated with more rapid disease progression and any intake of zinc supplements was associated with poorer survival. These results indicate that further research is necessary to determine optimal zinc intakes for HIV-infected individuals.[20]

Sources

Food Sources

Shellfish, beef, and other red meats are rich sources of zinc. Nuts and legumes are relatively good plant sources. Zinc bioavailability (the fraction of zinc retained and used by the body) is relatively high in meat, eggs, and seafood because of the relative absence of compounds that inhibit zinc absorption and the presence of certain amino acids (cysteine and methionine) that improve zinc absorption. The zinc in whole grain products and plant proteins is less bioavailable due to their relatively high content of phytic acid, a compound that inhibits zinc absorption.[5] The enzymatic action of yeast reduces the level of phytic acid in foods. Therefore, leavened whole grain breads have more bioavailable zinc than unleavened

Table 27–2   Food Sources of Zinc

Food	Serving	Zinc, mg
Oysters	6 medium, cooked	43.4
Beef	3 ounces,* cooked	5.8
Crab, Dungeness	3 ounces,* cooked	4.6
Turkey, dark meat	3 ounces,* cooked	3.5
Chicken, dark meat	3 ounces,* cooked	2.4
Pork	3 ounces,* cooked	2.2
Beans, baked	1/2 cup	1.8
Yogurt, fruit	1 cup (8 ounces)	1.8
Cashews	1 ounce	1.6
Chickpeas (garbanzo beans)	1/2 cup	1.3
Milk	1 cup (8 ounces)	1.0
Almonds	1 ounce	1.0
Cheese, cheddar	1 ounce	0.9
Peanuts	1 ounce	0.9

*A 3-ounce serving of meat or fish is about the size of a deck of cards.

whole grain breads. Recently, national dietary surveys in the United States estimated that the average dietary zinc intake was 9 mg/d for adult women and 13 mg/d for adult men.[4] The zinc content of some relatively zinc-rich foods is listed in milligrams in Table 27–2.

Supplements

A number of zinc supplements are available, including zinc acetate (30% elemental zinc), zinc gluconate (14% elemental zinc), zinc picolinate (35% elemental zinc), and zinc sulfate (23% elemental zinc). If not stated otherwise, all of the zinc doses discussed in this presentation represent elemental zinc. Zinc picolinate has been promoted as a more absorbable form of zinc, but there is little data to support this idea in humans. Limited work in animals suggests that increased intestinal absorption of zinc picolinate may be offset by increased elimination.[4]

Safety

Toxicity

Acute Toxicity. Isolated outbreaks of acute zinc toxicity have occurred as a result of the consumption of food or beverages contaminated with zinc released from galvanized containers. Signs of acute zinc toxicity are abdominal pain, diarrhea, nausea, and vomiting. Single doses of 225 to 450 mg of zinc usually induce vomiting. Milder gastrointestinal distress has been reported at doses of 50 to 150 mg/d of supplemental zinc. Metal fume fever has been reported after the inhalation of zinc oxide fumes. Profuse sweating, weakness, and rapid breathing may develop within 8 hours of zinc oxide inhalation and persist 12 to 24 hours after exposure is terminated.[4,5]

Chronic Toxicity. The major consequence of long-term consumption of excessive zinc is copper deficiency. Total zinc intakes of 60 mg/d (50 mg supplemental and 10 mg dietary zinc) have been found to result in signs of copper deficiency. To prevent copper deficiency, the Food and Nutrition Board of the Institute of Medicine recently set the upper level (UL) for adults at 40 mg/d, including dietary and supplemental zinc (Table 27–3).[4]

Drug Interactions

Concomitant administration of zinc supplements and certain antibiotics, specifically tetracyclines and quinolones, may decrease absorption of the antibiotic with potential reduction of its efficacy. Taking zinc supplements and these antibiotics at least 2 hours apart should prevent this interaction.[51] The therapeutic use of metal-chelating (binding) agents like penicillamine (used to treat copper overload in Wilson's disease) and diethylenetriamine pentaacetate or (DTPA) (used to treat iron overload) has resulted in severe zinc deficiency. Anticonvulsant drugs, especially sodium valproate, may also precipitate zinc deficiency. Prolonged use of diuretics may increase urinary zinc excretion, resulting in increased loss of zinc. The tuberculosis medication ethambutol has metal-chelating proper-

Table 27–3 Tolerable Upper Intake Level (UL) for Zinc

Life Stage	Age	UL, mg/d
Infants	0–6 months	4
Infants	6–12 months	5
Children	1–3 years	7
Children	4–8 years	12
Children	9–13 years	23
Adolescents	14–18 years	34
Adults	19 years and older	40

ties and has been shown to increase zinc loss in rats.[5]

LPI Recommendation

The RDA for zinc (8 mg/d for adult women and 11 mg/d for adult men) appears sufficient to prevent deficiency in most individuals, but the lack of sensitive indicators of zinc nutritional status in humans makes it difficult to determine the level of zinc intake most likely to promote optimum health. Following the Linus Pauling Institute recommendation to take a multivitamin/multimineral supplement containing 100 % of the daily values of most nutrients will generally provide 15 mg/d in of zinc in addition to that in foods.

Older Adults

Although the requirement for zinc is not known to be higher for adults over the age of 65, their average zinc intake tends to be considerably less than the RDA. A reduced capacity to absorb zinc, increased likelihood of disease states that alter zinc utilization, and increased use of drugs that increase zinc excretion may contribute to an increased risk of mild zinc deficiency in older adults. Because the consequences of mild zinc deficiency, such as impaired immune system function, are particularly relevant to the health of older adults, they should pay particular attention to maintaining adequate zinc intake.

References

1. Prasad AS, Halsted JA, Nadimi M. Syndrome of iron deficiency anemia, hepatosplenomegaly, hypogonadism, dwarfism, and geophagia. *Am J Med* 1961;31:532–546.
2. Prasad AS. Zinc deficiency in humans: a neglected problem. *J Am Coll Nutr* 1998;17(6):542–543.
3. Cousins RJ. Zinc. In: Ziegler EE, Filer LJ, eds. *Present Knowledge in Nutrition*. Washington, D.C.: ILSI Press; 1996:293–306.
4. Food and Nutrition Board, Institute of Medicine. Zinc. *Dietary Reference Intakes for Vitamin A, Vitamin K, Boron, Chromium, Copper, Iodine, Iron, Manganese, Molybdenum, Nickel, Silicon, Vanadium, and Zinc*. Washington, D.C.: National Academy Press; 2001:442–501.
5. King JC, Keen CL. Zinc. In: Shils M, Olson JA, Shike M, Ross AC, eds. *Nutrition in Health and Disease*, 9th ed. Baltimore: Williams & Wilkins; 1999:223–239.
6. O'Dell BL. Role of zinc in plasma membrane function. *J Nutr* 2000;130(5S Suppl):1432S–1436S.
7. Truong-Tran AQ, Ho LH, Chai F, Zalewski PD. Cellular zinc fluxes and the regulation of apoptosis/gene-directed cell death. *J Nutr* 2000;130(5S Suppl):1459S–1466S.
8. O'Brien KO, Zavaleta N, Caulfield LE, Wen J, Abrams SA. Prenatal iron supplements impair zinc absorption in pregnant Peruvian women. *J Nutr* 2000;130(9):2251–2255.
9. Fung EB, Ritchie LD, Woodhouse LR, Roehl R, King JC. Zinc absorption in women during pregnancy and lactation: a longitudinal study. *Am J Clin Nutr* 1997;66(1):80–88.
10. Wood RJ, Zheng JJ. High dietary calcium intakes reduce zinc absorption and balance in humans. *Am J Clin Nutr* 1997;65(6):1803–1809.
11. McKenna AA, Ilich JZ, Andon MB, Wang C, Matkovic V. Zinc balance in adolescent females consuming a low- or high-calcium diet. *Am J Clin Nutr* 1997;65(5):1460–1464.
12. Kauwell GP, Bailey LB, Gregory JF, 3rd, Bowling DW, Cousins RJ. Zinc status is not adversely affected by folic acid supplementation and zinc intake does not impair folate utilization in human subjects. *J Nutr* 1995;125(1):66–72.
13. Hambidge M. Human zinc deficiency. *J Nutr* 2000;130(5S Suppl):1344S–1349S.
14. Walravens PA, Hambidge KM, Koepfer DM. Zinc supplementation in infants with a nutritional pattern of failure to thrive: a double-blind, controlled study. *Pediatrics* 1989;83(4):532–538.
15. Hambidge M, Krebs N. Zinc and growth. In: Roussel AM, ed. *Trace Elements in Man and Animals 10: Proceedings of the Tenth International Symposium on Trace Elements in Man and Animals*. New York: Plenum Press; 2000:977–980.
16. MacDonald RS. The role of zinc in growth and cell proliferation. *J Nutr* 2000;130(5S Suppl):1500S–1508S.
17. Caulfield LE, Zavaleta N, Shankar AH, Merialdi M. Potential contribution of maternal zinc supplementation during pregnancy to maternal and child survival. *Am J Clin Nutr* 1998;68(2 Suppl):499S–508S.
18. Sandstead HH, Penland JG, Alcock NW, et al. Effects of repletion with zinc and other micronutrients on neu-
ropsychologic performance and growth of Chinese children. *Am J Clin Nutr* 1998;68(2 Suppl):470S–475S.
19. Black MM. Zinc deficiency and child development. *Am J Clin Nutr* 1998;68(2 Suppl):464S–469S.
20. Baum MK, Shor-Posner G, Campa A. Zinc status in human immunodeficiency virus infection. *J Nutr* 2000;130(5S Suppl):1421S–1423S.
21. Shankar AH, Prasad AS. Zinc and immune function: the biological basis of altered resistance to infection. *Am J Clin Nutr* 1998;68(2 Suppl):447S–463S.
22. Wapnir RA. Zinc deficiency, malnutrition and the gastrointestinal tract. *J Nutr* 2000;130(5S Suppl):1388S–1392S.
23. Bhutta ZA, Bird SM, Black RE, et al. Therapeutic effects of oral zinc in acute and persistent diarrhea in children in developing countries: pooled analysis of randomized controlled trials. *Am J Clin Nutr* 2000;72(6):1516–1522.
24. Bhutta ZA, Black RE, Brown KH, et al. Prevention of diarrhea and pneumonia by zinc supplementation in children in developing countries: pooled analysis of randomized controlled trials. Zinc Investigators' Collaborative Group. *J Pediatr* 1999;135(6):689–697.
25. Black RE. Therapeutic and preventive effects of zinc on serious childhood infectious diseases in developing countries. *Am J Clin Nutr* 1998;68(2 Suppl):476S–479S.
26. Shankar AH. Nutritional modulation of malaria morbidity and mortality. *J Infect Dis* 2000;182(Suppl 1):S37–S53.
27. Muller O, Becher H, van Zweeden AB, et al. Effect of zinc supplementation on malaria and other causes of morbidity in west African children: randomised double blind placebo controlled trial. *BMJ* 2001;322(7302):1567.
28. Salgueiro MJ, Zubillaga M, Lysionek A, et al. Zinc status and immune system relationship: a review. *Biol Trace Elem Res* 2000;76(3):193–205.
29. Fortes C, Forastiere F, Agabiti N, et al. The effect of zinc and vitamin A supplementation on immune response in an older population. *J Am Geriatr Soc* 1998;46(1):19–26.
30. Caulfield LE, Zavaleta N, Figueroa A, Leon Z. Maternal zinc supplementation does not affect size at birth or pregnancy duration in Peru. *J Nutr* 1999;129(8):1563–1568.
31. Osendarp SJ, van Raaij JM, Arifeen SE, Wahed M, Baqui AH, Fuchs GJ. A randomized, placebo-controlled trial of the effect of zinc supplementation during pregnancy on pregnancy outcome in Bangladeshi urban poor. *Am J Clin Nutr* 2000;71(1):114–119.
32. Jackson JL, Lesho E, Peterson C. Zinc and the common cold: a meta-analysis revisited. *J Nutr* 2000;130(5S Suppl):1512S–1515S.
33. Macknin ML, Piedmonte M, Calendine C, Janosky J, Wald E. Zinc gluconate lozenges for treating the common cold in children: a randomized controlled trial. *JAMA* 1998;279(24):1962–1967.
34. Prasad AS, Fitzgerald JT, Bao B, Beck FW, Chandrasekar PH. Duration of symptoms and plasma cytokine levels in patients with the common cold treated with zinc acetate: a randomized, double-blind, placebo-controlled trial. *Ann Intern Med* 2000;133(4):245–252.
35. Turner RB, Cetnarowski WE. Effect of treatment with zinc gluconate or zinc acetate on experimental and natural colds. *Clin Infect Dis* 2000;31(5):1202–1208.

36. Turner RB. Ineffectiveness of intranasal zinc gluconate for prevention of experimental rhinovirus colds. *Clin Infect Dis* 2001;33(11):1865–1870.

37. Belongia EA, Berg R, Liu K. A randomized trial of zinc nasal spray for the treatment of upper respiratory illness in adults. *Am J Med* 2001;111(2):103–108.

38. VandenLangenberg GM, Mares-Perlman JA, Klein R, Klein BE, Brady WE, Palta M. Associations between antioxidant and zinc intake and the 5-year incidence of early age-related maculopathy in the Beaver Dam Eye Study. *Am J Epidemiol* 1998;148(2):204–214.

39. Smith W, Mitchell P, Webb K, Leeder SR. Dietary antioxidants and age-related maculopathy: the Blue Mountains Eye Study. *Ophthalmology* 1999;106(4):761–767.

40. Cho E, Stampfer MJ, Seddon JM, et al. Prospective study of zinc intake and the risk of age-related macular degeneration. *Ann Epidemiol* 2001;11(5):328–336.

41. Newsome DA, Swartz M, Leone NC, Elston RC, Miller E. Oral zinc in macular degeneration. *Arch Ophthalmol* 1988;106(2):192–198.

42. Stur M, Tittl M, Reitner A, Meisinger V. Oral zinc and the second eye in age-related macular degeneration. *Invest Ophthalmol Vis Sci* 1996;37(7):1225–1235.

43. A randomized, placebo-controlled, clinical trial of high-dose supplementation with vitamins C and E, beta carotene, and zinc for age-related macular degeneration and vision loss: AREDS report no. 8. *Arch Ophthalmol* 2001;119(10):1417–1436.

44. Evans JR. Antioxidant vitamin and mineral supplements for age-related macular degeneration (Cochrane Review). *Cochrane Database Syst Rev* 2002(1):CD000254.

45. Blostein-Fujii A, DiSilvestro RA, Frid D, Katz C, Malarkey W. Short-term zinc supplementation in women with non-insulin-dependent diabetes mellitus: effects on plasma 5'-nucleotidase activities, insulin-like growth factor I concentrations, and lipoprotein oxidation rates in vitro. *Am J Clin Nutr* 1997;66(3):639–642.

46. Cunningham JJ, Fu A, Mearkle PL, Brown RG. Hyperzincuria in individuals with insulin-dependent diabetes mellitus: concurrent zinc status and the effect of high-dose zinc supplementation. *Metabolism* 1994;43(12):1558–1562.

47. Anderson RA, Roussel AM, Zouari N, Mahjoub S, Matheau JM, Kerkeni A. Potential antioxidant effects of zinc and chromium supplementation in people with type 2 diabetes mellitus. *J Am Coll Nutr* 2001;20(3):212–218.

48. Lai H, Lai S, Shor-Posner G, Ma F, Trapido E, Baum MK. Plasma zinc, copper, copper:zinc ratio, and survival in a cohort of HIV-1-infected homosexual men. *J Acquir Immune Defic Syndr* 2001;27(1):56–62.

49. Wellinghausen N, Kern WV, Jochle W, Kern P. Zinc serum level in human immunodeficiency virus-infected patients in relation to immunological status. *Biol Trace Elem Res* 2000;73(2):139–149.

50. Mocchegiani E, Muzzioli M. Therapeutic application of zinc in human immunodeficiency virus against opportunistic infections. *J Nutr* 2000;130(5S Suppl):1424S–1431S.

51. Minerals. *Drug Facts and Comparisons*. St. Louis: Facts and Comparisons; 2000:27–51.

Appendix 1

Nutrient–Nutrient Interactions

Nutrient	Nutrient	Interaction
Biotin	Pantothenic acid	High doses of pantothenic acid may compete with biotin for absorption
Folic acid	Vitamin B_{12}	Works synergistically with folate to lower homocysteine levels
	Vitamin B_6	Works synergistically with folate to lower homocysteine levels
Niacin	Tryptophan	Niacin can be synthesized from tryptophan, reducing the dietary niacin requirement
Pantothenic acid	Biotin	High doses of pantothenic acid may compete with biotin for absorption
Riboflavin	Vitamin B_6	Riboflavin deficiency may decrease conversion of vitamin B_6 to its coenzyme form
	Niacin	Riboflavin deficiency may increase the risk of niacin deficiency by decreasing niacin synthesis from tryptophan
	Folic acid	Works synergistically with folate to lower homocysteine levels
	Iron	Riboflavin deficiency may impair iron absorption or utilization
Vitamin A	Zinc	Zinc deficiency may interfere with vitamin A metabolism
	Iron	Vitamin A deficiency may exacerbate iron deficiency
Vitamin B_6	Folic acid	Works synergistically with vitamin B_6 to lower homocysteine levels
	Vitamin B_{12}	Works synergistically with vitamin B_6 to lower homocysteine levels
Vitamin B_{12}	Folic acid	Works synergistically with vitamin B_{12} to lower homocysteine levels
		High-dose folic acid therapy may mask the symptoms of vitamin B_{12} deficiency
	Vitamin B_6	Works synergistically with vitamin B_{12} to lower homocysteine levels
Vitamin C	Vitamin E	Vitamin C may regenerate vitamin E
	Iron	Concomitant intake increases the absorption of non-heme iron

Nutrient	Nutrient	Interaction
Vitamin D	Calcium	Active form of vitamin D increases intestinal calcium absorption and decreases urinary calcium excretion
Vitamin E	Vitamin C	Vitamin C may regenerate vitamin E
Vitamin K	Vitamin A	High doses of vitamin A may decrease vitamin K absorption
	Vitamin E	High doses of vitamin E may inhibit activity of vitamin K–dependent enzymes, resulting in functional vitamin K deficiency
Calcium	Vitamin D	Active form of vitamin D increases intestinal calcium absorption and decreases urinary calcium excretion
	Iron	Concomitant intake decreases nonheme iron absorption
	Sodium	Increases urinary calcium excretion
	Protein	Increases urinary calcium excretion
	Zinc	High calcium intakes may decrease zinc absorption
Chromium	Vitamin C	Concomitant intake may enhance the absorption of chromium
Copper	Iron	Copper deficiency may interfere with iron transport
		High-iron formula may decrease infant copper absorption
	Zinc	High supplemental zinc intakes may cause copper deficiency by decreasing intestinal copper absorption
Fluoride	Calcium	Concomitant intake of calcium may decrease absorption of sodium fluoride
	Magnesium	Concomitant intake of magnesium may decrease absorption of sodium fluoride
Iodine	Selenium	Selenium deficiency can exacerbate the effects of iodine deficiency
Iron	Vitamin A	Vitamin A deficiency may exacerbate iron deficiency
	Vitamin C	Concomitant intake increases nonheme iron absorption
	Calcium	Concomitant intake decreases nonheme iron absorption
	Copper	Copper deficiency may interfere with iron transport
		High-iron formula may decrease infant copper absorption
	Magnesium	Concomitant intake may decrease nonheme iron absorption
	Manganese	Concomitant iron intake may decrease manganese absorption
		Manganese absorption is increased in iron-deficient individuals
	Zinc	Supplemental doses of iron may decrease zinc absorption

Nutrient	Nutrient	Interaction
Magnesium	Iron	Concomitant intake may decrease nonheme iron absorption
	Manganese	Supplemental magnesium may decrease manganese absorption
	Zinc	High-dose zinc supplement intake may decrease magnesium absorption
Manganese	Calcium	Concomitant intake may decrease manganese absorption
	Magnesium	Supplemental magnesium may decrease manganese absorption
	Iron	Concomitant iron intake may decrease manganese absorption
		Manganese absorption is increased in iron-deficient individuals
Phosphorus	Potassium	Taking potassium supplements together with phosphates may cause hyperkalemia
Selenium	Vitamin C	Selenium-dependent enzymes catalyze the regeneration of vitamin C and function synergistically in antioxidant system
	Vitamin E	Selenium-dependent enzymes function synergistically in antioxidant system
	Iodine	Selenium deficiency can exacerbate the effects of iodine deficiency
Zinc	Calcium	High calcium intakes may decrease zinc absorption
	Copper	High supplemental zinc intakes may cause copper deficiency by decreasing intestinal copper absorption
	Iron	Supplemental doses of iron may decrease zinc absorption

Appendix 2

Drug–Nutrient Interactions

Drug classes are listed first, alphabetically, followed by specific drugs known to act with specific nutrients. Because there may be drug–nutrient interactions that are not listed in the table below, it is important to review the prescribing or patient information of any medication prior to its use for the possibility of clinically significant drug–nutrient interactions. This table does not address the potential for multiple drug–nutrient interactions in individuals taking more than one medication. *Note*: Medications that increase the risk of hyperkalemia and hypokalemia are listed in Tables 24–3 and 24–4, respectively. Medications that increase the risk of hyponatremia are listed in Table 26–4.

Drug Class	Nutrient	Interaction
Antacids	Copper	High doses may decrease copper absorption
	Fluoride	Concomitant intake may decrease fluoride absorption
	Iron	May decrease iron absorption
	Manganese	Concomitant intake of magnesium-containing antacids may decrease manganese absorption
	Phosphorus	Aluminum-containing antacids decrease phosphate absorption and may cause hypophosphatemia in high doses
Antibiotics	Biotin	Prolonged use of broad-spectrum antibiotics may decrease biotin synthesis by intestinal bacteria
	Vitamin K	Prolonged use of broad-spectrum antibiotics may decrease vitamin K synthesis by intestinal bacteria
		Cephalosporins may decrease vitamin K recycling
	Calcium	Concomitant use of calcium and quinolone or tetracycline classes of antibiotics may decrease antibiotic absorption
	Iron	Concomitant intake of iron supplements may decrease the efficacy of quinolone and tetracycline classes of antibiotics
	Magnesium	Concomitant intake of magnesium supplements may decrease the absorption of nitrofurantoin and quinolone and tetracycline classes of antibiotics
	Manganese	Concomitant intake of manganese and tetracycline classes of antibiotics may decrease manganese absorption
	Zinc	Concomitant intake of zinc supplements may decrease the efficacy of quinolone and tetracycline classes of antibiotics
Anticonvulsants	Biotin	Long-term therapy may increase dietary biotin requirement

Drug Class	Nutrient	Interaction
Anticonvulsants (continued)	Folic acid	May interfere with dietary folate absorption
	Riboflavin	Long-term therapy may increase riboflavin requirement by increasing hepatic metabolism
	Thiamin	Long-term therapy may increase dietary thiamin requirement
	Vitamin B_6	High doses of vitamin B_6 may decrease the efficacy of the anticonvulsants phenobarbitol and phenytoin
	Vitamin D	May decrease plasma levels of calcidiol
	Vitamin E	May decrease plasma levels of vitamin E
	Vitamin K	May increase the risk of neonatal vitamin K deficiency and hemorrhagic disease of the newborn when taken by pregnant women
	Selenium	Valproic acid use may decrease plasma selenium levels
	Zinc	Anticonvulsant use, especially valproic acid, may precipitate zinc deficiency
Anitplatelet drugs	Vitamin E	High doses of vitamin E may potentiate antiplatelet effects
Bisphosphonates	Calcium	Concomitant intake may decrease bisphosphonate absorption
	Iron	Concomitant intake of iron supplements may decrease bisphosphonate absorption
	Magnesium	Concomitant intake may decrease bisphosphonate absorption
	Zinc	Concomitant intake may decrease bisphosphonate and zinc absorption
Calcium channel blockers	Calcium	Calcium supplements may decrease the efficacy of calcium channel blockers
Diuretics	Thiamin	Loop diuretics may increase urinary thiamin excretion
	Calcium	Thiazide diuretics increase renal reabsorption of calcium
	Magnesium	Prolonged high doses of diuretics may result in magnesium depletion
	Phosphorus	Taking potassium-sparing diuretics together with phosphates may cause hyperkalemia
	Zinc	May increase urinary zinc excretion
H_2-receptor antagonists	Vitamin B_{12}	May decrease the absorption of food-bound but not supplemental vitamin B_{12}
	Calcium	May decrease the absorption of calcium salts (supplements)
	Iron	May decrease iron absorption

Drug Class	Nutrient	Interaction
Nonsteroidal anti-inflammatory drugs	Folic acid	High doses may interfere with folate metabolism
Oral contraceptives (estrogen-containing)	Pantothenic acid	May increase pantothenic acid requirement
	Vitamin C	May decrease plasma and leukocyte vitamin C levels
Phenothiazine derivatives	Riboflavin	May inhibit the incorporation of riboflavin into active coenzymes flavin adenine dinucleotide (FAD) and flavin mononucleotide (FMN)
	Magnesium	Magnesium supplements may decrease the efficacy of chlorpromazine
Proton pump inhibitors	Vitamin B_{12}	May decrease the absorption of food-bound but not supplemental vitamin B_{12}
	Calcium	May decrease the absorption of calcium salts (supplements)
	Iron	May decrease iron absorption
Retinoid drugs	Vitamin A	Supplemental vitamin A may add to the risk of toxicity of retinoid drugs
Tricyclic antidepressants	Riboflavin	May inhibit the incorporation of riboflavin into active coenzymes FAD and FMN

Specific Drug	Nutrient	Interaction
Alcohol	Vitamin A	Chronic alcohol consumption increases the risk of vitamin A–induced hepatotoxicity
Allopurinol	Iron	May increase iron storage in the liver; should not be used in combination with iron supplements
Aspirin	Vitamin C	High doses of aspirin may increase urinary excretion of vitamin C
	Vitamin K	May decrease vitamin K recycling
	Vitamin E	High doses of vitamin E may potentiate antiplatelet effects
Calcitriol	Phosphorus	High doses of calcitriol and some vitamin D analogs may cause hyperphosphatemia
Chloramphenicol	Vitamin B_{12}	May decrease the absorption of food-bound but not supplemental vitamin B_{12}
Cholestyramine and colestipol	Most vitamins and minerals	May decrease vitamin and mineral absorption when taken concomitantly
Colchicine	Vitamin B_{12}	May decrease the absorption of food-bound but not supplemental vitamin B_{12}
Cycloserine	Vitamin B_6	May cause functional vitamin B_6 deficiency by forming inactive complex with vitamin B_6

Specific Drug	Nutrient	Interaction
Digoxin	Calcium	High doses of supplemental calcium may increase the risk of arrhythmia
	Magnesium	Concomitant use may decrease the absorption of digoxin
Diethylenetri-amine pen-taacetate (DTPA)	Zinc	Treatment with DTPA has resulted in severe zinc deficiency
Doxorubicin (adri-amycin)	Riboflavin	May inhibit the incorporation of riboflavin into active coenzymes FAD and FMN
5-Fluorouracil (5-FU)	Niacin	Long-term therapy has resulted in niacin deficiency
	Thiamin	5-FU decreases phosphorylation of thiamin to its active form
	Iron	May decrease iron absorption
Isoniazid	Niacin	Niacin antagonist; niacin supplementation is recommended during long-term isoniazid treatment
	Vitamin B_6	May cause functional vitamin B_6 deficiency by forming inactive complex with vitamin B_6
	Vitamin E	May decrease absorption of vitamin E
	Vitamin K	May increase the risk of vitamin K deficiency and hemorrhagic disease of the newborn when taken by pregnant women
Ketoconazole (oral)	Vitamin D	May decrease blood levels of calcitriol, the active form of vitamin D
Levodopa	Vitamin B_6	May cause functional vitamin B_6 deficiency by forming inactive complex with vitamin B_6
		High doses of vitamin B_6 may decrease the efficacy of levodopa
	Iron	Concomitant intake of iron supplements may decrease the efficacy of levodopa
Levothyroxine	Calcium	Concomitant intake may decrease levothyroxine absorption
	Iron	Concomitant intake of iron supplements may decrease the efficacy of levothyroxine
Lithium	Iodine	Concomitant use of lithium and pharmacologic doses of potassium iodide may result in hypothyroidism
Lovastatin	Niacin	Coadministration of pharmacologic doses of nicotinic acid and lovastatin has resulted in cases of rhabdomyolysis
Metformin	Vitamin B_{12}	Decreases vitamin B_{12} absorption; may be corrected by taking vitamin B_{12} supplements with milk or calcium supplements

Specific Drug	Nutrient	Interaction
Methyldopa	Iron	Concomitant intake of iron supplements may decrease the efficacy of methyldopa
Methotrexate	Folic acid	Folate antagonist; may require folic acid supplementation during methotrexate therapy
Neomycin	Vitamin B_{12}	May decrease the absorption of food-bound but not supplemental vitamin B_{12}
Nitrous oxide	Vitamin B_{12}	Inhalation of nitrous oxide may result in functional vitamin B_{12} deficiency
Olestra	Fat-soluble vitamins	Inhibits the absorption of fat-soluble vitamins; vitamins A, D, E, and K are added to olestra for this reason
Orlistat	Fat-soluble vitamins	May decrease the absorption of fat-soluble vitamins (vitamins A, D, E, and K); take orlistat and vitamin supplements at least 2 hours apart
Penicillamine	Vitamin B_6	May cause functional vitamin B_6 deficiency by forming inactive complex with vitamin B_6
	Copper	Increases urinary excretion of copper; used to treat copper overload in Wilson's disease
	Iron	Concomitant intake of iron supplements may decrease the efficacy of penicillamine
	Magnesium	Concomitant intake may decrease the efficacy of penicillamine
	Zinc	Treatment with penicillamine has resulted in severe zinc deficiency
Pyrimethamine	Folic acid	Folate antagonist; may increase folate requirement
Quinocrine	Riboflavin	May inhibit the incorporation of riboflavin into active coenzymes FAD and FMN
Rifampin	Vitamin K	May increase the risk of vitamin K deficiency and hemorrhagic disease of the newborn when taken by pregnant women
Sucralfate	Vitamin E	May decrease vitamin E absorption
Sulfasalazine	Folic acid	Folate antagonist; may increase folate requirement
	Vitamin K	May decrease vitamin K recycling
Sulfinpyrazone	Niacin	Nicotinic acid may decrease the uricosuric effect of sulfinpyrazone
Triamterene	Folic acid	Folate antagonist; may increase folate requirement
Trimethoprim	Folic acid	Folate antagonist; may increase folate requirement
Warfarin	Vitamin C	High doses of vitamin C have been reported to decrease anticoagulant efficacy in a few cases
	Vitamin E	High doses of vitamin E may potentiate anticoagulant effects
	Vitamin K	High intake of dietary or supplemental vitamin K may decrease anticoagulant efficacy

Specific Drug	Nutrient	Interaction
Warfarin (continued)	Vitamin K (continued)	May increase the risk of neonatal vitamin K deficiency and hemorrhagic disease of the newborn when taken by pregnant women
	Iodine	Pharmacologic doses of potassium iodide may decrease the anticoagulant efficacy of warfarin
	Magnesium	Magnesium-containing antacids may decrease the anticoagulant efficacy of warfarin

Appendix 3

Quick Reference to Diseases

Disease	Chapter Section	Nutrient	Pages
Alzheimer's disease	Prevention	Folic acid	11
		Vitamin B_{12}	61
	Treatment	Thiamin	35
		Vitamin E	85–86
Asthma	Treatment	Magnesium	153
Autoimmune disease	Treatment	Vitamin D	78
Cancer (general)	Prevention	Folic acid	10–11
		Niacin	17–18
		Vitamin B_{12}	59–60
		Vitamin C	66–67
		Vitamin E	84
		Selenium	182–183
	Treatment	Thiamin	36
		Vitamin C	68
Breast cancer	Prevention	Folic acid	11
		Vitamin A	43
		Vitamin D	77
Colorectal cancer	Prevention	Folic acid	11
		Vitamin D	77
		Calcium	100
Gastric cancer	Prevention	Sodium chloride	191
Gastroesophageal cancer	Prevention	Molybdenum	164
Leukemia (acute promyelotic)	Treatment	Vitamin A	43
Lung cancer	Prevention	Vitamin A	42–43
Prostate cancer	Prevention	Vitamin D	77
	Treatment	Vitamin D	78
	Safety	Calcium	105–106
Thyroid cancer	Prevention	Iodine	133
Cardiovascular diseases	Prevention	Folic acid	10
		Vitamin B_6	49
		Vitamin B_{12}	59
		Vitamin C	66
		Vitamin E	83–84
		Vitamin K	94
		Chromium	111

Disease	Chapter Section	Nutrient	Pages
Cardiovascular diseases	Prevention	Copper	118–119
		Magnesium	150
		Selenium	183–184
	Treatment	Vitamin C	68
		Vitamin E	84–85
		Magnesium	151–152
Carpal tunnel syndrome	Treatment	Vitamin B_6	52
Cataracts	Prevention	Riboflavin	29–30
		Vitamin C	67
		Vitamin E	84
Common cold	Treatment	Vitamin C	69
		Zinc	200–201
Congestive heart failure	Treatment	Thiamin	35–36
Dementia	Prevention	Folic acid	11
		Vitamin B_6	50–51
		Vitamin B_{12}	61
	Treatment	Vitamin E	85–86
Dental caries (cavities)	Prevention	Fluoride	124
Depression	Prevention	Vitamin B_{12}	61
	Treatment	Vitamin B_6	51
Diabetes mellitus			
Type I (IDDM)	Prevention	Niacin	18
	Treatment	Biotin	3
		Zinc	201–202
Type II (NIDDM)	Prevention	Chromium	111
		Manganese	159
	Treatment	Biotin	3
		Vitamin C	68–69
		Vitamin E	85
		Chromium	112
		Magnesium	152
		Zinc	201–202
Growth/developmental delays	Prevention	Iron	140
		Zinc	199
HIV/AIDS	Treatment	Niacin	19
		Selenium	184
		Zinc	202
Hypercholesterolemia	Treatment	Niacin	18–19
		Pantothenic acid	24–25
Hypertension	Prevention	Magnesium	150
	Treatment	Vitamin C	68
		Calcium	102–103
	Treatment	Magnesium	150
		Potassium	175
		Sodium chloride	192–193

Disease	Chapter Section	Nutrient	Pages
Immunity, impaired	Prevention	Vitamin B$_6$	50
		Vitamin E	84
		Copper	119
		Iron	141
		Selenium	182
		Zinc	199–200
Kidney stones (nephrolithiasis)	Prevention	Vitamin B$_6$	51
		Calcium	101
		Potassium	174
		Sodium chloride	192
Lead toxicity	Prevention	Vitamin C	67
		Calcium	102
		Iron	140
Macular degeneration	Treatment	Zinc	201
Migraine	Treatment	Riboflavin	30
		Magnesium	153
Osteoporosis	Prevention	Vitamin D	76–77
		Vitamin K	93–94
		Calcium	100–101
		Copper	120
		Fluoride	124–125
		Manganese	158–159
		Potassium	174
		Sodium chloride	191–192
	Treatment	Vitamin D	78
		Fluoride	125
		Magnesium	152
Pregnancy complications (general)	Prevention	Iron	140–141
		Zinc	200
Gestational diabetes	Treatment	Chromium	112
Morning sickness	Treatment	Vitamin B$_6$	52
Neural tube defects	Prevention	Folic acid	8–9
		Vitamin B$_{12}$	60–61
Other birth defects	Prevention	Biotin	2–3
		Folic acid	10
Preeclampsia-eclampsia	Prevention	Calcium	101–102
	Treatment	Magnesium	151
Premenstrual syndrome	Treatment	Vitamin B$_6$	51
Restless legs syndrome	Treatment	Iron	141
Seizure disorders (epilepsy)	Prevention	Manganese	159
Stroke	Prevention	Potassium	173–174
		Vitamin C	66

Appendix 4

Glossary

Acetylation: the addition of an acetyl group (–COCH3) group to a molecule.

Acidic: having a pH of less than 7.

Acute: having a short and relatively severe course.

Adjunct: assisting in the prevention, amelioration, or cure of a disease.

Adrenal glands: a pair of small glands, located above the kidneys, consisting of an outer cortex and inner medulla. The adrenal cortex secretes cortisone-related hormones and the adrenal medulla secretes epinephrine (adrenaline) and norepinephrine (noradrenaline).

AI: adequate intake, set by the Food and Nutrition Board of the Institute of Medicine; a recommended intake value based on observed or experimentally determined approximations or estimates of nutrient intake by a group of healthy people that are assumed to be adequate. The AI is used when the recommended dietary allowance (RDA) cannot be determined.

AIDS: acquired immune deficiency syndrome. AIDS is caused by the human immunodeficiency virus (HIV), which attacks the immune system leaving the infected individual vulnerable to opportunistic infection.

Alkaline: basic; having a pH of more than 7.

Allele: one of a set of alternative forms of a gene. Diploid cells possess two homologous chromosomes (one derived from each parent) and therefore two copies of each gene. In a diploid cell, a gene will have two alleles, each occupying the same position on homologous chromosomes.

Alzheimer's disease: a neurological condition characterized by the degeneration of brain cells. Symptoms include memory loss, confusion, and physical decline. Alzheimer's disease usually occurs later in life and worsens over time.

Amino acids: organic (carbon-containing) molecules that serve as the building blocks of proteins.

Anaerobic: refers to the absence of oxygen or the absence of a need for oxygen.

Analog: a chemical compound that is structurally similar to another but differs slightly in composition (e.g., the replacement of one functional group by another).

Anaphylaxis: a rapidly developing and severe systemic allergic reaction. Symptoms may include swelling of the tongue, throat, and trachea, which can result in difficulty breathing, shock, and loss of consciousness. If not treated rapidly, anaphylaxis can be fatal.

Anemia: the condition of having less than the normal number of red blood cells or hemoglobin in the blood, resulting in diminished oxygen transport. Anemia has many causes, including: iron, vitamin B_{12}, or folate deficiency; bleeding; abnormal hemoglobin formation (e.g., sickle cell anemia); rupture of red blood cells (hemolytic anemia); and bone marrow diseases.

Anencephaly: a birth defect, known as a neural tube defect, resulting from failure of the upper end of the neural tube to close during embryonic development. Anencephaly is a devastating and generally fatal birth defect resulting in the absence of most or all of the cerebral hemispheres of the brain.

Angina pectoris: pain generally experienced in the chest, but sometimes radiating to the arms or jaw, due to a lack of oxygen supply to the heart muscle.

Angiography (coronary): a diagnostic test used to identify the exact location and severity of coronary artery disease. During angiography a small tube or catheter is inserted into an artery and guided with the assistance of a fluoroscope (X-ray) to the opening of the coronary arteries, which supply blood to the heart. A dye, visible on X-ray, is then injected into each coronary artery to reveal the extent and severity of blockages. Images produced by angiography are known as angiograms.

Anion: a negatively charged ion.

Antagonist: a substance that counteracts the cellular effects of a natural compound, for example, a nutrient or a hormone.

Antibodies: also known as immunoglobulins (Ig), antibodies are specialized proteins produced by white blood cells that circulate in the blood recognizing and binding to foreign proteins, microorganisms, or toxins to neutralize them. They are a critical part of the immune response.

Anticoagulant: a class of compounds that inhibit the formation of blood clots.

Anticonvulsant: a class of medication used to prevent seizures, commonly used in individuals with seizure disorders or epilepsy.

Antigen: a substance that is capable of causing an immune response.

Antihistamine: a chemical that blocks the affect of histamine in susceptible tissues. Histamine is released by immune cells during an allergic reaction and also during infection with viruses that cause the common cold. The interaction of histamine with the mucus membranes of the eyes and nose results in "watery eyes" and the "runny nose" often accompanying allergies and colds. Antihistamines can alleviate such symptoms.

Antioxidant: any substance that prevents or reduces damage caused by reactive oxygen species (ROS) or reactive nitrogen species (RNS). ROS and RNS are highly reactive chemicals that attack other molecules and modify their chemical structure. Antioxidants are commonly added to foods to prevent or delay their deterioration due to exposure to air.

Antiresorptive agents: medications or hormones that inhibit bone resorption.

Apoptosis: gene-directed cell death or programmed cell death that occurs when age, condition, or state of cell health dictates. Cells that die by apoptosis do not usually elicit the inflammatory responses that are associated with necrosis. Cancer cells are not able to undergo apoptosis.

Arrhythmia: an abnormal heart rhythm. The heart rhythm may be too fast (tachycardia), too slow (bradycardia), or irregular. Some arrhythmias, such as ventricular fibrillation, may lead to cardiac arrest if not treated promptly.

Ataxia: a lack of coordination or unsteadiness usually related to a disturbance in the cerebellum, a part of the brain that regulates coordination and equilibrium.

Atherosclerosis: also known as arteriosclerosis, atherosclerosis results from the accumulation of cholesterol-laden plaque in artery walls. Plaque accumulation causes a narrowing and a loss of elasticity of the arteries, sometimes referred to as hardening of the arteries.

ATP: adenosine triphosphate. ATP is an important compound for the storage of energy in cells, as well as the synthesis (formation) of nucleic acids.

Atrophic gastritis: a chronic inflammation of the lining of the stomach, which ultimately results in the loss of glands in the stomach (atrophy) and decreased stomach acid production.

Atrophy: decrease in size or wasting away of a body part or tissue.

Autoimmune disease: autoimmune diseases occur when the body's tissues are mistakenly attacked by its own immune system. The immune system is a complex organization of cells and antibodies designed normally to destroy pathogens, particularly viruses and bacteria that cause infections. Individuals with autoimmune diseases have antibodies in their blood that target their own body tissues.

Balance study: a nutritional balance study involves the measurement of the intake of a specific nutrient as well as the elimination of that nutrient in urine, feces, sweat, etc. If intake is greater than loss of a particular nutrient, the individual is said to be in "positive balance." If intake is less than loss, an individual is said to be in "negative balance" for the nutrient of interest.

Bile: a yellow-green fluid made in the liver and stored in the gall bladder. Bile may then pass through the common bile duct into the small intestine where some of its components aid in the digestion of fat.

Bile acids: components of bile, formed by the metabolism of cholesterol. Bile acid deficiency may lead to the formation of cholesterol gall-stones, because bile salts (formed from bile acids) are required to dissolve cholesterol in bile so that it may be eliminated via the intestines.

Bioavailable: the portion of a nutrient (or other chemical) that can be absorbed, transported, and utilized physiologically.

Biomarker: a physical, functional, or biochemical indicator (e.g., the presence of a particular metabolite) of a physiological or disease process.

Bone mineral density (BMD): a term used in quantifying the mineralization of bone. The mineral component of bone consists largely of calcium and phosphorus. BMD is positively associated with bone strength and resistance to fracture. BMD can be determined through a low radiation X-ray technique known as dual-energy X-ray absorptiometry (DEXA).

Bone remodeling: the continuous turnover process of bone that includes bone resorption and bone formation. An imbalance in the regulation of bone resorption and bone formation increases the fragility of bone and may lead to osteoporosis.

Buffer: a chemical used to maintain the pH of a system by absorbing hydrogen ions (which would make it more acidic) or absorbing hydroxyl ions (which would make it more alkaline).

Carboxylation: the introduction of a carboxyl group (–COOH) or carbon dioxide into a compound.

Carcinogen: a cancer-causing agent; adjective: carcinogenic.

Carcinogenesis: the formation of cancer cells from normal cells.

Carcinoid syndrome: the pattern of symptoms exhibited by individuals with carcinoid tumors. Carcinoid tumors secrete excessive amounts of the neurotransmitter serotonin. Serotonin causes blood vessels to dilate (widen). Symptoms include flushing, diarrhea, and sometimes wheezing.

Cardiomyopathy: literally, disease of the heart muscle that often leads to abnormal function.

Cardiovascular: referring to the heart and blood vessels.

Cardiovascular diseases: literally, diseases affecting the heart and blood vessels. The term has come to encompass a number of conditions that result from atherosclerosis, including myocardial infarction (heart attack), congestive heart failure, and stroke.

Carnitine: a compound that is required to transport long-chain fatty acids across the inner membrane of the mitochondria, in the form of acyl-carnitine, where they can be metabolized for energy.

Case-control study: a study in which the risk factors of people who have been diagnosed with a disease are compared with those without the disease. Because the risk factor (e.g., nutrient intake) is generally measured at the time of diagnosis, it is difficult to determine whether the risk factor was present prior to the development of the disease. Another potential drawback is the difficulty in obtaining well-matched control subjects.

Catalyze: to increase the speed of a chemical reaction without changing the overall reaction process. See enzyme.

Cataract: clouding of the lens of the eye. As cataracts progress they can impair vision and may result in blindness.

Catecholamines: substances with a specific chemical structure (a benzene ring with two adjacent hydroxyl groups and a side chain of ethylamine) that function as hormones or neurotransmitters. Examples include epinephrine, norepinephrine, and dopamine.

Cation: a positively charged ion.

Celiac disease: also known as celiac sprue, celiac disease is an inherited disease in which the intestinal lining is inflamed in response to the ingestion of a protein known as gluten.

Treatment of celiac disease involves the avoidance of gluten, which is present in many grains, including rye, oats, and barley. Inflammation and atrophy of the lining of the small intestine leads to impaired nutrient absorption.

Cell signaling: communication among individual cells so as to coordinate their behavior to benefit the organism as a whole. Cell-signaling systems elucidated in animal cells include cell-surface and intracellular receptor proteins, protein kinases and protein phosphatases (enzymes that phosphorylate and dephosphorylate proteins), and guanosine triposphate (GTP)-binding proteins.

Cerebrospinal fluid: the fluid that bathes the brain and spinal chord.

Cerebrovascular disease: disease involving the blood vessels supplying the brain, including cerebrovascular accident (CVA), also known as a stroke.

Chelate: the combination of a metal with an organic molecule to form a ringlike structure known as a chelate. Chelation of a metal may inhibit or enhance its bioavailability.

Chemotherapy: literally, treatment with drugs. Commonly used to describe the systemic use of drugs to kill cancer cells as a form of cancer treatment.

Cholestatic liver disease: liver disease resulting in the cessation of bile excretion. Cholestasis may occur in the liver, gall bladder, or bile duct (duct connecting the gall bladder, to the small intestine).

Cholesterol: a lipid used in the construction of cell membranes and as a precursor in the synthesis of steroid hormones. Dietary cholesterol is obtained from animal sources, but is also synthesized by the liver. Cholesterol is carried in the blood by lipoproteins [e.g., low-density lipoprotein (LDL) and high-density lipoprotein (HDL)]. In atherosclerosis, cholesterol accumulates in plaques on the walls of some arteries.

Cholinergic: resembling acetylcholine in action, a cholinergic drug for example. Cholinergic nerve fibers liberate or are activated by the neurotransmitter, acetylcholine.

Chorionic villus sampling (CVS): a procedure for obtaining a small sample of tissue from the placenta (chorionic villi) for the purpose of prenatal diagnosis of genetic disorders. CVS can be performed between 9 and 12 weeks of pregnancy.

Chromosome: a structure composed of a long DNA molecule and associated proteins that carries part of the hereditary information of an organism.

Chronic disease: an illness lasting a long time. According to the U.S. Center for Health Statistics, a chronic disease is a disease lasting 3 months or more.

Cirrhosis: a condition characterized by irreversible scarring of the liver, leading to abnormal liver function. Cirrhosis has a number of different causes, including chronic alcohol use and viral hepatitis B and C.

Clinical trial: a research study, generally used to evaluate the effectiveness of a new treatment in human participants. Clinical trials are designed to answer specific scientific questions and to determine the efficacy of new treatments for specific diseases or health conditions.

Coagulation: the process involved in forming a blood clot.

Coenzyme: a molecule that binds to an enzyme and is essential for its activity but is not permanently altered by the reaction. Many coenzymes are derived from vitamins.

Cofactor: a compound that is essential for the activity of an enzyme.

Collagen: a fibrous protein that is the basis for the structure of skin, tendon, bone, cartilage, and all other connective tissue.

Collagenous matrix (of bone): the organic (nonmineral) structural element of bone. Collagen is a fibrous protein that provides the organic matrix upon which bone minerals crystallize.

Colon: sometimes called the large bowel or intestine, the colon is a long, coiled, tubelike organ that removes water from digested food after it has passed through the small intestine. The remaining material, solid waste called stool, moves through the colon to the rectum and leaves the body through the anus.

Colorectal adenoma: a tumor of the colon or rectum that arises in glandular tissue. Although not cancer, colorectal adenomas may develop into colorectal cancer over time.

Colorectal cancer: cancer of the colon (large intestine) and/or rectum.

Congenital hypothyroidism: also known as cretinism, congenital hypothyroidism occurs in two forms, although there is considerable overlap. The neurologic form is characterized by mental and physical retardation and deafness. It is the result of maternal iodine deficiency that affects the fetus before its own thyroid is functional. The myxedematous or hypothyroid form is characterized by short stature and mental retardation. In addition to iodine deficiency, the hypothyroid form has been associated with selenium deficiency and the presence of goitrogens in the diet that interfere with thyroid hormone production.

Congestive heart failure (CHF): a disorder of the heart, resulting in the loss of the ability to pump blood efficiently enough to meet the demands of the body. Symptoms may include swelling, shortness of breath, weakness, and exercise intolerance.

Coronary artery: the vessels that supply oxygenated blood to the heart muscle itself, so named because they encircle the heart in the form of a crown.

Coronary artery bypass graft (CABG): a surgical procedure used in individuals with significant narrowings and blockages of coronary arteries to create new routes around narrowed and blocked arteries, permitting increased blood flow to the heart muscle. The bypass graft for a CABG can be a vein from the leg or an inner chest wall artery.

Coronary heart disease (CHD): also known as coronary artery disease and coronary disease, coronary heart disease is the result of atherosclerosis of the coronary arteries. Atherosclerosis may result in narrowing or blockage of the coronary arteries and is the underlying cause of myocardial infarction (heart attack).

Corticosteroid: any of the steroid hormones made by the cortex (outer layer) of the adrenal gland. Cortisol is a corticosteroid. A number of medications are analogs of natural corticosteroid hormones.

Creatine phosphate: a high-energy compound found in muscle cells that is used to convert adenosine diphosphate (ADP) into ATP by donating phosphate molecules to ADP. ATP is a molecule that releases energy when converted to ADP, which may be used for metabolic processes.

Crohn's disease: an inflammatory disease of the gastrointestinal tract, often affecting the small intestine and colon.

Cross-sectional study: a study of a group of people at one point in time to determine whether a risk factor or a level of a risk factor is associated with the occurrence of a disease. Because the disease outcome and the risk factor (e.g., nutrient intake) are measured at the same time, a cross-sectional study provides a "snapshot" view of their relationship. Cross-sectional studies cannot provide information about causality.

Cystic fibrosis (CF): a genetic (inherited) disease characterized by the production of abnormal secretions, leading to the accumulation of mucus in the lungs, pancreas, and intestine. This buildup of mucus causes difficulty breathing and recurrent lung infections, as well as problems with nutrient absorption due to problems in the pancreas and intestines. Without treatment, CF results in death for 95 % of affected children before age 5; however, the longest-lived CF patient survived into his late 30s.

Cytochrome P450: a family of enzymes that play an important role in the metabolism of drugs and toxins in the liver. They also play a role in the synthesis (formation) of steroid hormones in the adrenal cortex.

Cytokine: a protein made by cells that affects the behavior of other cells. Cytokines act on specific cytokine receptors in the cells they affect.

De novo synthesis: the formation of an essential molecule from simple precursor molecules.

Decarboxylation: a chemical reaction involving the removal of a carboxyl (–COOH) group from a compound.

Dementia: significant loss of intellectual abilities such as memory capacity, severe enough to interfere with social or occupational functioning. Criteria for the diagnosis of dementia include impairment of attention, orientation, memory, judgment, language, and motor and spatial skills. By definition, dementia is not due to major depression or psychosis. Alzheimer's disease is the most common cause of dementia. Other causes include but are not limited to: AIDS, alcoholism, insufficient blood flow to the brain (vascular dementia), brain injury, brain tumors, drug toxicity, multiple sclerosis, and infections of the central nervous system.

Dental caries: cavities or holes in the outer two layers of a tooth—the enamel and the dentin. Dental caries are caused by bacteria that metabolize carbohydrates (sugars) to form organic acids that dissolve tooth enamel. If allowed to progress, dental caries may result in tooth decay, infection, and loss of teeth.

Depletion–repletion study: a nutritional study designed to determine the requirement for a specific nutrient. Generally, subjects are placed on a diet designed to deplete them of a specific nutrient over time. Once depletion is achieved, gradually increasing amounts of the nutrient under study are added to the diet until the individual shows evidence of sufficiency or repletion.

Dermatitis: inflammation of the skin. This term is often used to describe a skin rash.

DEXA: dual-energy X-ray absorptiometry. A precise instrument that uses the energy from very small doses of X-rays to determine bone mineral density and to diagnose and follow the treatment of osteoporosis.

Diabetes (diabetes mellitus): a chronic condition associated with abnormally high levels of glucose (sugar) in the blood. The two types of diabetes are referred to as insulin-dependent (type 1) and non-insulin–dependent (type 2). Type 1 diabetes results from a lack of adequate insulin secretion by the pancreas. Type 2 diabetes (also known as adult-onset diabetes) is characterized by an insensitivity of the tissues of the body to insulin secreted by the pancreas (insulin resistance).

Diabetic ketoacidosis: a potentially life-threatening condition characterized by ketosis (elevated levels of ketone bodies in the blood) and acidosis (increased acidity of the blood). Ketoacidosis occurs when diabetes is not adequately controlled.

Diastolic blood pressure: the lowest arterial blood pressure during the heartbeat cycle. The diastolic blood pressure is measured while the heart muscle is filling with blood.

Differentiation: changes in a cell resulting in its specialization for specific functions, such as those of a nerve cell. In general, differentiation of cells leads to a decrease in proliferation.

Diffusion: a process, which does not require energy expenditure, by which particles in solution move from a region of higher concentration to one of lower concentration.

Dimer: a complex of two protein molecules. Heterodimers are complexes of two different proteins, and homodimers are complexes of two of the same protein.

Diuretic: an agent that increases the formation of urine by the kidneys, resulting in water loss from the individual using the diuretic.

DNA: deoxyribonucleic acid. A long threadlike molecule made up of large numbers of nucleotides. Nucleotides in DNA are composed of a nitrogen containing base, a five-carbon sugar (deoxyribose), and phosphate groups. The sequence of bases in DNA serves as the carrier of genetic (hereditary) information.

Double-blind: refers to a study in which neither the investigators administering the treatment nor the participants know which participants are receiving the experimental treatment and which are receiving the placebo.

DRI: dietary reference intake. Refers to a set of at least four nutrient-based reference values (RDA, AI, UL, EAR), each with a specific use in defining recommended dietary intake levels for individual nutrients in the United States. The DRIs are determined by expert panels appointed by the Food and Nutrition Board of the Institute of Medicine.

EAR: estimated average requirement, set by the Food and Nutrition Board of the Institute of

Medicine; a nutrient intake value that is estimated to meet the requirement of half of the healthy individuals in a particular life stage and gender group.

Echocardiography: a diagnostic test that uses ultrasound to make images of the heart. It can be used to assess the health of the valves and chambers of the heart, as well as to measure cardiac output.

Electroencephalogram (EEG): a recording of the electrical activity of the brain, used to diagnose neurological conditions such as seizure disorders (epilepsy).

Electrolytes: ionized (dissociated into positive and negative ions) salts in the body fluids. Major electrolytes in the body include sodium, potassium, magnesium, calcium, chloride, bicarbonate, and phosphate.

Electron: a stable atomic particle with a negative charge.

Electron transport chain: a group of electron carriers in mitochondria that transport electrons to and from each other in a sequence to generate ATP.

Element: one of the 103 chemical substances that cannot be divided into simpler substances by chemical means. For example, hydrogen, magnesium, lead, and uranium are all chemical elements. Trace elements are chemical elements that are required in very small (trace) amounts in the diet to maintain health. For example, copper, selenium, and iodine are considered trace elements.

Enamel: the hard, white, outermost layer of a tooth.

Endocrine system: the glands and parts of glands that secrete hormones that integrate and control the body's metabolic activity. Endocrine glands include the pituitary, thyroid, parathyroids, adrenals, pancreas, ovaries, and testes.

Enzyme: a biological catalyst. That is, a substance that increases the speed of a chemical reaction without being changed in the overall process. Enzymes are vitally important to the regulation of the chemistry of cells and organisms.

Epidemiologic study: a study examining disease occurrence in a human population.

Epilepsy: also known as seizure disorder. Individuals with epilepsy experience seizures, which are the result of uncontrolled electrical activity in the brain. A seizure may cause a physical convulsion, minor physical signs, thought disturbances, or a combination of symptoms.

Esophagus: a soft muscular tube that connects the throat to the stomach. When a person swallows, the muscular walls of the esophagus contract to push food down into the stomach.

Etiology: the causes or origin of a disease.

Excretion: the elimination of wastes from blood or tissues.

Extracellular fluid (ECF): the volume of body fluid excluding that in cells. ECF includes the fluid in blood vessels (plasma) and fluid between cells (interstitial fluid).

Familial adenomatous polyposis: a hereditary syndrome characterized by the formation of many polyps in the colon and rectum, some of which ultimately develop into colorectal cancer.

Fatty acid: an organic acid molecule consisting of a chain of carbon molecules and a carboxylic acid (COOH) group. Fatty acids are found in fats, oils, and as components of a number of essential lipids, such as phospholipids and triglycerides. Fatty acids can be utilized by the body for energy.

Femoral neck: a portion of the thighbone (femur). The femoral neck is found near the hip, at the base of the head of the femur, which makes up the ball of the hip joint. Fractures of the femoral neck sometimes occur in individuals with osteoporosis.

Fibrocystic breast condition (FCC): a benign (noncancerous) condition of the breasts, characterized by lumpiness and discomfort in one or both breasts.

Fortification: the addition of nutrients to foods to prevent or correct a nutritional deficiency, to balance the total nutrient profile of food, or to restore nutrients lost in processing.

Free radical: a very reactive atom or molecule typically possessing a single unpaired electron.

Fructose: a very sweet six-carbon sugar abundant in plants. Fructose is increasingly common in sweeteners such as high-fructose corn syrup.

Gall bladder: a small pear-shaped sac adjacent to the liver. The gall bladder stores bile, which is secreted by the liver, and releases bile into the small intestine through the common bile duct.

Gallstones: "pebbles" formed by the precipitation (crystallization) of cholesterol (most common in the United States and Europe) or bilirubin (most common in Asia) in the gall bladder. Gallstones may be asymptomatic (without symptoms) or they may result in inflammation and infection of the gall bladder.

Gastroesophageal reflux disease (GERD): a condition in which stomach contents, including acid, back up (reflux) into the esophagus, causing inflammation and damage to the esophagus. GERD can lead to scarring of the esophagus and may increase the risk of cancer of the esophagus in some patients.

Gastrointestinal: referring to or affecting the stomach and intestines (small and large bowel).

Gene expression: the full use of the information in a gene through transcription and translation leading to production of a protein.

Genome: all of the genetic information (encoded in DNA) possessed by an organism.

Gluconeogenesis: the production of glucose from noncarbohydrate precursors, such as amino acids (the building blocks of proteins).

Glucose: a six-carbon sugar that plays a major role in the generation of energy for living organisms.

Glycogen: a large polymer (repeating units) of glucose molecules, used to store energy in cells, especially muscle and liver cells.

Goiter: enlargement of the thyroid gland. Goiter is one of the earliest and most visible signs of iodine deficiency. Thyroid enlargement may also be caused by factors other than iodine deficiency, especially in iodine sufficient countries, such as the United States.

Goitrogen: a substance that induces goiter formation by interfering with thyroid hormone production or utilization.

Gout: a condition characterized by abnormally high blood levels of uric acid (urate). Urate crystals may form in joints, resulting in inflammation and pain. Urate crystals may also form in the kidney and urinary tract, resulting in kidney stones. The tendency to develop elevated blood uric acid levels and gout is often inherited.

GTP: guanosine triposphate. A high-energy molecule, required for a number of biochemical reactions, including nucleic acid and protein synthesis (formation).

Hartnup's disease: a genetic disorder resulting in defective absorption of the amino acid tryptophan.

HDL: high-density lipoproteins. HDL transport cholesterol from the tissues to the liver where it can be eliminated in bile. HDL cholesterol is considered good cholesterol, because higher blood levels of HDL cholesterol are associated with lower risk of heart disease.

Heme: compounds of iron complexed in a characteristic ring structure known as a porphyrin ring.

Hemodialysis: a medical procedure that uses a specialized machine to filter waste products from the blood and restore its normal constituents. Hemodialysis is needed to perform the work of the kidneys if they can no longer function effectively.

Hemoglobin: the oxygen-carrying pigment in red blood cells.

Hemolysis: rupture of red blood cells.

Hemolytic anemia: anemia resulting from hemolysis (the rupture of red blood cells).

Hemorrhage: excessive or uncontrolled bleeding.

Hepatitis: literally, inflammation of the liver. Hepatitis caused by a virus is known as viral hepatitis. Other causes of hepatitis include toxic chemicals and alcohol abuse.

Hereditary spherocytosis: a hereditary form of anemia characterized by abnormally shaped red blood cells, which are spherical and abnormally fragile. The increased fragility of these red blood cells leads to hemolytic anemia (anemia caused by the rupture of red blood cells).

Heterodimer: a dimer or complex of two different molecules, usually proteins.

Heterozygous: possessing two different forms (alleles) of a specific gene.

HIV: human immunodeficiency virus. The viruses that cause AIDS.

Homocysteine: a sulfur-containing amino acid, which is an intermediate in the metabolism of another sulfur-containing amino acid, methionine. Elevated homocysteine levels in the blood have been associated with increased risk of cardiovascular diseases.

Homodimer: a dimer or complex of two of the same molecule, usually a protein.

Homologous: having the same relative position, value, or structure.

Homozygous: possessing two identical forms (alleles) of a specific gene.

Hydroxyapatite: a calcium phosphate salt. Hydroxyapatite is the main mineral component of bone and teeth and is what gives them their rigidity.

Hydroxylation: a chemical reaction involving the addition of a hydroxyl (–OH) group to a compound.

Hyperparathyroidism: excess secretion of parathyroid hormone by the parathyroid glands resulting in the disturbance of calcium metabolism. Symptoms may include increased blood levels of calcium (hypercalcemia), decreased blood levels of phosphorus, loss of calcium from bone, and kidney stone formation.

Hypertension: high blood pressure, defined as a systolic blood pressure greater than 140 mm Hg and/or diastolic blood pressure greater than 90 mm Hg.

Hyperthyroidism: an excess of thyroid hormone, which may result from an overactive thyroid gland or nodule, or from taking too much thyroid hormone.

Hypoparathyroidism: a deficiency of parathyroid hormone, which may be characterized by low blood calcium levels (hypocalcemia).

Hypothalamus: an area at the base of the brain that regulates bodily functions, such as body temperature, hunger, and thirst.

Hypothesis: an educated guess or proposition that is advanced as a basis for further investigation. A hypothesis must be subjected to an experimental test to determine its validity.

Hypothyroidism: a deficiency of thyroid hormone that is normally made by the thyroid gland, located in the front of the neck.

Idiopathic: of unknown cause.

Impaired glucose tolerance: a metabolic state between normal glucose regulation and overt diabetes. Generally, blood glucose levels are higher than normal but lower than those accepted as diagnostic for diabetes.

Insulin: a peptide hormone secreted by the β cells of the pancreas required for normal glucose metabolism.

Insulin resistance: diminished responsiveness to insulin.

Intracellular fluid (ICF): the volume of fluid inside cells.

In vitro: literally "in glass," referring to a test or research done in the test tube, outside a living organism.

In vivo: "inside a living organism." An in vivo assay evaluates a biological process occurring inside the body.

Ion: an atom or group of atoms that carries a positive or negative electric charge as a result of having lost or gained one or more electrons.

Ion channel: a protein embedded in a cell membrane that serves as a crossing point for the regulated transfer of an ion or a group of ions across the membrane.

Isomers: compounds that have the same numbers and kinds of atoms but that differ in the way the atoms are arranged.

Jaundice: a yellowish staining of the skin and whites of the eyes due to increased bilirubin (a bile pigment) levels in the blood. Jaundice can be an indicator of red blood cells rupturing (hemolysis) or of disease of the liver or gall bladder.

Ketone bodies: any of three acidic chemicals (acetate, acetoacetate, and beta-hydroxybutyrate). Ketone bodies may accumulate in the blood (ketosis) when the body has inadequate glucose to use for energy and must increase the use of fat for fuel. Ketone bodies are acidic, and very high levels in the blood are toxic and may result in ketoacidosis.

Kidney stones: also known as renal calculi, kidney stones are the result of crystallization of certain substances found in urine, including calcium, phosphate, oxalic acid, and uric acid. Stones may form in the urine-collecting area (pelvis) of the kidney, as well as the ureters (narrow tubes connecting the kidney to the urinary bladder).

LDLs: low-density lipoproteins. Lipoproteins (particles composed of lipids and protein) are the form in which fats are transported throughout the body, in the bloodstream. LDLs transport cholesterol from the liver to the tissues of the body. A high proportion of cholesterol carried in LDL (LDL cholesterol) is associated with an increased likelihood of developing cardiovascular diseases (heart disease and stroke). Oxidized LDLs appear to play an important role in the development of atherosclerosis.

Left ventricular hypertrophy (LVH): abnormal thickening of the wall of the left ventricle (lower chamber) of the heart muscle. The ventricles have muscular walls to pump blood from the heart through the arteries, but LVH occurs when the ventricle must pump against abnormally high volume or pressure loads. LVH may accompany congestive heart failure (CHF).

Leukemia: an acute or chronic form of cancer that involves the blood-forming organs. Leukemia is characterized by an abnormal increase in the number of white blood cells in the tissues of the body with or without a corresponding increase of those in the circulating blood and is classified according to the type of white blood cell most prominently involved.

Lipids: different types of fat molecules. For example, phospholipids, cholesterol, triglycerides.

Lipoic acid: a coenzyme, essential for the oxidation of alpha-keto acids, such as pyruvate, in metabolism.

Lipoproteins: particles composed of lipids and protein that allow for transport of fat and cholesterol through the blood. A lipoprotein particle is composed of an outer shell of phospholipid, which renders the particle soluble in water; a fatty core; and a surface apoprotein molecule that allows tissues to recognize and take up the particle.

Lipoprotein(a) [Lp(a)]: a lipoprotein particle in which the protein (apolipoprotein B-100) is chemically linked to another protein apolipoprotein(a). Increased blood levels of Lp(a) are associated with an increased risk of cardiovascular diseases.

Lupus: also known as systemic lupus erythematosus (SLE). Lupus is a chronic inflammatory condition caused by an autoimmune disease. An autoimmune disease occurs when the body's tissues are attacked by its own immune system. Individuals with lupus have unusual antibodies in their blood that are targeted against their own body tissues.

Lymphocyte: a white blood cell that creates an immune response when activated by a foreign molecule (antigen). T lymphocytes or T cells develop in an organ called the thymus and are responsible for cell-mediated immunity, and B lymphocytes develop in the bone marrow and are responsible for the production of antibodies (immunoglobulins).

Macrocytic anemia: low red blood cell count, characterized by the presence in the blood of larger than normal red blood cells.

Macula: a small area of the retina where vision is the keenest. The macula is located in the center of the retina and provides central vision. Activities that require central vision include driving, reading, and other activities that require sharp, straight-ahead vision.

Magnetic resonance imaging (MRI): a special imaging technique that uses a powerful magnet and a computer to provide clear images of soft tissues. Tissues that are well visualized using MRI include the brain and spinal cord, abdomen, and joints.

Malabsorption syndrome: a disease or condition that results in poor absorption of nutrients from food.

Malaria: an infectious disease caused by parasitic microorganisms called plasmodia. Malaria can be spread among humans through the sting of certain types of mosquitoes (anopheles) or by a contaminated needle or transfusion. Malaria is a major health problem in the tropics and subtropics, affecting over 200 million people worldwide.

Malignant: cancerous.

Megaloblastic anemia: low red blood cell count, characterized by the presence in the blood of large, immature, nucleated cells (megaloblasts) that are forerunners of red blood cells. Red blood cells, when mature, have no nuclei.

Melanin: a dark brown pigment found in the skin.

Membrane potential: the electrical potential difference across a membrane. The membrane potential is a result of the concentration differences between potassium and sodium across cell membranes, which are maintained by ion pumps. A large proportion of the body's resting energy expenditure is devoted to maintaining the membrane potential, which is critical for nerve impulse transmission, muscle contraction, heart function, and the transport of nutrients and metabolites in and out of cells.

Meta-analysis: a mathematical or statistical analysis, used to pool the results of all studies investigating a particular effect (e.g., the effect of folic acid supplementation on homocysteine levels) and provide an overall estimate of that effect.

Metabolism: physical and chemical processes within the body involving energy production and utilization.

Metabolite: a compound derived from the metabolism of another compound is said to be a metabolite of that compound.

Metastasize: to spread from one part of the body to another. Cancer is said to metastasize when it spreads from the primary site of origin to a distant anatomical site.

Methionine: an indispensable, sulfur-containing amino acid, required for protein synthesis and other vital metabolic processes.

Methylation: a biochemical reaction resulting in the addition of a methyl group ($-CH_3$) to another molecule.

Minerals: nutritionally significant elements. Elements are composed of only one kind of atom. Minerals are inorganic (i.e., they do not contain carbon) as do vitamins and other organic compounds.

Mitochondria: energy-producing structures within cells. Mitochondria possess two sets of membranes, a smooth continuous outer membrane and an inner membrane arranged in folds. Among other critical functions, mitochondria produce energy via the electron transport chain.

mm Hg: millimeters of mercury. The unit of measure for blood pressure.

Mole: the fundamental unit for measuring chemical compounds (abbreviated *mol*). One mole equals the molecular weight of a compound in grams. The number of molecules in a mole is equal to 6.02×10^{23} (Avogadro's number).

Multifactorial: refers to a disorder or condition that has a number of different causes.

Multiple sclerosis (MS): an autoimmune disorder that results in the demyelinization of nerves. In MS, the myelin sheath that allows for efficient transmission of nerve impulses is damaged, resulting in progressive neurological symptoms such as, numbness, tingling, loss of control of certain bodily functions, and paralysis.

Myelin: the fatty substance that covers myelinated nerves. Myelin is a layered tissue surrounding the axons or nerve fibers. This sheath acts as a conduit in an electrical system, allowing rapid and efficient transmission of nerve impulses. Myelination refers to the process in which nerves acquire a myelin sheath.

Myocardial infarction (MI): commonly known as a "heart attack," a myocardial infarction refers to changes that occur in the heart muscle due to an interruption in its blood supply. An MI is often the result of a clot that lodges in a coronary artery, resulting in deprivation of oxygen to a portion of the heart muscle (ischemia) and ultimately the death (necrosis) of a portion of the heart muscle if the oxygen supply is not restored within a few minutes.

Myocarditis: an inflammation of the heart muscle.

Myoglobin: a heme-containing pigment in muscle cells that binds and stores oxygen.

Necrosis: cell death due to infection or injury.

Neural tube defect (NTD): a birth defect caused by abnormal development of the neural tube, the structure that gives rise to the central nervous system. Neural tube defects include anencephaly and spina bifida.

Neurologic: or neurological; involving nerves or the nervous system (brain, spinal cord, and all sensory and motor nerves).

Neuropathy: malfunction or disease pathology of nerves. Peripheral neuropathy refers to a disease or degenerative state of peripheral nerves resulting in pain, numbness, and sometimes muscle weakness.

Neurotoxic: toxic or damaging to nervous tissue (brain and peripheral nerves).

Neurotransmitter: a chemical that is released from a nerve cell, which transmits an impulse from that nerve cell to another nerve cell or to another organ (a muscle, for example). Neurotransmitters are chemical messengers that transmit neurological information from one cell to another.

Neutrophils: also called polymorphonuclear leukocytes because they are white blood cells with a multilobed nucleus. Neutrophils combat infection by internalizing and destroying disease-causing organisms such as bacteria.

NIH: The National Institutes of Health are U.S. health agencies, devoted to medical research. Administered under the Department of Health and Human Services, the NIH consist of more than 20 separate institutes and centers.

Nucleic acids: DNA (deoxyribonucleic acid) and RNA (ribonucleic acid). Long threadlike molecules made up of large numbers of nucleotides. Nucleotides are composed of a nitrogen-containing base, a five-carbon sugar, and one or more phosphate groups. The sequence of bases in DNA or RNA represents the genetic (hereditary) information of a living cell.

Nucleotides: molecules composed of a nitrogen–containing base, a five-carbon sugar, and one or more phosphate groups. Long strands of nucleotides form nucleic acids (see above). The sequence of bases in DNA or RNA represents the genetic (hereditary) information of a living cell.

Nucleus: a membrane-bound cellular organelle that contains DNA organized into chromosomes.

Observational study: a study in which no experimental intervention or treatment is applied. Participants are simply observed over time.

One-carbon unit: a biochemical term for functional groups containing only one carbon in addition to other atoms. One-carbon units transferred by folate coenzymes include methyl ($-CH_3$), methylene ($-CH_2-$), formyl ($-CH=O$), formimino ($-CH=NH$), and methenyl ($-CH=$) groups. Many biosynthetic reactions involve the addition of a one-carbon unit to a precursor molecule.

Organic: refers to carbon-containing compounds, generally synthesized by living organisms.

Osteoarthritis: a degenerative joint condition that is characterized by the breakdown of articular cartilage (cartilage within the joint). Symptoms of osteoarthritis include pain and stiffness in the affected joint(s), particularly after activity.

Osteoblasts: cells associated with bone that are responsible for the new formation of bone in the bone remodeling process.

Osteoclasts: cells associated with bone that are responsible for the breakdown or resorption of bone. Bone remodeling is a continuous process of resorption and formation.

Osteomalacia: a disease of adults that is characterized by softening of the bones due to loss of bone mineral. Osteomalacia is characteristic of vitamin D deficiency in adults, although children with vitamin D deficiency suffer from rickets.

Osteoporosis: a condition of increased bone fragility and susceptibility to bone fracture due to a loss of mineral density (BMD).

Oxidation: a chemical reaction that removes electrons from an atom or molecule.

Oxidative stress: an organism is said to experience oxidative stress when the effects of pro-oxidants (e.g. free radicals, reactive oxygen and reactive nitrogen species) exceed the ability of antioxidant systems to neutralize them.

Pancreas: a small organ located behind the stomach. The head of the pancreas is connected to the duodenum (the first section of the small intestine). The pancreas makes enzymes that help digest food in the small intestine and hormones, including insulin, that control the amount of glucose in the blood.

Parathyroid glands: glands located behind the thyroid gland in the neck. The parathyroid glands secrete parathyroid hormone (PTH), which is critical to calcium and phosphorus metabolism.

Parkinson's disease: a disease of the nervous system caused by degeneration of a part of the brain called the basal ganglia and by low production of the neurotransmitter dopamine. Symptoms include muscle rigidity, tremors, and slow voluntary movement.

Pathogen: disease-causing agent, such as a virus or a bacterium.

Peptic ulcer disease: a disease characterized by ulcers or breaks in the inner lining (mucosa) of the stomach or duodenum (region of the small intestine closest to the stomach). The three major causes of peptic ulcer disease are nonsteroidal anti-inflammatory drugs, chronic *Helicobacter pylori* infection, and states of acid hypersecretion, like Zollinger-Ellison syndrome.

Peptide: a chain of amino acids. A protein is made up of one or more peptides.

Peptide hormones: hormones that are proteins, as opposed to steroid hormones, which are made from cholesterol. Insulin is an example of a peptide hormone.

Peripheral vascular diseases: diseases of the vessels of the extremities such as atherosclerosis, resulting in diminished circulation, pain (claudication), or a blood clot, for example.

Pernicious anemia: the end stage of an autoimmune inflammation of the stomach, resulting in destruction of stomach cells by one's own antibodies. Progressive destruction of the cells that line the stomach cause decreased secretion of acid and enzymes required to release food-bound vitamin B_{12}. Antibodies to intrinsic factor (IF) bind to IF, preventing formation of the IF-B_{12} complex, further inhibiting vitamin B_{12} absorption.

PET scan: positron emission tomography. An imaging technique that uses a sophisticated camera and computer to produce images that allow the analysis of metabolic function in organs such as the brain.

pH: a measure of acidity or alkalinity.

Pharmacologic dose: the dose or intake level of a nutrient many times the level associated with the prevention of deficiency or the maintenance of health. A pharmacologic dose is generally associated with the treatment of a disease state and considered to be a dose at least 10 times greater than that needed to prevent deficiency.

Phenylketonuria (PKU): an inherited disorder resulting in the inability to process the amino acid phenylalanine. If not treated, the disorder may result in mental retardation. Treatment is a diet low in phenylalanine. Newborns are screened for PKU to determine the need for treatment before brain damage occurs.

Phlebotomy: the removal of blood from a vein. Phlebotomy may be used to obtain blood for diagnostic tests or to treat certain conditions, for example, iron overload in hemochromatosis.

Phospholipids: lipids (fat molecules) in which phosphoric acid as well as fatty acids are attached to a glycerol backbone. Phospholipids are found in all living cells and in the bilayers of cell membranes.

Phosphorylation: the creation of a phosphate derivative of an organic molecule. This is usually achieved by transferring a phosphate group ($-PO_4$) from ATP to another molecule.

Physiologic dose: the dose or intake level of a nutrient associated with the prevention of deficiency or the maintenance of health. A physiologic dose of a nutrient is not generally greater than that which could be achieved through a conscientious diet, as opposed to the use of supplements.

Pituitary gland: a small oval gland located at the base of the brain that secretes hormones regulating growth and metabolism. The pituitary gland is divided into two separate glands, the anterior and posterior pituitary glands, which each secrete different hormones.

Placebo: a sugar pill or false treatment that is given to a control group while the experimental group is given the experimental treatment. Placebo-controlled studies are conducted to make sure that significant outcomes of a trial are due to the experimental treatment rather than another factor associated with participating in the study.

Placenta: a temporary organ joining the mother and unborn child (fetus). The placenta transfers oxygen and nutrients from the mother to the fetus and permits the release of carbon dioxide and waste products from the fetus.

Placental abruption: premature separation of the placenta from the wall of the uterus. Abruption is a potentially serious problem for both the mother and the baby.

Plasma: the liquid part of blood (as opposed to blood cells) that makes up about half its volume. Plasma differs from serum in that the blood sample has not clotted. A centrifuge is used to separate plasma from cells in the laboratory.

Platelet: irregularly shaped cell fragments that assist in blood clotting. During normal blood clotting, platelets aggregate (group together) to prevent hemorrhage.

Pneumonia: a disease of the lungs characterized by inflammation and accumulation of fluid in the lungs. Pneumonia may be caused by infectious agents (e.g., viruses or bacteria) or by inhalation of certain irritants.

Polymorphism: the existence of two (or more) forms of a gene with each form being too common to be due merely to new mutation.

Precursor: a molecule that is an ingredient, reactant, or intermediate in a synthetic pathway for a particular product.

Preeclampsia: a condition characterized by a sharp rise in blood pressure during the third trimester of pregnancy. High blood pressure may be accompanied by edema (swelling) and kidney problems, as evidenced by protein in the urine. Although preeclampsia is relatively common, occurring in about 5 % of all pregnancies and more frequently in first pregnancies, it can be a sign of serious problems. In some cases, untreated preeclampsia can progress to eclampsia, a life-threatening situation for both mother and baby.

Prevalence: the proportion of a population with a specific disease or condition at a given point in time.

Proliferation: rapid cell division.

Pro-oxidant: an atom or molecule that promotes oxidation of another atom or molecule by accepting electrons. Examples of pro-oxidants include free radicals, ROS, and nitrogen species (RNS).

Prophylaxis: prevention; often refers to a treatment used to prevent a disease.

Prospective study: a study in which participants are initially enrolled, examined, or tested for risk factors (e.g., nutrient intake) and then followed up at subsequent times to determine their status with respect to the disease or condition of interest.

Prostaglandin: any of a class of hormone-like, regulatory molecules constructed from polyunsaturated fatty acids such as arachidonate. These molecules participate in a number of functions in the body, such as smooth muscle contraction and relaxation, vasodilation, and kidney regulation.

Prostate: a gland situated at the beginning of the urethra (passage through which urine leaves the body) in men. It secretes an alkaline fluid that is the major component of semen (ejaculatory fluid). Prostate cancer is the second leading cause of death due to cancer in men in the United States.

Proteoglycan: a large compound composed of protein and polysaccharide units known as glycosaminoglycans (GAGs). GAGs are polymers of sugars and amino sugars, such as glucosamine or galactosamine. Proteoglycans are integral components of structural tissues such as bone and cartilage.

Psoriasis: a chronic skin condition often resulting in a red, scaly rash located over the surfaces of the elbows, knees, scalp, and around or in the ears, navel, genitals, or buttocks. Approximately 10 to 15 % of patients with psoriasis develop joint inflammation (psoriatic arthritis). Psoriasis is thought to be an autoimmune condition.

Pyruvate kinase deficiency: a hereditary deficiency of the enzyme pyruvate kinase. Pyruvate kinase deficiency results in hemolytic anemia.

Quartile: one fourth of a sample or population.

Quintile: one fifth of a sample or population.

Radiation therapy: the local use of radiation to destroy cancer cells or stop them from dividing and growing.

Randomized controlled trial (RCT): a clinical trial that involves at least one test treatment and one control treatment, in which the treatments administered are selected by a random process (e.g., coin flips or a random-numbers table).

Randomized design: an experiment in which participants are chosen for the experimental and control groups at random to reduce bias caused by self-selection into experimental and control groups. This type of study design can provide evidence of causality.

RDA: recommended dietary allowance. Set by the Food and Nutrition Board of the Institute of Medicine, the RDA is the average daily dietary intake level sufficient to meet the nutrient requirements of nearly all (97 to 98 %) healthy individuals in a specific life stage and gender group (e.g., women from 19 to 30 years of age).

It is intended as a goal for daily intake of specific nutrients by individuals.

Reactive nitrogen species (RNS): highly reactive chemicals, containing nitrogen, that react easily with other molecules, resulting in potentially damaging modifications.

Reactive oxygen species (ROS): highly reactive chemicals, containing oxygen, that react easily with other molecules, resulting in potentially damaging modifications.

Receptor: a protein on or protruding from the cell surface to which select chemicals can bind. Binding of a specific molecule (ligand) may result in a cellular signal or the internalization of the receptor and the ligand.

Recessive trait: a trait that is expressed only when two copies of the gene responsible for the trait are present.

Redox reaction: another term for an oxidation–reduction reaction. A redox reaction is any reaction in which electrons are removed from one molecule or atom and transferred to another molecule or atom. In such a reaction one substance is oxidized (loses electrons) while the other is reduced (gains electrons).

Reduction: a chemical reaction in which a molecule or atom gains electrons.

Renal: refers to the kidneys.

Resorption: the process of breaking down or assimilating something. With respect to bone, resorption refers to the breakdown of bone by osteoclasts that results in the release of calcium and phosphate (bone mineral) into the blood.

Response element: a sequence of nucleotides in a gene that can be bound by a protein. Proteins that bind to response elements in genes are sometimes called transcription factors or binding proteins. Binding of a transcription factor to a response element regulates the production of specific proteins by inhibiting or enhancing the transcription of genes that encode those proteins.

Retina: the sensory membrane that lines most of the back of the eye. The retina is composed of several layers including one containing the rods and cones. It receives the image formed by the lens and converts it into chemical and nervous signals that reach the brain by way of the optic nerve.

Rheumatoid arthritis: an autoimmune disease that causes chronic inflammation of the joints, the tissue around the joints, as well as other organs in the body. Rheumatoid arthritis is a systemic illness and is sometimes called rheumatoid disease.

Riboucelotide: a molecule consisting of a five-carbon sugar (ribose), a nitrogen-containing base, and one or more phosphate groups.

Rickets: often the result of vitamin D deficiency. Rickets affects children while their bones are still growing. It is characterized by soft and deformed bones and is the result of impaired incorporation of calcium and phosphate into the skeleton.

RNA: ribonucleic acid; a chain of nucleotides, which are composed of a nitrogen-containing base, a five-carbon sugar (ribose), and phosphate groups. RNA functions in the translation of the genetic information in DNA for protein synthesis.

Ruminant: an animal that chews cud. Ruminant animals include cattle, goats, sheep, and deer.

Scavenge (free radicals): to combine readily with free radicals, preventing them from reacting with other molecules.

Scurvy: a disorder caused by lack of vitamin C. Symptoms include anemia, bleeding gums, tooth loss, joint pain, and fatigue. Scurvy is treated by supplying foods high in vitamin C as well as with vitamin C supplements.

Seizure: uncontrolled electrical activity in the brain, which may produce a physical convulsion, minor physical signs, thought disturbances, or a combination of symptoms.

Serotonin: a hormone also known as 5-hydroxytryptamine. Serotonin functions as both a neurotransmitter and a vasoconstrictor (substance that causes blood vessels to narrow).

Serum: the liquid part of blood (as opposed to blood cells) that makes up about half its volume. Serum differs from plasma in that the blood sample has clotted. A centrifuge is used in the laboratory to separate serum from cells after blood has clotted.

Short bowel syndrome: a malabsorption syndrome resulting from the surgical removal of an extensive portion of the small intestine.

Sickle cell anemia: a hereditary disease in which a mutation in the gene for one of the proteins that constitutes hemoglobin results in the formation of defective hemoglobin molecules known as hemoglobin S. Individuals who are homozygous for this mutation (possess two genes for hemoglobin S) have red blood cells that change from the normal discoid shape to a sickle shape when the oxygen supply is low. These sickle-shaped cells are easily trapped in capillaries and damaged, resulting in severe anemia. Individuals who are heterozygous for the mutation (possess one gene for hemoglobin S and one normal hemoglobin gene) have increased resistance to malaria.

Sideroblastic anemia: a group of anemias that are all characterized by the accumulation of iron deposits in the mitochondria of immature red blood cells. These abnormal red blood cells do not mature normally, and many are destroyed in the bone marrow before reaching the circulation. Sideroblastic anemias can be hereditary, idiopathic (unknown cause), or caused by such diverse factors as certain drugs, alcohol, or copper deficiency.

Small intestine: the part of the digestive tract that extends from the stomach to the large intestine. The small intestine includes the duodenum (closest to the stomach), the jejunum, and the ileum (closest to the large intestine).

Sorbitol: the polyol (sugar alcohol) corresponding to glucose.

Spina bifida: a birth defect, also known as a neural tube defect, resulting from failure of the lower end of the neural tube to close during embryonic development. Spina bifida, the most common cause of infantile paralysis, is characterized by a lack of protection of the spinal cord by its membranes and vertebral bones.

Sprue: also known as celiac sprue and celiac disease, it is an inherited disease in which the intestinal lining is inflamed in response to the ingestion of a protein known as gluten. Treatment of celiac disease involves the avoidance of gluten, which is present in many grains, including rye, oats, and barley. Inflammation and atrophy of the lining of the small intestine leads to impaired nutrient absorption.

Status: the state of nutrition of an individual with respect to a specific nutrient. Diminished or low status indicates inadequate supply or stores of a specific nutrient for optimal physiological functioning.

Steroid: a molecule related to cholesterol. Many important hormones such as estrogen and testosterone are steroids.

Steroid hormone receptor: a protein within a cell, which binds to a specific steroid hormone. Binding of the steroid hormone changes the shape of the receptor protein and activates it, allowing it to activate gene transcription. In this way, a steroid hormone can activate the synthesis of specific proteins.

Stress fracture: a hairline or microscopic break in a bone, usually due to repetitive stress rather than trauma. Stress fractures are usually painful and may be undetectable by X-ray. Though they can occur in almost any bone, common sites of stress fractures are the tibia (lower leg) and metatarsals (foot).

Stroke: the sudden death of some brain cells due to lack of oxygen, when blood flow to the brain is impaired by the blockage (usually due to a blood clot) or rupture of a blood vessel in the brain. A stroke is also called a cerebrovascular accident (CVA).

Subclinical: without clinical signs or symptoms; sometimes used to describe the early stage of a disease or condition, before symptoms are detectable by clinical examination or laboratory tests.

Substrate: a reactant in an enzyme catalyzed reaction.

Supplement: a nutrient or phytochemical supplied in addition to that which is obtained in the diet.

Systolic blood pressure: the highest arterial pressure measured during the heartbeat cycle.

It occurs when the heart muscle is contracting (pumping).

Tannins: a large group of plant-derived compounds. Tannins tend to be bitter tasting and may function in pigment formation and plant protection.

Tertile: one third of a sample or population.

Tetany: a condition of prolonged and painful spasms of the voluntary muscles, especially the fingers and toes (carpopedal spasm) as well as the facial musculature.

Thalassemia major: beta thalassemia is a genetic disorder that results in abnormalities of the globin (protein) portion of hemoglobin. An individual who is homozygous for the beta thalassemia gene (has two copies of the beta thalassemia gene) is said to have thalassemia major. Infants born with thalassemia major develop severe anemia a few months after birth, accompanied by pallor, fatigue, poor growth, and frequent infections. Blood transfusions are used to treat thalassemia major but cannot cure it.

Thalassemia minor: individuals who are heterozygous for the beta thalassemia gene (carry one copy of the beta thalassemia gene) are said to have thalassemia minor or thalassemia trait. These individuals are generally healthy but can pass the beta thalassemia gene to their children and are said to be carriers of the beta thalassemia gene.

Threshold: the point at which a physiological effect begins to be produced, for example, the degree of stimulation of a nerve that produces a response or the level of a chemical in the diet that results in a disease.

Thyroid: a butterfly-shaped gland in the neck that secretes thyroid hormones. Thyroid hormones regulate a number of physiologic processes, including growth, development, metabolism, and reproductive function.

Thyroid follicular cancer: a cancer of the thyroid gland that constitutes about 30% of all thyroid cancers. It has a greater rate of recurrence and metastasis (spreading to other organs) than thyroid papillary cancer.

Thyroid papillary cancer: the most common form of thyroid cancer, which most often affects women of childbearing age. Thyroid papillary cancer has a lower rate of recurrence and metastases (spreading to other organs) than thyroid follicular cancer.

Total parenteral nutrition (TPN): intravenous feeding that provides patients with essential nutrients when they are too ill to eat normally.

Transcription: DNA transcription; the process by which one strand of DNA is copied into a complementary sequence of RNA.

Transcription factor: generally a protein that functions to initiate, enhance, or inhibit the transcription of a gene. Transcription factors can regulate the formation of a specific protein encoded by a gene.

Transient ischemic attack (TIA): sometimes called a small or mini-stroke. TIAs are caused by a temporary disturbance of blood supply to an area of the brain, resulting in sudden, brief (usually less than 1 hour) disruptions in certain brain functions.

Translation: RNA translation; the process by which the sequence of nucleotides in a messenger RNA molecule directs the incorporation of amino acids into a protein.

Triglycerides: a triglyceride consists of three molecules of fatty acid combined with a molecule of the alcohol glycerol. Triglycerides serve as the backbone of many types of lipids (fats). Triglycerides are the major form of fat in our diets and are also produced by the body.

Tuberculosis: an infection caused by the bacterium *Mycobacterium tuberculosis*. Many people infected with tuberculosis have no symptoms because it is dormant. Once active, tuberculosis may cause damage to the lungs and other organs. Active tuberculosis is also contagious and is spread through inhalation. Treatment of tuberculosis involves taking antibiotics and vitamins for at least 6 months.

Typhoid: an infectious disease, spread by the contamination of food or water supplies with the bacterium *Salmonella typhi*. Food and water can be contaminated directly by sewage or indirectly by flies or poor hygiene. Though rare in the United States, it is common in some parts of the world. Symptoms include fever, abdominal pain, diarrhea, and a rash. It is treated with antibiotics and intravenous fluids. Vaccination is recommended for those traveling to areas where typhoid is common.

UL: tolerable upper intake level, set by the Food and Nutrition Board of the Institute of Medicine; the highest level of daily intake of a specific nutrient likely to pose no risk of adverse health effects in almost all individuals in the specified life stage and gender group.

Ulcerative colitis: an inflammatory disease of the colon of an unknown cause. Symptoms include abdominal pain and cramping, diarrhea, and rectal bleeding.

Vascular dementia: dementia resulting from cerebrovascular disease, for example, a cerebrovascular accident (stroke).

Vasoconstriction: narrowing of a blood vessel.

Vasodilation: relaxation or opening of a blood vessel.

Vertebral: of or pertaining to a vertebra, one of the 23 bones that make up the spine.

Vesicle: literally a small bag or pouch. Inside a cell, a vesicle is a small organelle surrounded by its own membrane.

Virulent: marked by a rapid, severe, or damaging course.

Vitamin: an organic (carbon-containing) compound necessary for normal physiological function that cannot be synthesized in adequate amounts and must therefore be obtained in the diet.

Zollinger-Ellison syndrome: a rare disorder caused by a tumor called a gastrinoma, most often occurring in the pancreas. The tumor secretes the hormone gastrin, which causes increased production of gastric acid leading to severe recurrent ulcers of the esophagus, stomach, and upper portions of the small intestine.

The Linus Pauling Institute Prescription for Healthy Living

Healthy Eating

- Eat at least five servings of fruits and vegetables every day.
- Reduce your intake of saturated and hydrogenated (trans) fat, such as butter, stick margarine, cheese, animal fat, and vegetable shortening.
- Use oils high in polyunsaturated fat, such as soy, corn, and safflower oils, or oils high in monounsaturated fat, such as olive, canola, and nut oils, for cooking and salad dressings.
- Eat fish high in omega-3 fatty acids, such as salmon, tuna, and trout, at least once a week.
- Reduce your intake of refined carbohydrates, such as sugar, white flour, and white rice.
- Eat unrefined foods high in complex carbohydrates and fiber, such as brown rice, and whole-grain breads, cereals, and pasta.
- Drink plenty of healthful fluids, such as water, fruit juices and tea.
- Limit your intake of overcooked or charred meat, and eat meat or fish with ample portions of vegetables.

Supplements

- Take a multivitamin/multimineral supplement with 100% of the Daily Value (DV) of most vitamins and minerals. Men and postmenopausal women don't need iron in their supplement unless they are at risk of iron deficiency.
- Consume at least 200 mg/day of vitamin C. Five servings/day of most fruits and vegetables should provide at least 200 mg/day of vitamin C.
- Men should take an extra selenium supplement of 100 µg/day.
- Take an extra vitamin E supplement of 200 mg/day, either natural source or d-alpha-tocopherol (with a meal).
- No multivitamin/multimineral supplement contains 100% of the DV for calcium. If you don't consume at least 1000 mg of elemental calcium/day in your diet, add a calcium supplement (with a meal) to make up the difference.

Lifestyle

- Maintain a healthy weight.
- Exercise consistently. Work up to at least 30 minutes of aerobic exercise 4-5 days a week. To improve muscular strength and minimize bone loss, include resistance exercise (weights)–a set of 8-10 exercises involving the major muscle groups at least twice a week.
- Moderate alcohol consumption is associated with reduced risk of cardiovascular diseases but increased risk of some cancers. If you drink alcohol,

limit your consumption to one alcoholic drink per day for women and two for men. Avoid alcohol if you have a personal or family history of breast or colon cancer or alcoholism.

- If you smoke, make the effort to quit. Even if you have smoked many years, quitting will result in dramatically decreased risk of chronic diseases.

Index

Note: Page numbers followed by f and t refer to figures and tables respectively.

B

C

E

D

J

K

L

Q